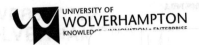

A Textbook of
Gerontological Nursing

A Textbook of
Gerontological Nursing

PERSPECTIVES ON PRACTICE

Edited by

Lesley Wade MA, RGN, RNT, RCNT, Cert Ed
Lecturer in Nursing, School of Nursing Studies,
University of Manchester, UK, and Nurse Tutor,
Manchester College of Midwifery and Nursing

and

Karen Waters PhD, BSc, RGN
Senior Lecturer in Nursing, School of Nursing Studies,
University of Manchester, UK, and
Rehabilitation Manager,
Barnes Hospital, Cheadle, Cheshire.

Baillière Tindall
London • Philadelphia • Toronto • Sydney • Tokyo

BAILLIERE TINDALL

24–28 Oval Road, London NW1 7DX

The Curtis Center, Independence Square West
Philadelphia, PA 19106–3399, USA

Harcourt Brace & Company

55 Horner Avenue, Toronto, Ontario, M8Z 4X6, Canada

Harcourt Brace & Company, Australia

30–52 Smidmore Street, Marrickville
NSW 2204, Australia

Harcourt Brace & Company, Japan

Ichibancho Central Building, 22–1 Ichibancho, Chiyoda-ku, Tokyo 102, Japan

A catalogue record for this book is available from the British Library

ISBN 0-7020-1603-9

Typeset by Phoenix Photosetting, Chatham, Kent

Printed and bound in Great Britain by

The Bath Press, Avon

Contents

Contributors vii

Foreword *Professor Mike Nolan* ix

Editors' Introduction xi

SECTION 1: PERSPECTIVES ON AGEING

1 New Perspectives on Gerontological Nursing *Lesley Wade* 3

2 The Social World of Older People *Lesley Wade* 27

3 The Impact of Ageing *Helen Jones* 49

4 Promoting Health in Older People *Gillian Granville* 73

SECTION 2: INDIVIDUAL PERSPECTIVES

5 Gender, Race and Social Responses to an Ageing Client *Helen Jones* 107

6 Loss and Bereavement in Later Life *Margaret Foulkes* 135

7 Individual Responses *John Dean, Glenys Dean and Mary Savage* 168

SECTION 3: NURSING PERSPECTIVES

8 Developments in Nursing Older People: Past, Present and Future *Lesley Wade* 187

9 Developing a Knowledge Base in Gerontological Nursing: A Critical Appraisal
   Mike Nolan 210

10 Rehabilitation *Karen Waters* 238

11 Advanced Practice: The Case of Leg Ulcers *Yvonne Awenat* 258

12 The Challenge of Advocacy: A Moral Response *Kevin Kendrick* 281

SECTION 4: EUROPEAN PERSPECTIVES

13 European Perspectives *Tom Keighley* 299

Appendix: Useful Addresses 320

Index 325

Contributors

EDITORS

Lesley Wade MA, RGN, RNT, RCNT, Cert Ed, Lecturer in Nursing, School of Nursing Studies, University of Manchester, UK, and Nurse Tutor, Manchester College of Midwifery & Nursing.

Karen Waters PhD, BSc, RGN, Senior Lecturer in Nursing, School of Nursing Studies, University of Manchester, UK, and Rehabilitation Manager, Barnes Hospital, Cheadle, Cheshire.

CONTRIBUTORS

Yvonne Awenat BSc, RGN, ONC, Clinical Nurse Specialist at Barnes Hospital, Stockport and Honorary Lecturer in Nursing, University of Manchester.

Glenys Dean BEd, SRN, SCM, QN, Retired Teacher and Carer, Mid-Glamorgan, Wales.

John Dean BA, Cert Ed, RGN, RNT, Head of Vocational and Professional Studies, North Yorkshire College of Health Studies, York District Hospital, York.

Margaret C Foulkes BA (Hons), MA, DASS, CQSW, Hospice Social Worker/Trainer at St John's Hospice in Wirral.

Gillian Granville BA, MA, RGN, RM, RHV, CPT, Development Officer (SCIPSHA – Senior Citizens Involved in Public Services, Health and Advocacy), Beth Johnson Foundation, Hartshill, Stoke-on-Trent.

Helen M Jones BSc(Hons), RGN, Cert Ed FE, RNT, MA (Gerontology) Senior Nurse, Research and Development Institution, The Glenfield Hospital NHS Trust, Leicester.

Tom Keighley RGN, RMN, NDN Cert, RCNT, DN (Lond), BA Hons, Director, Institute of Nursing at the University of Leeds.

Kevin Kendrick MSc, BA(Hons), Dip Soc Admin (Oxon), Cert Ethics & Theol (Oxon), FETC, Cert Ed, RGN, EN(G), OTN, Senior Lecturer in Philosophy and Nursing Ethics, School of Health Care, Liverpool John Moores University, Liverpool.

Mike Nolan BEd, MA, MSc, PhD, RGN, RMN, FRSH, Professor of Gerontological Nursing, University of Sheffield.

Mary Savage RGN, RCNT, RNT, Cert Ed, Residential Care Home Owner/Manager, Thornage Residential Care Home, Denton, Manchester.

Publisher's Acknowledgements

Figures 1.1, 1.2, 2.1, 2.2 and 5.4 reproduced with kind permission from Sally & Richard Greenhill Photo Library, London.

Figure 1.4, by Val Wilmer, reproduced with kind permission of Format Photographers Photo Library, London.

Figure 3.1 and 5.1, by Ulrike Preuss, reproduced with kind permission of Format Photographers Photo Library, London.

Table 4.1, from *Health and Health Care in Later Life*, Victor (1991). Reproduced with kind permission of Open University Press, Bucks.

Table 4.2, Health Promotion – Shifting the Emphasis, from *Health Visiting and Elderly People*, McClymont M et al. Reproduced with kind permission of Churchill Livingstone, Edinburgh.

Table 4.3, Looking at your communication style from *Promoting Health*, Ewles & Simnett (1988). Reproduced with kind permission of Scutari Press, London.

Figure 4.1, Ottawa Charter for Health Promotion, from *Promoting Health Among Elderly People*. Reproduced with kind permission from King's Fund Centre, London.

Figures 1.3, 4.2, 4.5, 10.1 and 13.2 by Brenda Prince, reproduced with kind permission of Format Photographers Photo Library, London.

Figure 4.6 reproduced with kind permission of PictureBank Photo Library, Kingston-Upon-Thames.

Figure 6.1, Cones of Awareness: How the dying person's view of the world may change, reprinted from Ainsworth-Smith & Speck (1982). Reproduced with kind permission of SPCK Publishing, London.

Figure 6.2, reproduced with kind permission of Barnaby Picture Library, London.

Figure 13.1, by Joanne O'Brien, reproduced with kind permission of Format Photographers Photo Library, London.

Foreword

GERONTOLOGICAL NURSING COMES OF AGE?

It is both a pleasure and a privilege to have been asked to write the Foreword for this important book, which simultaneously marks a point of arrival and a point of departure for nurses working with older people.

It is a point of arrival because for the first time a major British nursing text focuses attention on gerontological nursing and all that entails. As is highlighted in Chapter 1, gerontological nursing draws upon a number of perspectives including gerontology, geriatrics and geriatric nursing, and in so doing is more than a sum of its parts, creating a new and exciting direction for work with older people and their family carers. Arriving at this point has been the result of a process of growth and maturation over many years, much like ageing itself.

The point of departure will become apparent as soon as readers become engaged with the book and its contents. For this is no standard nursing text which reduces individuals to a set of systems and diseases or applies a functional approach, based around a particular conceptual model of care. Nor is there any attempt to provide an all-encompassing tome which purports to cover every eventuality. Instead a more individual and developmental approach is adopted which acknowledges the unique contribution both of the older person and the nurse, whilst also recognizing the societal and group pressures which shape the world in which we live.

Readers will therefore not find accounts of how to nurse individuals with communication problems or how to deal with the effects of a stroke. Something far more fundamental is attempted. To me this book is about exploring parameters and about challenging nurses to think critically and creatively about their work with older people. It is about identifying key concepts and developing, testing and applying these in order to improve the services older people receive.

Inevitably a book which breaks new ground is, by definition, incomplete. It can be no other way. Our knowledge base is as yet sparse, we are only just beginning to appreciate the subtleties of ageing and to consider their implications for nursing. There can be no doubt therefore that this volume is timely and necessary. Read it, enjoy it, but most of all act upon it. Only then will gerontological nursing begin to come of age.

MIKE NOLAN
Professor of Gerontological Nursing
University of Sheffield

Editors' Introduction

Nursing older people appears to be at a crossroads. Changes in the structure and delivery of health and social services to older people in the community, alongside emergent trends in geriatric medicine, combine to cloud our vision of nursing older people.

'Long-stay' care has largely left the confines of the hospitals, and been replaced predominantly by private sector nursing homes; acute care seems to be merging into the background of general medicine; while post acute care is emerging as the core component of hospital care for older people. Outside the institutions, radical changes in community care have led to the attempt to distinguish between health and social care for older people. What was once defined as district nursing (bathing, washing and dressing) is now often considered to be under the remit of the personal social care agencies, both public and private. The shift from health to social sector fudges the boundaries of gerontological nursing and makes its identification more complex.

Shifting boundaries can sometimes mask the fact that the number of older people who need or who are directed to health care services is ever increasing, thus although the specialty is perhaps more fragmented in the 90s, the challenge to deliver appropriate and effective health care to this client group is mounting. The numbers and types of agencies involved in the assessment, planning, delivery and evaluation of services for and with older people are increasing, rendering the definition of health care for older people ever more complex and intricate. A text could be written on 'Gerontological Nursing – What it is and What it is not': our main concern is not to be preoccupied by definition, but rather to paint broad brush strokes of gerontological nursing and to examine some aspects of it in detail. Gerontological nursing concepts are not viewed as static or solid, but dynamic and fluid, being influenced by and influencing the context in which they occur.

Nursing is one of many components of health care for older people, one of many threads which weave together to form the cloth of health care, but it is one which needs to be picked out and carefully examined. Recent changes in nursing education mean that students of nursing do not always study gerontological nursing, care of older people may be subsumed under the generic title of adult nursing, but we contend that there is a specialty of gerontological nursing which deserves to be highlighted.

So, this book aims to put gerontological nursing on the podium, to explore the background scenery against which it is set, and to explore in detail some of the parts which make up its character. In sharpening our focus onto gerontological nursing we hope to broaden your horizons and widen your perspective of nursing older people.

This book is written neither from a hospital nor a community standpoint, but embraces both. We believe that older people need nurses who are cognizant of the similarities and the differences between hospital and community and who can function effectively in any health care setting. It is not based on a specific model, but is underpinned by the themes introduced in the first chapter.

Ageing Matters	New Social World	Lifespan Perspective	Health and Old People
Illness and Dependency	Quality Nursing Care	Therapeutic Intervention	Politicizing Gerontological Nursing

These themes reflect the underlying framework of the book: the effects of ageing on individuals; the context in which it occurs; the emotional and social impact of ageing; the wellness–illness continuum; health and social interventions; and finally the emergence of elderly people as a political force. Throughout the book these issues are addressed and highlighted, enabling the reader to gain a broad insight into gerontological nursing in its many guises.

The book is divided into four sections; the first, Perspectives on Ageing, focuses on the themes of the book, the context of ageing and its effects on life and health. In the second section we focus in more detail on the influence of race and gender on older people, the experience of loss and bereavement, and the impact of changes in health care provision on carers.

Against the backdrop of health and social care the focus moves onto gerontological nursing, tracing its inception, its theory, its practice and finally its moral context. The chapter on advanced practice demonstrates how a previously unpopular field of practice – chronic wound care – provided the opportunity to implement effective health care and at the same time enhance the nursing role, analogous with gerontological nursing as a whole.

Finally in the fourth section we take a European perspective to place the British experience into a wider context and enable us to consider the future of gerontological nursing within the Community.

WHY HAS THE BOOK BEEN WRITTEN?

The book was born out of the desire to bring gerontology into nursing practice, whilst recognizing that they are two separate disciplines, gerontology has much to inform the practice of nursing older people.

WHO IS IT WRITTEN BY?

The editors of the book have both had long experience in elderly care nursing and both have been Joint Appointees between educational and health care institutions and are therefore well placed to edit this text. Similarly many of the contributors are experienced educators, practitioners and/or researchers and are therefore able to marry together the theory, the research findings and the practice.

WHO IS IT FOR?

This book is aimed at students of nursing on P2000 courses and qualified nurses eager to enter the world of gerontological nursing. It may also be useful to teachers of nursing to use as a resource book.

HOW TO USE IT

Each chapter is designed to be complete in its own right, and therefore readers may wish to pick out certain topics to study one at a time. Each section also has its own focus which may provide structure to the reader.

Like most editors, I suspect, we hope you will read all the book, which has been designed to be a complete whole.

At the beginning of this introduction we wrote that various changes had clouded our vision of gerontological nursing: our hope is that this book will enable you to see more clearly what gerontological nursing is and can be in the future.

KAREN WATERS and LESLEY WADE
1995

Section 1

Perspectives on Ageing

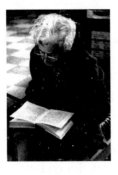

New Perspectives on Gerontological Nursing
Lesley Wade

The Social World of Older People
Lesley Wade

The Impact of Ageing
Helen Jones

Promoting Health in Older People
Gillian Granville

"*Age is an opportunity no less
Than youth itself, though in other dress
And as the evening twilight fades away
The sky is filled with stars, invisible by day*"

Longfellow (1874), *Marituri Salutamus*

The first section of this text introduces the reader to new ways of seeing and new ways of practising gerontological nursing. This way of perceiving is rather like the satisfaction one gains from decoding three-dimensional illusions. The skill in seeing the hidden picture of gerontology nursing appear out of the embedded complexities of health care commences when nursing concentrates on older people themselves. Once this focal point is mastered myriad images emerge that energize nursing. In creating new perspectives, each writer's background as a nurse or health visitor, counsellor or researcher provides the backcloth that enhances this vision of gerontological nursing.

Lesley Wade begins this process by introducing the reader to a simple gerontological framework that helps to inform practice. The need for such a framework has materialized whilst teaching degree and pre- and post-registration students. This new way of knowing is supported with a detailed account of creating a reflective culture within gerontological nursing. The importance of having this level of reflection and broad framework is reiterated in the following chapter on the social world of older people. By using this perspective, Lesley verifies that the social world of older people emerges to challenge negative stereotyping, emphasizing that growing old is in fact a new age of discovery. Within Chapter 3, Helen Jones emphasizes that the impact of ageing is a convoluted process of living and evolving. Throughout this chapter the reader is challenged to see that ageing is an integrated web that affects the older person in an exclusive way. Helen's chapter exemplifies how gerontological nursing requires depth and breadth within biological and social sciences. The concluding chapter by Gillian Granville continues this exploration of new perspectives by addressing health promotion for older people. This section ends as it begins: with a positive, dynamic, optimistic approach to ageing. Amalgamating gerontological knowledge to creative, sensitive health promotion, Gillian increases the dimensions of gerontological nursing.

Chapter One

New Perspectives on Gerontological Nursing

Lesley Wade

Core Themes in Gerontological Nursing

Ageing Matters	*New Social World*	*Lifespan Perspective*	*Health and Old People*
Illness and Dependency	*Quality Nursing Care*	*Therapeutic Intervention*	*Politicizing Gerontological Nursing*

Key Words

Gerontological Perspective • Positive Ageing • Changing Roles • Reflective Practice

INTRODUCTION

Few people know how to be old
Duc De La Rochefoucauld (1613–1680)

Society and nursing's response to old age has, paradoxically, been influenced by the assumption that older people abdicate their personhood by virtue of growing old. Gerontological nursing contradicts this assumption, believing that many of the population know how to be old. In return, nursing is gaining insights into the needs of older people from a very different perspective. As older people grow in their ability to express themselves, so will nursing. Old age is not a disease, it is strength and survivorship and triumph over all kinds of vicissitudes. Positive self expression about ageing is demonstrated by the need to be creative and develop. The French writer Collette thought that to be 'astonished' was one of the surest ways of not growing old, while Virginia Woolf believed ageing was forever altering one's aspect to the sun. Older people *do* know how to be old and the study of how older people experience ageing in its totality is known as gerontology.

Why should nurses use this perspective? The profession needs to employ a system and an understanding of nursing that responds to the needs of older people. Clarity of strategy and clarity on how nursing responds to these challenges requires some frames of reference. In helping gerontological nursing itself 'come of age', a number of core themes are addressed. These themes serve as a rudimentary guide in developing a framework that informs nursing practice. They serve as a menu, a sophisticated 'smorgasbord' that helps you in your nursing. Often nursing undersells itself by not stating explicitly what is meant by gerontological nursing, considering it tacit knowledge, marginalizing its importance within the profession. This chapter demonstrates how reflective practice within gerontological nursing can shape and construct new approaches in nursing older people that as yet lie dormant. The central remit of this chapter and subsequent chapters is to identify what constitutes gerontological nursing. The depth and breadth of that content is explored in various chapters, assisting us to advance our practice.

This Chapter aims to look at the advancement of practice by:

Identifying core gerontological nursing knowledge, recognizing that nursing has to become more responsive to older people's needs

---

Reviewing some of the delivery and practice of nursing using a gerontological nursing framework

---

Developing the concept of reflective practice.

NEW POSITIONS, NEW VANTAGE POINTS

In advancing our nursing practice, how conscious are we of our body of knowledge and the frameworks we use to give care? Are we totally accepting of the use of models, the adoption of a systematic approach, or the introduction of primary nursing as the panacea to cure all? In moving towards a gerontological nursing perspective we first need to define what we mean by this term and how it relates to those we care for. A gerontological perspective moves away from an illness-dependency model of care towards a biographical developmental, positive approach. This is not to say older people are not ill, but the focus of nursing is to assist the individual to maximize and adapt according to their own potential, within varied settings. This approach recognizes the older person as a consumer of care, requiring varied skills from nursing. Gerontological nursing frameworks focus upon the person and the environment, and the process between the two that produces health and wellness. Gerontological nursing encompasses the definition of *gerontology* (the study of ageing) *geriatrics* (medical treatments of old age and disease) and *geriatric nursing* (care of an older person during wellness and illness). It is the growing awareness of the need simultaneously to use all three areas of knowledge as distinct from elderly care nursing, with its more hospital-dominated approach, that moves nursing towards a gerontological perspectives. Nolan (1994) questions how holistic the term *elderly care* nursing actually is, and develops a reasoned argument for the development of gerontological knowledge within nursing in Chapter 9. Reappraising the concept of elderly care nursing is not a slight on the immense progress made in this area, but as a mature discipline, the term gerontology opens up discussion on the future direction of nursing older people.

To move the debate forward, nursing needs to reassess its direction. When Norton (1962) and Wells (1980) sought to investigate and improve *geriatric nursing*, research focused very much within hospitals and professional perspectives. The context of care and on whom it will focus, has changed dramatically. Gerontological nurses recognize that older people are not a homogenous group. Seventy-year-olds are very different from 90-year-olds, whilst well people in their 60s have very different needs from frail people in their 80s. Gerontological nursing recognizes the diversity among functionally impaired older people while recognizing the impact of environment and life events. Older women and older persons from ethnic backgrounds need to be researched and incorporated into gerontological nursing programmes, alongside nursing home residents and the sick older person. Positive nursing models on ageing that incorporate a developmental approach to nursing older people such as those of Rodgers (1970) Roy (1976) and Neuman (1982) may be of some practical use as they stress the potential for human growth. However, searching for the ideal model of care may be as fruitless as searching for the holy grail. It must be reiterated that one of the key ideas of gerontological nursing is the recognition of the heterogeneity of older people. Also, the knowledge used in nursing older people is not found within single ideas. The practice of gerontological nursing is not closed, it is open to outside influences. Therefore the skills encompassed within gerontological nursing go beyond the confines of a model of nursing. Nursing needs new ways of seeing, new ways of doing, cognizant of social and political change.

Whom are we Targeting?

Accurate knowledge must be gained about who old people are, their health status and their particular needs. This information is important when we consider that the number of older people in our population will increase while resources will continue to be limited. Needs will vary according to life courses, gender, class and dependency level. Nurses will increasingly be giving care to a complex diverse group of older people. It is important that the delivery and practice of that care are age- and needs-related. An important point is that gerontological nursing occurs in virtually all areas of nursing; it is at the very interface of hospital and community care. Therefore practitioners and educationalists who are interested in the development of nursing older people must respond to care needs. This is best achieved by strengthening ties between education and practice, preparing nurses to advanced levels of practice. I hope I have set out very briefly an agenda that continues this dialogue throughout this book. In your reading, reflection and practice, many of these unknown elements of gerontological nursing will be recognized, practised or sought for.

REFLECTIVE PRACTICE

New perspectives on ageing within nursing therefore require new ways of thinking and knowing. Contemplating new thought processes requires ways of internalizing knowledge that has individual and professional significance. Reflective practice is a way of thinking and acting which has a tangible reality. This way of thinking is pertinent and realistic for gerontological nursing. Schon (1991), one of its exponents, candidly states that any professional practice is 'messy' and 'complex' and compares it to a swamp. Gerontological nursing is acknowledged as highly complex (RCN, 1993) and the context in which it takes place is varied and transitional.

On what issues must gerontological nurses reflect? They must reflect on health needs as well as on medical care, the needs of the frail and aspects of promoting health. They need to reflect *on, in* and *around practice.* An important aspect of reflective practice within gerontological nursing is the personal dimension this approach explores. This is vitally important within gerontological nursing where attitude, role modelling and conducive environments influence practice. James (1994) acknowledges that reflection can take place in a variety of domains. Gerontological nursing can reflect on the *social, political* and *economic* aspects of practice, for example financial constraints may create complex messy problems complicating discharge planning, rehousing and admissions into nursing and residential homes. Changes in health care funding will require rethinking and alternative approaches to nursing. A second area for reflection is on the everyday aspects of *practice.* This may include aspects like routines, roles and unwritten rules that are familiar occurrences. Here the nurse can consider the appropriateness of actions, such as assisting with mobility or a patient who has a pressure sore. Third, the *technical* aspects of gerontological nursing need to be considered, for example the effects of specific drugs or the introduction of new cardiac monitoring equipment that may require extra resources. A major purpose of reflection is that it enables gerontological nurses to make sense of new experiences, drawing on their vast array of professional knowledge.

Testament of Experience

Reflecting brings its own intrinsic and professional rewards but can appear very detached from practice. Reflecting on my own practice, are three examples of how I used journal writing at different points in practice. My reflective journal was very important to me; it recorded the highs and lows of my personal development, from a ward and unit sister, clinical nurse specialist and a joint appointment to nurse teacher within a nursing development unit. I found it easier to write about positive things, although the journal is scattered with self indulgent episodes of misery. The diary was started in 1985 and written weekly. It travelled with me to Malta, where I worked alongside Mediterranean nurses successfully changing nursing practice. Sometimes I wrote in smooth prose but often I doodled or drew cartoons. Over the last 10 years I often look back and am surprised by my failures as well as my progress. The faces of the people I have nursed are embedded within the scenarios and case studies, and all levels of reflection are incorporated within the pages. Recently, I started to use a hand-held microphone to record my experiences and find this useful. What follows are exemplars from my journal. I usually divide the page in half, one half for the description and the other for my analysis, which is highly personal. I have selected examples that demonstrate a wide range of reflection and illustrate my different roles. I was taught to use this method of reflection by my 94-year-old grandmother who was my confidant whenever I needed advice. She herself had been taught this from her grandmother. I consider my journal keeping as the most important developmental process during my nursing career, taught to me from older people who value reciprocity.

Case Study: Reflecting in practice

APRIL 1986

I'm increasingly getting upset by the number of older clients with black heels. I'm quite sure that at weekends care plans are not being looked at and correct physical assessments are not being made. The problem is the staff are so tired; the Easter break and sickness on other wards are not helping. Mr Corscadden's heels, slightly red on Friday, are quite black. This has happened over 3 days! As Mr Corscadden is my client I feel responsible and guilty, after all I'm supposed to be setting an example.

We had a team meeting this week and I stressed the need to examine people physically, especially if they had mobility problems. Black heels have become my personal nightmare. After preaching about this I examined two other men who had different degrees of heel redness. One has a known problem of cardiac failure with peripheral oedema and the other man wears shoes bought for him by his deceased wife in 1955! Ill-fitting they may be, but we will need to consult tactfully with other members of the team about this problem. I've used every method I can find to resolve the black heel problem, then in a lull, I gaze down the ward and suddenly see the reason. Unbelievably, it was staring me in the face. From the top of the ward I can see clearly that Mr Corscadden and fellow men are lounging in their chairs. They are tall men and the chairs are totally ill-fitting; the only way they are comfortable is sitting with their feet outstretched – a consequence, their heels are taking a great deal of pressure.

Comments

Insights into solving such problems in nursing, if not recorded and reflected upon, can be lost for ever. As a consequence, the ward team looked into the ergonomics of equipment used in gerontological units, talking with commissioning bodies and acquiring various sizes of chairs for the opening of a new ward. We were all more critical of care planning and our ability to make appropriate assessments on pressure sores. I learned a valuable lesson – that at times you have to 'stand back' in gerontological nursing and now I believe more in gestalt psychology.

Case Study: Reflection on practice

MAY 1990

Today I had an uneasy feeling that what we see as progress within our new medical unit for older people may not be so. The consultant told me that he had ordered three new monitors for the cardiac patients, but when I asked him who was to read the monitors and act upon any cardiac arrhymias, particularly defibrillation, the reply was unclear. This reminds me of the time as an intensive care sister I defibed Mr Parks five times. I clearly remember the rest of the staff disapproving of this action, many of them ignoring that this was a simple conduction problem. I felt totally alone initiating this action, until the pacing team arrived. I see Mr and Mrs Parks shopping sometimes 5 years after the event, and he shyly reminds me that all he remembers is my voice apologizing, as I kept placing the paddles on his chest.

Comments

This reflection is an example of how an experience had unwittingly informed my understanding and advanced my thinking about the problems of equipment, resources and ethical implications regarding resuscitation. Both incidents had a very positive effect on my approach towards resuscitation. The episode emphasized that in-depth knowledge about cardiac problems and skilled actions were also needed as well as equipment to improve care. Ethical issues surrounding resuscitation have now a deep significance.

Case Study: Reflection around practice

OCTOBER 1993

I have been asked to head a team designing a new curriculum in the care of older people. Despite my protest that the course should use the term gerontology my seniors insist it is called elderly. Also they want the ageing process to be covered at the beginning of the course. For 7 years working alongside development and practice units I have endorsed the idea that nursing must start from health in old age. My ward experiences and clinical and theoretical teaching have been directed towards the need to recognize the actual needs of older people. I have presented a plan to my managers that produces a pathway through gerontological nursing up to Masters level. But I feel very alone with my ideas, although I am sure of my knowledge. I need a fellow professional to talk my ideas over with.

Comments

This aspect of reflection demonstrates a willingness to challenge, and because of the deep level of reflection this needs to be shared. Challenging and changing a curriculum appears surprisingly just as difficult as challenging practice!

ESTABLISHING A REFLECTIVE CULTURE

Establishing a reflective culture, particularly in practice, can be performed in diverse ways. Aesthetic forms of developing reflection can be encouraged through poetry, drawings and narratives. These reflective processes can reveal emotional and spiritual dimensions within the nursing of older people. Creative ways of exploring relationships and professional frustration can be facilitated. A poignant narrative a nursing student shared with me showed gerontological nursing's potential for creativity.

Case Study: Susan's story

I had been caring for Amy for 4 weeks. Amy was a stroke patient, with a right-sided weakness. Although some improvement had been made I felt we were not getting through to her. All the physical and emotional problems as per care plan were being addressed; the physiotherapist and other members of the team worked closely together, but still something was missing. Amy's husband brought photographs of his wife to show me the beautiful garden she had nurtured. The next day I bought Amy a gardening magazine and all through her process of rehabilitation used the metaphor of the garden and its need of water to help her understand what had happened to her. I felt I gave Amy some control, self respect and power back. I gave her information and she reciprocated with her gardening knowledge. I don't really know how beneficial this was but I felt I reached out to her, and she to me.

A second narrative that illustrates how we can learn from older people, to the benefit of gerontological nursing, is Kate's story of her patient's reaction to triage in an accident and emergency department. Kate was a sister who had implemented a very successful triage system in her A and E department. As a member of a continual educational course (ENB 298) she used a reflective journal.

Case Study: Kate's story

I was on night duty and, as usual, it was a very busy night. Mr Lubinski, a 78-year old, had slipped coming home from the pub. After assessing him, the triage nurse explained about our system. Friday nights in casualty are notoriously busy so he was made comfortable in a side room until we could find him a bed. Walking passed the cubicle I found Mr Lubinski in a very emotional state. He was very agitated and after talking to him I noticed some tattoos on his forearms. Seemingly, Mr Lubinski had been in a concentration camp during the war and the only time he had received medical treatment was after an attempted escape, when he was shot in the same ankle he had fallen over. A further complication was that his triage nurse was in fact German, compounding his anxiety.

All these forms of reflected practice demonstrate the process of how gerontological nurses arrive at certain levels of knowledge.

The following hints may help you start off the process of reflection. Select a significant situation concerning your practice and ask your self:

- *What was your role in the situation?*
- *What actions did you and other colleagues take?*
- *How appropriate was the action taken?*
- *What knowledge from theory and practice within gerontological nursing could you apply to similar situations?*
- *What are the broader issues related to this situation?*

CORE THEMES AND THEIR RELATIONSHIP IN DEVELOPING NURSING OF OLDER PEOPLE

New perspectives require the scope of gerontological nursing to expand and extend from within and laterally. A number of core themes have been identified that may help to develop this breadth of practice. In accordance with the philosophy of gerontological nursing, these themes emphasize health and wellbeing, health promotion, disability postponement and the role of the recipient of care, the older person within these processes. Theoretical content covers such areas as demography and the epidemiology of ageing, health, social and community policies, resources, ethical and legal issues, and teaching and counselling. Nurses reading this book are advised to reflect on their ability to link theory to practice. To develop this ability to think critically about practice, nurses need to use a variety of problem-solving methods. Nursing older people has many dimensions, relating to other disciplines, generations and cultures. For example, it was formerly seen that we cared *for* older people, now we care *with* older people.

Theme One

Ageing Matters: Age-appropriate Practice

New ways of seeing and doing must start by questioning whether our practice is age appropriate. In developing perspectives towards age-appropriate practice we need to examine a number of issues. We need to be selective in using sociological, psychological and biological theories that are gerontologically based. We need to look at the changing nature of nursing older people and the role of the nurse as a career. Pearson (1994) states that scholarship in nursing begins by examining the relationship, between the nurse and the nursed. Therefore, we need to look at our own personal attitudes towards growing old, recognizing the real world of older men and women according to class, gender and ethnicity. We need to examine critically influential theories on ageing, understanding the meaning of loss in old age including abuse, dignity power and choice. We need to understand how the role of the nurse is changing, as we work alongside social services, voluntary services and self-help groups. Last, we need to examine whether a gerontological perspective enhances the nursing of older people.

Gerontological nursing requires nurses to have both depth and breadth within their repository of skills. For example, it is not only a matter of understanding population changes, but also of reviewing demographic trends by drawing distinction between needs of older people in urban or rural areas, differing age groups and diverse health expectations. Where the nurse lives and works will influence the very nature of how care is delivered, and what resources are available.

When reflecting whether you give specific age-appropriate practice it is important to avoid blanket statements on the needs of all older people as though they were one homogeneous mass. The Medical Research Council is conscious of the degree of potential error in the projections of older people and their health needs (Medical Research Council, 1994). Therefore, we need to incorporate scientific data and older people's self-assessed and lay beliefs into mutually agreed care plans. In responding to culture, gender and loss as related to older people we need to act as role models, combating ageism, racism and other forms of stereotyping. Co-ordination of care within multidisciplinary and interdisciplinary teams requires liaison skills and the ability to assess if other practice is age-appropriate. The use of language, as in the terms 'orthopaedic' or 'cot sides' does not reflect an orientation towards older people. A particular gerontological nursing skill is to enable carers of older people, who increasingly are taking care of relatives, towards this perspective. The changing roles of relatives from being cared for by father and mother, to becoming the main carer is not simply role reversal. Age-appropriate practice in aspects of feeding and helping and moving should be taught by nurses to various caregivers who may have to continue this care.

An essential skill needed within this area of practice is to evaluate and promote gerontological nursing within a health care service undergoing political and economic change. It is therefore imperative to use knowledge of local as well as central social policies as we decentralize decision making. Gerontological nursing is increasingly performed outside of a hospital setting and agencies other than professional nursing may play their part in delivering care. The United Kingdom Central Council report on professional misconduct (UKCC, 1994) is testimony to differing areas of practice within gerontological homes Inadequate induction and training are cited as one of the major reasons for poor practice. It would seem that in these developing areas of practice there is an absence of age-appropriate practice.

Theme Two

Nursing in the New Social World of Older People

Exploring the actual social world of older people might alter nursing approaches altogether. Some of my best friends are older people and they bear no resemblance to the images portrayed on television. The chapter on the social world of older people emphasizes the positive aspects of growing old with the freedom and opportunities it can bring. The changing

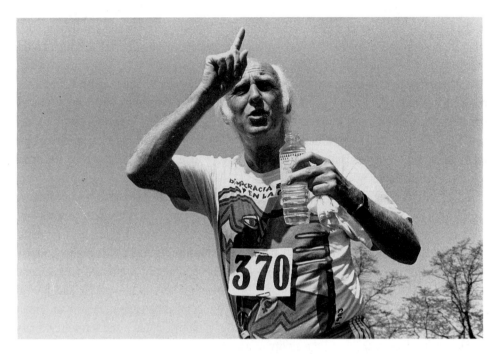

Fig. 1.1 *The individual older person should be allowed to go at their own pace*

world of older people is as varied as the people who live there. Equally, it is important not to exceptionalize this world. Throughout this book great emphasis is made in asking nurses to recognize the social world of older people. Consider the passage below. Does this produce a negative or positive image about ageing in Britain today?

> *If a space ship with friendly natives asked to take one passenger back to their planet to examine what life was like on earth who do you think they would take? A current popstar; a politician? What about an old woman or man shopping at Woolworths? They have worked hard all their life in jobs such as cleaning, cooking and bringing up children. Never educated to their capacity, they have wit and much common sense. They have faced death many times, perhaps coping with all these hardships in a more resilient way than you or I could imagine. When we superficially take their history they have nothing to say, not being used to voicing an opinion, especially with nurses.*

At first this imaginary scene could appear negative, particularly if we apply the standards of professional people. Housework, shopping and facing hardship may not be some professionals' idea of a good time and a reluctance to voice an opinion may not fit within a politically correct compaign to improve the image of older people. However, not every older person will want or feel able to ski in France this winter, or articulate their health needs. Professional ideas regarding the social world of older people therefore need to recognize the banal as well as the exciting. Nurses too often see only the social world of older people, from

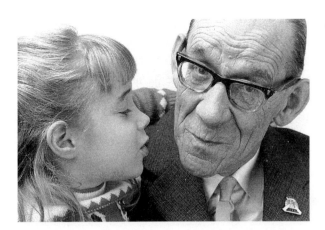

Fig. 1.2 *Intergenerational sharing*

contact with hospital patients or through relatives. Many of the sociological theories on ageing ignore the new developing social world of older people. In developing clinical gerontological nursing skills, it is important to consider how far some of these theories still influence nursing practice. These themes are more extensively examined in Chapters 4 and 12.

Theme Three

Recognizing Lifespan Perspectives within Gerontological Nursing

This theme recognizes the positive aspects of growing old, including the emotional needs of older people. This omission in our practice is often demonstrated by inadequate communication and interviewing skills. In looking at the positive aspects of growing and developing in old age the nurse may draw on aspects such as:

■ *the use of a lifespan perspective;*

■ *emotional needs of older people;*

■ *communication skills;*

■ *sexuality in old age;*

■ *relationships with significant others;*

■ *the social and occupational life of older people;*

■ *changing living arrangements for older people with learning disabilities or lost independence.*

Looking at the stages of psychosocial development, the work of Erikson (1963) emphasizes the interdependence of generations; the old needing the young and vice versa. If gerontological nursing is to examine the therapeutic nature of this aspect of nursing then human development is central in nursing older people. In Erikson's theory, with its recognition of development in old age, the actions of the nurse can be planned and organized around establishing a trusting relationship and finding ways of assisting the client to become as autonomous as possible. Johnson (1976) argued that one specific way of making care more individualized is to adopt a biographical approach that includes a lifespan development. At the very minimum, the biographical approach can help to establish rapport between an older person and somebody who has suddenly come into their life to 'assess' them. The benefit of this approach lies in listening to the life stories of older people, gaining different pictures of the person and their needs from others. Therefore self esteem can be enhanced by skilful encouragement of reminiscence, thus helping older people to use their coping mechanisms related to their life experiences.

Reflecting on my own practice, two significant incidents demonstrate this specific gerontological perspective.

Case Study: Albert and the War

According to Albert's care plan that morning the primary and associate nurse were going to help him bathe. Albert did not have a bathroom of his own and whilst recovering from his chest infection in hospital agreed this would be refreshing. The nurse ran the bath water and because Albert had poor mobility sat him on a hoist and began lowering him into the water. Albert began to panic showing signs of anxiety and quickly was taken out of the water. A warm towel was placed over him. The primary nurse, who had formed a trusting relationship with Albert comforted him as the tears came rolling down his face. As they talked the primary nurse remembered that on television that night there had been a documentary on the Second World War. She asked 'Albert you were in the war weren't you?' Albert confirmed this 'yes love, the navy.' 'Did you do the Atlantic runs?' Albert nodded. 'Did you ever get torpedoed?' again Albert nodded. She gently asked how many survived. Albert told her just nine, including himself. 'We were hours in the water.'

Now the nurse understood Albert's reaction to entering the water. This immersion, married with the television coverage the night before, brought out levels of unresolved grief and terror to what appeared to be a commonplace procedure. This example recognizes complex emotional needs and the corresponding sensitive response to these needs required from gerontological nursing. This significant incident demonstrates the need for a lifespan perspective in providing systematic care.

Case Study: Betty and her diet

The primary nurse of Betty, a newly diagnosed diabetic, was consulting the multidisciplinary team about diet. Although the dietician had seen Betty on a number of occasions, it was clear to the nurse that Betty did not fully understand the carbohydrate exchange treatment. The learning pack used to help older people understand about dietary control in diabetes appeared to be orientated towards younger people. Food examples like chilli con carne and hamburgers did not fit into the culture or life course of this 80-year-old client. At the next joint planning meeting the primary nurse acting as Betty's advocate put forward a proposal. Using a life course perspective, she suggested drawing on Betty's life skills as a mother, having to weigh and measure rationed food during the late 1940s and early 1950s. In this way she suggested to the team they could enhance her self esteem by relating the control of diet to a previously successful time. To an extent the recognition of Betty's skills as a housewife and the incorporation of this within her newly diagnosed diabetes is an example of enabling the client to be empowered.

Reflecting on these examples of practice, could the primary nurse have been more aware of Albert's and Betty's needs that day? Do models of nursing used in gerontological settings look at older peoples' biographies and coping mechanisms?

Theme Four

The Healthy Older Person and their Nursing Needs

Health promotion and maintenance have only recently been addressed within gerontological nursing. It is not just a question of displaying leaflets or making sure certain age groups have health screening. The health status of older people, their illness behaviour and uptake is difficult to ascertain. This may well be due to a lack of knowledge combined with ageist

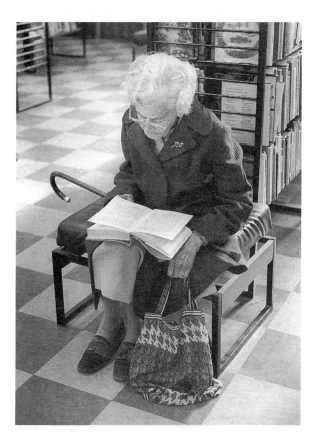

Fig. 1.3 *A potential consumer of care accessing knowledge*

attitudes that inhibits appropriate health-promoting nursing activities. The Healthy Active Life Expectancy (HALE) is a tool measuring the expectation of life before disability (Medical Research Council, 1994). Measurements as these have drawbacks, needing sensitive questioning and non-valuing judgements. The gerontological literate nurse could be in an ideal position to undertake this research, increasing her scholarship which in turn benefits older people. Areas needing to be addressed within health care and its promotion must centre on assessing, planning and meeting needs of older people to maintain their health. The application of teaching and learning skills that facilitate effective health education is a vital gerontological nursing requirement. Chapter 3 looks comprehensively at health and older people, demonstrating the increasing scope of gerontological nursing.

Understanding the differences and dichotomies that arise between professional and lay beliefs is a fundamental gerontological nursing skill. An example of this is demonstrated by the problems surrounding continence promotion, particularly as so often the sexual needs of the older incontinent patient are ignored. How encouraging are we in our nursing practice in suggesting intermittent self catheterization to this group? Initiatives like Well Women and Well Men clinics or 'pop in' health shops perhaps offer more consumer choice. Therefore nurses may have to be prepared to take on new roles, which may be more effective and better accomplished in unconventional settings. Leisure and exercise in old age are an underdeveloped aspect of health promotion within gerontological nursing. Increases in osteoporosis can be related to changes not only in hormones in both sexes but reduced exercise patterns. Without an understanding of how older people engage in exercise, this health promoting activity lies dormant. Applying nursing strategies that incorporate cultural needs and maximize older people's self worth is an integral part of assisting older people to stay healthy.

Theme Five

Illness and Dependency

Fries (1980) made a significant contribution to the focus of nursing within the care of older people. In suggesting that chronic illness, so often associated with older people, may be postponed by changes in lifestyle, he should have alerted nursing to changing much of their focus. Extending adult vigour far into a fixed lifespan, compressing the period of ageing near the end of life, will and has changed practice. So the longer an individual can live an independent life, the shorter the period of subsequent dependency. For gerontological nursing this contradicts the conventional anticipation of an ever older, even more feeble patient.

However, for older people who do not have good health, it is important to recognize that chronic disease has replaced acute illness as a major health threat. The growing prevalence of chronic illness is due both to control of infectious diseases and to technology. The major causes of mortality in older people are heart disease, strokes, neoplasms and respiratory problems. Yet older people are omitted from clinical trials for new cancer therapies, or coronary bypass surgery. Less overt inequalities stem from policies excluding older age groups from admission to specialist coronary care units or some thrombolytic therapy. Screening programmes exclude women from regular invitation to breast screening or regular cervical screening. One of the key questions we as nurses should be asking is whether it should be physiological status and not health that determines health care and nursing. Quite simply, what is needed is a gerontological nursing perspective guiding practice.

Further chapters within this section look directly at the ageing process. Up-to-date epidemiological studies must be digested and acted upon by nurses. The relevance of biological studies lies in the prevention and possible reversibility of age-associated disease and disability. This is especially important in wound healing, autoimmune disease and osteoporosis. The Medical Research Council has set up a number of research initiatives looking at a variety of issues. The General Practice Research Framework (GPRF) has undertaken research into cardiovascular and osteoporotic disease. The Medical Research Council's Institute on Hearing has been undertaking research on this aspect, looking at such varied aspects as sensory neural loss to the prevision of hearing aids. The Dunn Nutritional Unit has focused on nutritional status. Assessing older people within the community and the social and cultural impact of strokes are other pertinent research aspects relating to mortalities and morbidities. As stated earlier, there is a huge gap in gerontological nursing knowledge, so where is nursing within this fact-finding mission? How much research money goes into funding specific nursing of older people? Encouraging greater collaboration between existing researchers and attracting high-quality nurse researchers into this area are of paramount urgency. Nurses need to analyse the prevalence of chronic and acute illness within the specific locality of their practice. Quite clearly, they need to liaise with other health care professionals, the relationship being symbiotic.

Theme Six

Quality within Gerontological Nursing

The core theme of quality in gerontological nursing should begin by defining what this means for both practitioner and the older person. Using this perspective, this theme should then be examined when ever clinical and educational audits are performed, standards are set and new initiatives are introduced into nursing. In particular, the abstract word 'quality' needs to be embedded within gerontological nursing in disseminating research and evaluating its practice. In evaluating the nursing care given to older people some areas have been identified from the Department of Health paper: *The Vision for the Future* (Department Of Health, 1993), helping nurses develop their practice.

Individual Client Care All clinical nurses, whether in statutory, private or voluntary sectors, will wish to ensure there are systems in place to encourage and facilitate development of individual client care. In gerontological nursing, this may take the form of primary nursing and collaborative care plans. Evaluation is needed on the development of shared protocols, shared care planning with consumers, professional colleagues and managers.

Partnership It is important to elicit whether clients have been involved as fully as possible in the planning and delivery of care. Gerontological nursing perspectives would very much see the older person as the co-leader within such partnerships; examples are given within Chapter 8 on developments in gerontological nursing on educational partnerships and their effectiveness.

Standards and Quality Nurses and health visitors should ensure that their work is based on good practice, is well documented and continuously evaluated both with process and outcome. Factors to include in such evaluations will be the appropriateness, effectiveness, acceptability and cost of care. Evaluation of care will require nurses to participate in both multidisciplinary clinical audits. According to these audits, standards of practice must be amended, in relation to their pertinence to older people. The setting of standards and the undertaking of audits is another opportunity to work alongside and recognize specific issues raised by older people themselves. Assisting older people to participate by sitting on committees or vetting audit tools affords gerontological nursing opportunity to listen and learn what the consumer wants.

Resource Management The provision of high quality cost effective health care should take account of resource management and value for money initiatives. To do so the management structure must be evaluated in order to deliver an effective mix of nursing skills. This is specially important within care of older people. This group's vulnerability lies in a gerontological naïve population that often assumes that anyone can carry out this care.

Innovation Emphasis on the evaluation here is to look at innovation and development in new approaches in gerontological nursing. New ways of delivering care, development and practice units, art and music and drama therapy and new roles linking community and hospitals should be explored. Examples of good practice especially within day hospitals and links with the voluntary sector such as 'Age Exchange' demonstrate the leading role of nurses caring for older people. Chapter 8 recognizes the innovation and boundary crossing that has been the hallmark of nursing older people.

Patients' Charter Each nurse caring for older people should ensure that their own individual practice meets the requirements of the Patient's Charter.

Tripartite Liaison The dialogue among commissioners of professional education, health care providers and educational institutions, must evaluate how pre- and postregistration meets the needs of older people. Specifically, the evaluation should examine the skills of assessment, care management, health education and promotion. Educational programmes should include the healthy older person, research application in practice and management skills. In many ways gerontological nursing has been the leader in interprofessional working, partnerships and empowerments. Access to clients' notes has been a normal part of my nursing practice for the last 8 years, yielding positive results in client education and communication.

Recognizing Excellence Regional nurse directors and trust nurse executive directors working in partnership with academic departments should establish networks to identify and promote examples of good practice. Good areas evaluated should have their ideas disseminated.

Clinical Research Regional directors of nursing should liaise closely with regional directors of research and development to evaluate the development of clinical research within gerontological nursing. All purchasing organizations should review their arrangements, ensuring that informed professional advice recognizes the contribution nurses skilled in gerontological case bring to an organization. Critical examinations of research in gerontological nursing in relation to nursing practices need to be evaluated efficiently. Complaints procedures and joint consultative committees need to include voluntary bodies and older people themselves. Nursing standards groups must meet regularly with a remit to improve care. Maximizing the use of human and other resources is needed to benefit both nursing and older people.

Theme Seven

Nursing Interventions that are Therapeutic within Gerontological Nursing

The therapeutic approach emphasizes the future potential of the older person. If we wish to advance the therapeutic approach we need to reinstate the older client's autonomy. Gerontological nursing must equip the older person with new skills, physically and socially. Rehabilitation is central to the care of older people, therefore we need to evaluate packages of care that appear to be effective. The organization and delivery of nursing have been cited as therapeutic in itself (Ersser and Tutton, 1991). If this is so, then the way we deliver care through a systematic approach needs to be examined within a gerontological nursing framework.

The last quarter of the twentieth century has seen an emphasis on individualized nursing care, but what do we mean by this within gerontological nursing? The approach the nurse must take is to build up a relationship of trust rather than bluntly asking a set of questions about the person's functional abilities and current circumstances. The nurse encourages the older person to describe their past life, putting it in relationship to their present circumstances. This approach can yield much information about the older person's coping abilities, changing circumstances and the role relationships play in their life. This approach requires time to be spent and, to some extent, the formation of a contract between the nurse and older client. Chapter 7 extends this example in relation to chronic leg ulcers. The feeling of identity could be strengthened by means of conversation with the clients about his or her present and future.

Primary nursing, with its emphasis on the one patient one nurse concept and its emphasis on continuity of care, may be an ideal vehicle where this approach could be used. As we move in Britain towards the named nurse concept, nurses giving systematic care to older people will need many new skills. Nurses specializing in the care of older people have already demonstrated how the use of primary nursing assumes responsibility and a degree of accountability for client management and improving quality (Wright, 1990). New approaches to managing care, for example interviewing skills, very much depend on the nurse adopting a gerontological perspective. The RCN guidelines (1990) provide a useful framework for the assessment of older people. They are based upon the activities of a daily living model. Within the broad heading of the model, problems and needs can be identified and goals set with the client to overcome or meet them. In looking at examples of assessments, specific criteria could be used to examine how effective they are in providing systematic nursing. The process of assessment and its documentation should address many of the issues listed below. We need to ask is the process:

- *User friendly?*
- *Easily accessible information?*
- *Needs led?*
- *Holistic/comprehensive?*
- *Addresses the needs of carers?*
- *Addresses the needs of black and ethnic minority consumers?*
- *Multi- and interdisciplinary?*
- *Leads to identifiable outcome?*
- *Allows ongoing review and evaluation?*

The skills required by an experienced, knowledgeable gerontological nurse practitioner in planning care emphasize that this is an interactive process. As previously stated, if we are to provide a needs-based nursing service, planning should be decentralized otherwise care will revolve around professional need. One approach adopted by the nursing development unit at Tameside gerontological unit in Lancashire emphasizes the need for older clients to have access to nursing records. A statement of rights is given in a booklet. These rights include such things as knowing how and why you are being treated, what is being done, and having a choice in your care, so that you can make an informed decision.

In demonstrating a number of issues that can and do arise and cause problems when planning services, nurses have to be aware of conflict of interest, competing power groups and disciplinary rivalries. In looking at assessment, nurses need knowledge about older people – who they are, where they are, their health status, their desires, their needs. For example, are all nurses able to provide advice about sex in later life? To deliver nursing care to older people in a systematic way, nurses need increased levels of knowledge and skills.

Summarizing, we want to give care that meets the needs of older people from different backgrounds and which recognizes and encourages participation if desired. Are the tools you use, for example nursing models, the nursing process, clinical and learning audits, and standard settings, appropriately set within the gerontological perspective described?

In helping you reflect on and then evaluate your care, consider some of these issues:

- *Are you a knowledgeable, skilled accountable practitioner?*

- *Do you work in partnership with other professionals, working with users of services, cares and other agencies towards common goals?*
- *Does the type of specialized nursing you deliver secure improvement in the health and wellbeing of older people?*
- *Does the specialized care that you give reduce premature death; reduce the adverse effects of illness and disability; promote healthy lifestyles, and improve the quality of life?*

Theme Eight

Politicizing Gerontological Nursing

Trends within health care and nursing are often overlooked when we examine practice. How viable are issues in consumer choice, decision making and self assessed needs within the everyday life of all older people? The need for nurses to acquire a business imperative within their practice has a long history in British nursing (Procheska, 1992). Using the example of the market economy, importing and exporting ideas from other specialities and countries is essential for advancing practice. But initially we have to look within our own backyard. The challenges for nursing have been identified clearly within The Heathrow Debate (1993). The challenge for gerontological nursing is to look at changing demands, improved scientific and technological knowledge and policy changes and become involved within them. Changes in society since the 1950s, in how people relate to each other, their families and work, will affect how able and willing people are to support others, especially the frail and old. Unsteady work careers within nursing and society will make the systematic planning of care not as predictable as previously thought. Minimally invasive techniques within surgery are already transforming diagnostics and operations, and the implication of genetic research may be profound. In turn, gerontological nursing will have to face new ethical challenges, which may compromise an unprepared profession. Deciding what is right will not get any easier and gerontological nursing will be at the forefront. Services once offered automatically by the nurse now need to compete; having a treasury of skill is no good if skills have lost their currency. The benchmarks that the Heathrow Debate marked out for the year 2002 are highly significant and they include these points:

- *everyone over 85 will have a key worker;*
- *referrals from GPs to specialist medical services will be reduced by 20%;*
- *40% of outpatients' consultations with specialist medical staff will occur in locations other than a district general hospital;*
- *80% of surgical intervention will be by minimal access;*
- *60% of surgery will be day cases;*
- *hospital acute beds in DGHs will be reduced by at least 40%.*

These benchmarks will change the nature of gerontological nursing. If services polarize between high technology centres and community, what will the role of gerontological nurses be? They will have to bridge the boundaries, perhaps becoming the human counterweight in an increasingly technical era. An example of new skills that gerontological nursing can develop is demonstrated using new initiatives that have been developed in collaboration with other agencies.

The first initiative is the Advocacy in Action (1991) project supported by the Beth Johnson Foundation project, partly funded by the Department of Health. The origin of the Advocacy in Action project lies in the Foundation's increasing awareness of the sense of powerlessness that could overcome an older person who is frail and finds it difficult to contribute to decisions that are being made on their behalf. Its aim is to:

- *help older people to become more effective at self advocacy;*
- *where necessary advocate for care that meets wishes and preference.*

Advocacy occurs when a private citizen enters into a relationship with and represents the interests of an older person.

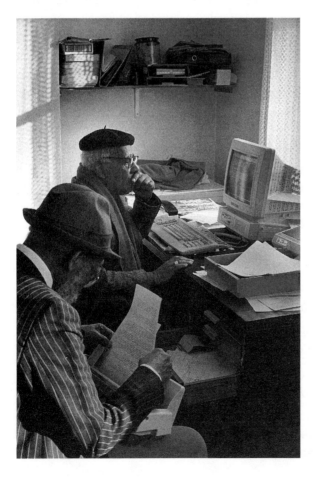

Fig. 1.4 *New age discovers travelling via the internet*

How Advocacy Works After negotiating with managers of hospitals or nursing or residential homes, an advocacy training/support officer visits each establishment regularly. Clients and residents receive a small clear written card. Once the advocacy officer has made contact and established that an advocate would be welcomed, a volunteer advocate outside the mainstream of professional health care workers is found. These volunteer advocates are encouraged to do all they can to help their partners on a personal level. There are times when the problems experienced seem to originate from the organization concerned and these issues are then discussed at monthly meetings with an advisory panel.

Interactive Decision Making A similar initiative in promoting interactive decision making has been aimed solely at carers. In facilitating care involvement in community care planning, a project in Birmingham from 1987 to 1990 looked at carers' contributions within this area (Barnes, 1991). In helping nurses plan care within the community, this project identified that those carers looking after older people needed specific help in nursing them at home and the chance of getting a break. Because of the emphasis on joint planning, the weekly meetings between the two groups helped to expose district general managers of hospitals to the raw pain of caring at home. Resulting from the planning initiative, specific needs were addressed. The carers wanted:

- *more health information;*
- *better respite care;*
- *help if a crisis arose;*
- *more day care;*
- *availability of incontinence pads.*

From the initiative it was clear that nurses must understand that carers are not just a named resource, but have specific needs.

If initiatives like these help gerontological nursing to become increasingly cognizant of health trends, what more can we do? We can begin by asking the right sort of questions. Health trends, either politically, socially or demographically driven, will alter the public's opinion towards nursing. It will be increasingly important that the care older people experience is first class. Nurses need to be able to evaluate health care trends and their relationship to gerontological nursing. They need to examine the impact of community care on professional care givers and unpaid carers. They must consider what role they will play as agents of change. We need to examine critically whether there are professional gatekeepers in various parts of the health service; for example what is the impact of age on the clinical decision making processes within various nursing practices? Nursing research needs to examine how effective we are in responding to older people's needs. This research could take the form of case studies, ethnographic studies or structured surveys on the behaviour of nurses and other allied professionals.

CONCLUSIONS

This chapter goes some way in assisting in a development programme that generates learning, raises questionable issues, demanding growth in the individuals. One of the key suggestions throughout the chapter is for the individual to reflect on the issues arising in relation to their practice. Benner (1984) demonstrated how nurses operate on very different levels of experience and knowledge. The core themes identified can be used at various levels of knowledge and exposure. What do these core gerontological themes bring to nursing older people? We can say they reflect the current perspective on the role of the older person as a consumer. They recognize the shifting focus from institutional care towards community-based health. But more importantly they require specialized nursing practice.

With more people reaching an older age we need well-educated gerontologically orientated nurses. However, many nurses are unfamiliar with this concept. Since unknown is unloved, it is important to make clear what we mean by this. For those who nurse older people, new perspectives within gerontological nursing will create a clinical environment that has appropriate role models, educators and researchers. With an ability to focus equally on the community as well as institutions, this career structure is attractive to both nurse and manager. It offers the development of multiskilled, innovative roles, whether in intensive nursing units or nursing clinics within the community.

CLINICAL DISCUSSION POINTS

Spend some time thinking about your personal and physical developments since childhood. What events have influenced your development, and what do you think the rest of your life will be like?

Convene a meeting with nurses and other members of the multidisciplinary team to discuss shared ideas on care. Agree on and mutually adopt shared philosophies.

How could you contribute to curricula that teach not only nurses but other groups that provide and give direct care?

Produce a business plan for your clinical area that incorporates the development of new skills and nursing roles. Share this with senior management and those interested in allocating money for nursing research.

SUGGESTIONS FOR FURTHER READING

Bains, E. (1991). **Perspectives on Gerontological Nursing.** Newbury Park Sage, California. *This is an American text that requires the reader to translate terms and concepts to their own culture and area of practice. It is a well organized and comprehensive book.*

Redfern, S. (Ed.) (1991). **Nursing Elderly People.** Churchill Livingstone, London.

This second edition combines the expertise of social sciences, doctors and nurses, in an excellent, well-referenced text.

Palmer, A., Burns, S. and Bulman, C. (1994). **Reflective Practice in Nursing.** Blackwell Scientific, London.
This is a very well thought out book, clearly illustrating levels and uses of reflected practice. It offers practical advice to nurses developing reflective skills. Recommended as essential reading in developing the reflected skills needed within gerontological nursing.

REFERENCES

Advocacy in Action, Bulletin (1991), No. 1. Beth Johnson Foundation, Staffordshire, England.

Barnes, M. (1991). **Carer's Contribution to Care.** Paper given to the Master of Art in Gerontology. Keele University, July.

Benner, P. (1984). **From Novice to Expert: Excellence and Power in Clinical Nursing Practice.** Menlo Park, California. Addison Wesley.

Department of Health (1993). **The Nursing, Midwifery and Health Visiting Contribution to Health and Health Caring.** DOH, London.

Erikson, E. H. (1963). **Childhood and Society.** W. W. Norton, New York. (Penguin, Harmondsworth, 1965).

Ersser, S. and Tutton, L. (1991). **Primary Nursing in Perspective.** Oxford University Press, Oxford.

Fries, J. (1980). Ageing, natural death and the compression of morbidity. **New England Journal of Medicine, 303,** 130–135.

James, J. (1994). Reflective Practice: Broadening the scope. Paper presented to the Clinical Nurse Specialism Conference. Nottingham, May 1994.

Johnson, M. L. (1976). That was your life: a biographical approach to later life. In: J. M. A Munnichs and W. J. A Van Den Heuval (Eds) **Dependency and Independancy in Old Age.** The Hague.

Medical Research Council (1994). **The Health of the UK's Elderly People.** MRC, London.

Neuman, B. (1982). **The Neuman Systems Model: Application to Nursing, Education, and Practice.** Appleton-Century-Crofts, Norwalk CT.

Nolan, M. R. (1994). Geriatric nursing: An idea whose time has gone: A polemic. **Journal of Advanced Nursing, 20,** 989–996.

Norton, D., McLaren, R. and Exton-Smith, A. N. (1962). **An Investigation of Geriatric Nursing Problems in Hospital.** Churchill Livingstone, Edinburgh.

Pearson, A. (1994). **Scholarship in Nursing.** Paper given to Manchester College of Nursing, Stepping Hill Hospital, Stockport.

Procheska, F. (1992). **Philanthropy and the Hospitals of London**. Oxford University Press, Oxford.

Rodgers, M. E. (1970). **An Introduction to the Theoretical Basis of Nursing.** F. A. Davis, Philadelphia.

Royal College of Nursing (RCN) (1990). **Guideline for Assessment of Elderly People.** Royal College of Nursing, London.

Royal College of Nursing (RCN) (1993). **Older People and Continuing Care: The Skill and Value of the Nurse.** RCN, London.

Roy, C. (1984). **An Introduction to Nursing: An Adaptation Model.** Prentice Hall, Englewood Cliffs, NJ.

Schon, D. A. (1991). **The Reflective Practitioner.** Temple Smith, London.

The Heathrow Debate (1993). **The Challenge for Nursing and Midwifery in the 21st Century.** HMSO, London.

United Kingdom Central Council (1994). **Professional Conduct Occasional Report on Standards of Nursing in Nursing Homes.** UKCC, Portland Place, London.

Wells, T. (1980). **Problems in Geriatric Nursing Care.** Churchill Livingstone, Edinburgh.

Wright, S. G. (1990). **My Patient, My Nurse.** Scutari Press, London.

Chapter Two

The Social World of Older People

Lesley Wade

Core Themes in Gerontological Nursing

Ageing Matters	*New Social World*	*Lifespan Perspective*	*Health and Old People*
Illness and Dependency	*Quality Nursing Care*	*Therapeutic Intervention*	*Politicizing Gerontological Nursing*

Key Words

Golden Age Myth • Ageism • Intergenerational Tensions • Networks

INTRODUCTION

The advancement of nursing practice lies deep within the uncharted waters of the social world of older people. This advancement and development are determined by how much nursing understands and accepts the diverse needs of this group. One of the great pleasures in nursing older people lies in the mutual benefit gained from sharing and interacting within this ever-developing society. This chapter emphasizes the need for nursing to challenge accepted stereotypes, understand the new character of old age, discuss population issues and review aspects of professional knowledge. Although turbulent, the social world of older people is a positive world. It is confident, anticipatory and hopeful. It is hopeful because of the intrinsic qualities that old age brings. The assurance old age can give is served by the opportunities age gives to receive and give help. This mutual reciprocity has hidden benefits. Older people have faced a life of continual goal setting and forward planning within diverse and often unclear health care structures and resilience and risk is their hallmark.

Proactive and becoming increasingly powerful, older people are the *new age travellers, spenders, carers and technocrats of the new millennium*. The varied 'group' society calls ageing is the inheritor of a post-war European identity, travelling further socially and physically than any previous generation. If nursing is to contribute to positive ageing it needs to re-examine its views, relationships and roles, recognizing the pioneering spirit of this varied group. To achieve this aim of positive ageing, gerontological nurses must also be risk takers, moving away from the supportive environment of hospitals, clinics and established nursing structures.

This Chapter has three broad aims enabling the nurse to:

Acquire up-to-date information on the social world of older people

---

Challenge social perceptions that may adversely effect older people whether in hospital, institutions or other community settings

---

Create a positive image of older people

RISK TAKING

Migration, house ownership, car driving and smoking may not seem risky from the perspective of the 1990s, but for older persons these apparent innocuous activities constituted initial forms of risk taking. Moving locality and home is a risk for any person but often age compounds this stress. Whether it be to a nursing home or to a warmer climate, migration may be a calculated risk worth taking. The plight of expatriates living in either Spain, France and Italy who, with illness and growing dependency, face unknown risk demonstrates the adventurous nature of age. The risks older people take may surprise some nurses and the general public. Consider some of the intolerance demonstrated towards older people's lifestyles and risk taking in the newspaper article below:

Case Study: Changing smoking habits

The drug squad thought it was just another bust of a small time dealer. Detectives were amazed when the suspect turned out to be a 70-year-old retired engineer, growing cannabis for himself and friends, many running foul of the law for the first time in their lives as they try to obtain supplies. The demand for the drug stunned doctors, police and suppliers. The sudden demand has alarmed regional drug advisory services. 'At the moment we are at a loss in helping this group' quotes an expert, while Dame Jill Knight, member of the Conservative Home Affairs Committee said, 'The idea of drug crazed pensioners ram raiding, to get money for this habit is a horrendous one.' (Sunday Times, July 5th, 1994).

This group of older people and their activities appears to challenge accepted norms. Before reading this chapter, reflect on the image this information portrays about older people, considering these points:

- *Why was the drug squad 'amazed' by the group?*
- *What assumptions are being made about class, gender, retirement and health within this article?*
- *Why was Jill Knight so repulsed by the thought of 'drug crazed pensioners'?*

If this image shocks members of society such as politicians and the police force, how do we, the nursing profession stand? Could it be that the image nursing has about how older people live and feel ignores the real world of older people? A further example of growing risk taking is the increasing growth of car ownership and licence-holding, particularly among women (Warnes, 1992). In the future there may be a greater amount of car dependency within this group and, compounded by changes in peripheral vision and psychomotor speed, rehabilitation nursing programmes need to address this issue. If older people are responsible drivers and are conscious of risks, an increasingly motorized population will require its health needs to be directed around this form of mobility. Redistribution of the population from towns to rural suburbs may in fact create a dependency that presently the nursing profession has not monitored and not planned for. Risk taking among older people is not unusual – it has been and remains a part of everyday life.

There are many myths surrounding old age that are perpetuated by television, radio, popular magazines and even by professionals involved in care of older people. The vast amount of prejudice shown towards older people is not premeditated and is a result of a lack of knowledge about their social world. In making some sense of our limited knowledge, we make sweeping generalizations. Inadvertently, we may have seen old people as all alike, socially isolated, having ill health, unproductive and senile. Lack of knowledge of older people's lives leads to myth, prejudice and discrimination and thus we need to examine the social world of older people to dispel some of this ignorance.

AGEISM WITHIN NURSING: A CASE OF REFLECTIVE PRACTICE?

One of the greatest threats to an individual's self esteem lie in how that person's self image is perceived by others. This is particularly so within nursing. If those caring for older people are treated and feel undervalued, then the client being cared for may feel the same. Phillipson (1982) stated that the low status and value given to caring for older people was linked to the low social value given to this age group. In changing contemporary attitudes towards older people, the fears and anxieties often held by nurses as well as the general public must be challenged. Stereotypes about older people as inflexible, hypochondriac self-preoccupied people abound, even within powerful professional groups. So nurses need to understand the social world of older people by asking what kind of activities do they pursue? How do they spend their time? What kind of relationships do they form? How do relationships and activities differ; for example, according to social class, age and gender? It is important to emphasize that older people actively reconstruct their lives and nursing must keep abreast of this and move away from custodial patterns of care.

Forms of Ageism

According to Butler (1969), *ageism* is a process of systematic stereotyping of people just because they are old. This *ageism* allows younger generations to see older people as different, thus they subtly cease to identify with their elders as human beings.

Sheppard (1988) coined the phase *new ageism* to describe the specific form of discrimination that makes older people the scapegoat for the alleged ills of society. Ageism or the process of systematic stereotyping and discrimination of people because of age, can be seen and heard among nurses. The nurse – whether in accident and emergency, intensive care or specialized gerontological units – may have to confront various forms of ageism within their practice; therefore, it is important to clarify what this term means within a nursing context.

Compassionate ageism emphasizes the problems of old age. This problem-orientated approach has too often been applied to nursing models and systematic approaches to care. Nolan (1994) questioned whether imposing a model of nursing which alienates gerontological nursing actually benefits older people. An emphasis on the problems experienced by older people is a legitimate concern, especially as gerontological nursing aims to develop services and provision of care. But if there is too much focus on the disadvantages of old age, this can constitute a stereotype of older people as weak, dependent and burdensome, reinforcing low self esteem.

Nursing within the consumer society of the 1990s brings us into contact with another form of ageism, *conflictual ageism*. The nature of ageism here limits resources to older people who appear to be an avaricious group of health consumers. Older persons may be seen as the 'nouveaux riches' who consume resources at the expense of families with children. Intergenerational tension does not take into account the essential need for the gerontological nurse to differentiate needs according to class, race and culture. Age is not the great leveller of inequalities. This point will be discussed later in this chapter.

Negative views towards older people are compounded by *medical ageism*; that is, the erroneous belief that older people do not benefit from technology and varied medical interventions (Grimley Evans, 1994). All these views of ageing have faults, particularly as they ignore the fact that many older people are in good health and making a valuable contribution to society.

Optimistic ways of viewing age emphasize the expansion of opportunities for older people. Greater consumption power and increasing personal development benefit society. Positive ageing mean that life is optimistic and worth living.

If nursing is to avoid some of these new aspects of ageism we need to reassess the status of this group. This may pay dividends; the wellbeing of older people and of nursing is a symbiotic relationship. In the future, it is this group that, as the major consumers of care, may determine the future of nursing. Nursing can influence stereotypes pertaining to ageing by developing gerontological nursing courses that help to change attitudes. Teaching and learning styles need to be creative in producing positive images of ageing.

The Status of Older People: The 'Golden Age' Mythology

At present the debate within gerontology still inclines to view preindustrial society as a 'golden age'. Stearns (1985) claims that this view is based on a great number of inaccuracies. One attractive claim, made by the supporters of the preindustrial 'golden age' myth, is the emphasis on the educational role of older people. In dispelling this myth, we must recognize that preindustrial society was largely illiterate; learning depended on word of mouth therefore the older person, because their memories ran the longest, served as society's mentors. However, as learning became stored in books instead of minds, older people automatically lost status and function. We also make assumptions about the older person's role in the family. First, we assume a functioning role between grandparents and grandchildren, but European marriage patterns within preindustrial societies preclude this mixing. Many couples married in their late twenties and with an average life expectancy of 56 years the average person would overlap the first-born grandchild by only 1 year, hardly any time to exert an influence. In an analysis of old age in Western cultures, Minosis (1989) suggests that the conditions of the old were determined by several components each acting independently, or occasionally together. He sees that each civilization has its own unique model of the older person, and judges all its old accordingly. In reality, there has never been a 'golden age' for the old, more of a chaotic evolution at the whim of various civilizations' values. The 'golden age' myth does not address how older men and particularly how older women were treated, it ignores class or those that were highly dependent.

However, some late twentieth century attitudes towards older people are being challenged. This challenge comes from a variety of sources. Historical perspective on older peoples lives are showing increasingly that older people worked to maintain themselves within a variety of systems of social support, whether family or larger communities (Pelling and Smith, 1991). Chapter 8 on the development of gerontological nursing looks at previous models of care within the community, a heritage which nursing has only just started to explore.

POPULATION CHANGES: FEARS AND SOCIAL CONSTRUCTION

The demography of Britain is undergoing dramatic reshaping. The ageing of the population has been a gradual process throughout the century. Among the most elderly – those aged at least 85, this change is more evident. We should see the numbers of older people as a reason to celebrate, the implications of these demographic changes being the basis for positive debate by policy makers to work with and for older people. In clarifying what the population changes mean to nursing it is important to look at the projected age of the population.

There have been significant changes in both population and household structures throughout this century. The dominant trend in Europe has been to smaller households and more people living alone. Much public debate has reflected ageist attitudes, which cast older people as a dependent, burden on society. Myths abound about the part of the life cycle known as old age, older people are usually portrayed as a mass of dependent has beens. Worse, they are often seen as a possible threat to the living standards of younger age groups because they are seen as a 'burden' or as consumers who are non-productive. Let us consider an alternative view, one that sees the older population as a positive force.

Intergenerational Tension

The effect of an increasing population, as in Africa, tends to focus on famine and the very young. However, Newsome (1994) asked that the plight of the older citizens in Africa should be given equal consideration. Here older people are seen a type of intergenerational glue that allows communities to survive, especially in war-torn areas like central Africa and eastern Europe. Help the Aged looks towards the older generation to foster some of the orphans in Rwanda and Romania and Bosnia. This is in direct contrast to established industrialized countries such as Germany's reaction to welfare reform. In Germany today, the proportion of over 60s is 20%; by the year 2030 it will be over a third. In a report on the future of older people, the German government have said that there will be just 100 people working to sustain benefits for 80 pensioners in 35 year's time (*The Independent*, 21 September 1994). Using information on population figures in isolation from factual accounts about older people, produces intergenerational tensions. The idea that within countries such as Britain and Germany older people are going to drain resources because of dependency has been criticized by and Phillipson and Walker (1986). They believe that long-term economic and social policies, fostered by retirement, income maintenance residential domiciliary and institutionalized care have created this. The question nursing must ask is whether developments in gerontological nursing have influenced dependency practices. Reflecting on the sociological theories of ageing, Cummings and Henry (1961), present the view that older people withdraw from society. How far nursing contributes to this disengagement theory remains unresearched. Nursing needs to examine the way it provides care to this community.

Over the past decade the definition of what the NHS provides in terms of continuity of care has been narrowed and tightened. The security of a publicly funded health care system in old age now seems unlikely. The future may involve a NHS free at the point of entry, but with a new national insurance covering long-term non-medical care.

What Do Different Generations Feel About Growing Old?

Interviewing a sample of older people over 55, who were differentiated according to gender, household structure, tenure and income, Midwinter (1991) identified active, lively, sexy older citizens. Interviews were also obtained from a younger age group of 16–24-year-olds, helping to produce a cross-generational picture of how generations see each other. In summary, there was room for moderate and qualified optimism.

OLDER PEOPLE AND THEIR RELATIONSHIPS

Concentration in the past on the centrality of the family in old age has steered us away from the importance of friendship in older people's lives. Jerrome (1990) argues, along with

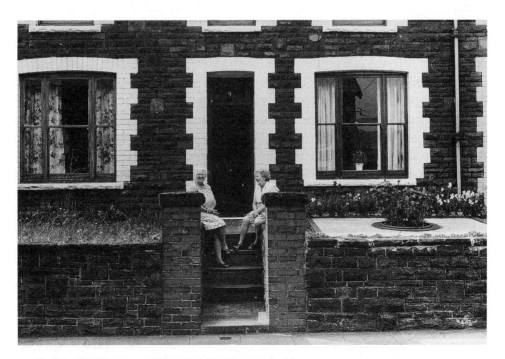

Fig. 2.1 Friendships are essential in maintaining self esteem and social support

33

American gerontologists, that friendships with peers are often more important influences than marriage, work roles and relationships with children. The very fact that friendship rests on mutual choice and mutual needs and involves a voluntary exchange of sociability between equals, often sustains a person's usefulness and self esteem more effectively than filial relationships. Thus the social world of older people – their networks, kinship patterns and friends – is important if we want to know more about the real world of older people. Qureshi and Walker (1989) looked critically at the research on social support and commitment by relatives, and showed that families continue to care, keeping in touch even at a distance. However, we lack information on the value of these relationships and may ignore the importance of infrequent contact, such as the chat in the corner shop or library, which may be invaluable to older people.

An image that is slowly being dispelled is that older people no longer require love, affection or sexual pleasure. Stereotypes attributed to the sex lives of older people consisted of:

- *sexual desire and activity cease to exist with the onset of old age;*
- *sexual desire and activity should cease to exist with the onset of old age;*
- *those who say they are still active sexually are morally perverse;*
- *overt expressions of affection or sexual interest are to be ridiculed and to be disapproved of.*

There are several reasons why sexuality in older people is difficult to discuss. First, professionals have not historically been trained to cope with sexuality, professional group training more often being about maintaining purity and asexuality. Second, there is the problem of ageism in a youth-orientated Britain. Hockey and James (1993) take an anthropological view on ageing, seeing older people reduced to infants, ignoring their sexual needs. Often older people themselves are reluctant to verbalize their sexual feelings for fear of being seen as depraved or lecherous, so myths about this group's sexuality are internalized. Iddedens (1987) finds it sad that referrals for sexual counselling are often given to people well below 50. White (1982), in an extensive literature search on sexuality and ageing, concluded that cohort studies to date suggest that males are more sexually active in later life than females; this, however, was due to the declining attitude of male partners. He also concluded that there was often a significant difference between individuals starting their sexual life between the wars. Masters and Johnson (1981) support the idea that older people are victims of ageism, which ultimately discourages sexual activity in later life. Starr and Wiener (1981) collected questionnaire data from 800 respondents between the age of 60 and 90. When asked how they felt about older people who were not married living together, 91% approved of the practice. This evidence suggests that older people's sexual norms may have more in keeping with those of the younger generation.

Contrary to the popular notion that passion and romance are only for the young, the fact is that older people date, fall in love, and behave romantically. O'Connor and Rodin's (1986) findings clearly show that older people falling in love physiologically and psychologically demonstrate the usual tell-tale signs. A 65-year-old man stated 'love is when you look across the room and your heart goes pitter patter'. The pursuit of intimacy causes special problems for older people and often they feel they have to hide intimate aspects of their dating. In O'Connors and Rodin's study, a 61-year-old female stated 'my boyfriend spends three nights a week with me but when the grandchildren come I hide his shoes'. Khun (1976) argued that Victorian values are perpetuated by many health workers, who may have unspoken anxieties about older people expressing sexuality. Homosexual relationships are seldom discussed, and especially not in institutions. Harris (1990) found that, in general, male and female homosexuals tend to have stronger friendship ties. Kelly (1977) revealed that male homosexuals did not perceive themselves as ageing as quickly as heterosexuals. It is interesting to ponder whether homosexuality may in some way facilitate adjusting to ageing.

COMMUNITIES

Where they live, as well as their gender, also plays an important part in how the older person interacts within their social world. Living in the inner city is often more isolating than living in rural communities. Some old people are likely to have more friends than others – poverty, ill health and gender governing their ability to play a part in social activity. A theoretical model by Kahan and Antonucci (1987), called the notion of the convoy, shows how the older person may lose contact with other people. The convoy theory suggests that each person moves through the life cycle surrounded by a convoy, a set of other people to whom he or she is related by the giving or receiving of social support. The specific people who make up the individual's social network may change over time as properties of the person such as age, health and situational forces shape the convoy.

If we accept that contemporary knowledge about the normal social world of older people is little understood or researched, we may be able to replace our half-baked notions about older people with fact. As Bond and Coleman (1990) state, one of the most influential factors in all of our lives is the environment in which we live. In this context, although the stereotype of old age may be that people as they age lose control over aspects of their environment, we can in fact see these people reconstructing their physical world. For example, older people's desires to improve aspects of their physical environment are well established: retirement migration, for example, can be traced back for centuries. In the 1920s the University of Chicago developed a model of city life that may help us understand why and how older people may feel isolated. This model of the average city of the twentieth century consists of zones of transition. The richer you are the more you may be able to move outside the city, while the upwardly mobile may select an inner city penthouse. Between these two zones older people may live in decaying pre-Second World War neighbourhoods. Tonnies (1955) described how living in a city produces different types of community spirit. He calls these relationships Gemeinschaft and Gesellschaft. Gemeinschaft city relationships are of friendship, mutual co-operation and mutual respect for others. Gesellschaft relationships in the city are based on rationality and calculation. Here action does not occur on the basis of personal ties. If this theory of city life is accurate, where does it leave older people who may be retired, single and poorer? The social world of the older person is therefore changing. As it changes, will new stereotypes emerge to replace the old hackeneyed ones?

Hepworth (1993) noted that positive images of ageing are emerging crime fiction. Although frail, white-haired and appealing, the outer appearance of Agatha Christie's 'Miss Marple' is deceptive. Miss Marple is a formidable criminal investigator who brings high intellectual skills into play. This example of positive ageing has enthralled audiences for the last four decades. Townsend (1989) sees that during the twentieth century the dependency of older people has been structured by long-term economics and social policies. As a result, he argues that older people are perceived and treated by the state as more dependent than they are or need to be. The developing institutions of retirement, income maintenance, residential and domiciliary care are cited as examples of the structures creating dependency within the older population. Although recognizing this, the perception of older people as vulnerable may be dated and too pessimistic. As Kuhn (1976), an American activist for her generation, has stated 'we are a new breed of old people'.

Living in the community, whether in one's own home, with or without the help of family, neighbours and friends, or in the home of close family, is the reality for most older people. There are three to four times as many older people living in the community as in residential care (Department of Health, 1992). Although the practice of community care has a history and is especially topical at present, the terminology is comparatively recent. In general, it has been used in vague and imprecise ways to mean different things to different groups of people. Indeed, its very diffuseness has made it an immensely useful idea with a wide appeal and strong emotional overtones. It is difficult for anyone to be against an idea that carries so positive a charge. But what does the notion mean to the different groups of people involved?

For most older people needing help with their everyday lives it is an ideal, offering the possibility of maintaining autonomy in as many aspects of life as possible, maintaining continuity with their earlier way of life and integration within their social network. Community care likewise appeals as an ideal to members of the general public; it suggests the picture of a caring society, respecting traditional values of mutual concern. For service providers and professionals, community care represents a pragmatic solution to the problem of deploying scarce resources to meet increasing need. But the reality of provision lags far behind the rhetoric. Services such as home helps, meals on wheels, social work assistance, friendly visiting, laundry provision and social clubs are still embryonic. Many writers, notably Phillipson and Walker (1986) have criticized the use of the term 'community care' and the kinds of policies that have been pursued in its name. Walker argues that the term is imprecisely defined in official documents. Does it mean providing care in the community in the sense of being non-residential or does it mean that care should be provided by the community? If the latter, are the providers to be members of the community or the employees of local authorities acting on behalf of the community? More realistically, is the term simply a euphemism for care by the family?

A second point of criticism concerns the inadequacy of provision about need. Community care for older people has normally been restricted to a narrow range of services, providing practical help with the basic, daily tasks of living, rather than an overall programme to cope with social, recreational and emotional needs as well as physical survival. Individuals have had to adjust to what is available and there has been little opportunity to exercise choice in putting together a package of services to suit either older people or their carers. Therefore planning for implementation of community care policy has been unequal to the task. Too much reliance has been placed on gentle persuasion of local authorities and health authorities rather than on the setting of specific goals. The result is an uneven, inequitable distribution of provision. There has also developed a range of innovatory developments in the provision of community care that attempts to take account of and make use of the care already provided by family and friends. For example, many Social Services departments have reorganized their services on 'patch' lines, with small teams of social workers, social work assistants, home care workers and sometimes community nurses, providing flexible, responsive help within a clearly defined territory. An essential part of this approach is developing local knowledge of what are known in the social work jargon as 'natural helping networks'. Other local authorities have developed chains of resource centres for older people and their carers. The Kent Community Care Project (Challis and Davies, 1986) devolved responsibility for 'case management' to individual social workers. Each social worker has access to a budget for frail older clients and this can be used to buy in a range of services (from public, private, voluntary and informal sectors) thus meeting the needs of those in different social situations. Chapters in Section 3 explore this view of nurses acting as case managers within and outside hospital settings. Henwood (1992) warned of the danger to the essential character of the informal sector, particularly if its liveliness and spontaneity was usurped by local authorities and the NHS. In an attempt to take them over, they may 'colonize' neighbourhood caring and welfare initiatives for their own purposes. Many see the new found favour in which the informal sector now basks as a thinly disguised rationale for cost cutting, especially in areas of provision that have been starved of the resources needed for an adequate level of service.

ENTERING THE SOCIAL WORLD

Improving their skill in obtaining personal accounts of life experiences (Ford and Sinclair, 1987; Bernard and Meades, 1993) helps nurses develop a realistic picture of the previous experiences of ageing. This is important for the nursing profession, emphasizing an individualistic approach to care. As advocated by Arber and Evandrous (1993), listening, talking, reflection and counselling are central skills in adopting a life course perspective. The gap in our knowledge about older people in the past leaves people open to nostalgia that may be harmful to those growing old in the present day. We need to move away from this nostalgia and ask ourselves a number of things. How, for example, will nursing combat and shape key attitudes about old age within the next century?

With allies such as oral historians and gerontologists Gearing and Dant (1990), who support the biographical approach and research, gerontological nurses are in a unique position to gather accurate detail about older people's pasts. Using oral histories brings three advantages. First, they help create a more rounded picture of the past, hence the direct voice of marginalized groups such as ethnic groups and working class people can be heard. An example of this within our own profession of nursing is the oral history project which is being undertaken by the History Society at the Royal College of Nursing. This is revealing important innovative practice related to all spheres of gerontological nursing and care. Second, we can explore crucial areas which the written record scarcely touches; the private world of family relationships or the informal culture of work. Last, we can examine policies relating to gerontological nursing and care through new perspectives, for example how previous skills from past life styles assist in maintaining self esteem. Use can be made of the National Sound Archives, a part of the British Library, to obtain older people's life biographies and thus enhance our understanding.

Application to Practice

Within your locality, there may be a variety of interest groups collecting oral histories supported by libraries and local history centres. The use of oral history is an ideal platform from which to develop gerontological skills in qualitative research methods. These fundamental skills form the basis of reminiscence, life review and skills of assessment. Coleman (1986) argues for a greater understanding of the biographical approach to perform assessments. As nursing is equally concerned with promoting health in the older population, well older persons may also benefit from life histories. More importantly, it should be seen as the basis of any assessment and a continuous link with the previous and present world of the older person. The nurse adopting this approach must be familiar with the ethical and methodological skills required. Some of these skills are:

- *to understand the nature of memory in old age;*
- *to be aware of ethical implications and obtain permission to interview if using recording equipment;*
- *to use a thematic approach, like family and early life, work, later family life and leisure;*
- *to keep all questions simple and to the point.*

For more information consult Thompson and Perks (1993) or the National Sound Archives either in London, Yorkshire or Devon.

Developing Effective Social Support Skills within Gerontological Nursing

Although nursing recognizes that social networks are a positive force as one grows old, nursing has to analyse the quality and type of relationships these networks offer for social support. Valuable networks that improve coping, esteem and specific aid at the appropriate time, are attributed to meaningful interactions with friends, peers and health care providers. As part of older people's networks, gerontological nursing has numerous new roles to fulfil. It needs to assess support needs, plan interventions, intervene at a variety of levels, evaluating the effectiveness of interventions. Acting as surrogate supporter, gerontological nursing can replace inadequate support in times of stress, by educating, facilitating and co-ordinating between lay and professional groups. It can identify who is important in the older person's network, and mobilize networks by referrals offering further support. Listening, informing, valuing and validating are skills needed to give support. Within practice, nursing can use a systematic approach giving social support within a gerontological framework. First, nurses can learn to assess complexities around social support systems. The strength, intimacy and timing of support has to be assessed, recognizing over use as well as under use of resources. The planning phase will look at the stressors and the context of the concern. Planning may be around social isolation or ineffective coping and this must be collaborative, including the client's social networks. Interventions may assist in increasing network size, or reinforcing existing relationships. These interventions will vary according to the location of the older person. Increasing success in nursing acutely ill older people will extend the need for nursing to ease the stress of families, who possibly will be giving care. Caregivers of mentally impaired older people, who provide care without social support, risk distress and depression. Gerontological nursing must offer tangible, emotional support and mobilize caregivers' networks. Community care programmes could also teach older people social skills to reduce loneliness and isolation. All these skills should be incorporated into gerontological nursing curricula. Students can be guided to reflect on their own experience of informal help, mapping their own and an older relative's social support. Using a social support framework within gerontological nursing would emphasize professional collaboration between lay person networks while also recognizing that older people cope differently and take different risks when seeking and selecting support.

Equal Opportunities

Why do older people need equal opportunities? The short answer to this question is because opportunities are unequal. Butler (1969) coined the phrase 'ageism' to explain the specific discrimination older people suffer because of age. For some groups of older people this is magnified according to gender, ethnicity, and health status. Why is this? The main reason is stereotyping, the assumptions that are made about people on the basis of the group that people belong to rather than the individual. The type of comment that is based on stereotype could be: older women are more emotional than men; all older people are senile or incontinent. A good example of stereotyping that harms young and older people alike is the way old people are portrayed in advertising. Older people's image, mobility, spending power and lack of choice in not being part of the 'fast lane', is demonstrated in advertising on television and in magazines. As far as advertising is concerned, old people and their purchasing power are just not worth the effort of promoting. Whether on television or in magazines, older people are seen to have no disposable income, and what little they have each week is spent on cat food and tinned salmon. That is assuming that arthritic fingers and demented minds can deal with new money! The most optimistic adverts show grandparents dispensing toffees to grandchildren, in sepia-tinted images of gentile poverty. The image of older people in Britain seems to have been locked behind the doors of Ealing Studios. The obligatory cat (naturally always with grandmother) and the awaited telephone calls appear to dominate this world.

In every commercial break, a finger leaps out of the screen announcing 'Hey you, you with the tartan shopping trolley and slippers with zips on. Don't you dare buy that car, you're not the generation that first learned to drive'. Despite a car like the Volvo being a safety-conscious selling commodity, it is aimed at the young middle aged, despite its boot fitting a dozen zimmer frames and its seats being ideal for osteoporotic spines. Perhaps the older driver does not fit easily within the accepted stereotypes of lonely, frail, asexual beings. Therefore advertisers are missing the spending power of older people.

Discrimination within Patient Care

With a change of emphasis towards earlier discharge policies, it is important to consider whether relatives are able to accept responsibility for clients when they are discharged from hospital. It is unwise to assume that all relationships within families are happy ones, and so families who seem reluctant to care for relatives should not be criticized without knowledge of their domestic situation and other responsibilities. Although equal pay may seem remote from the economic situation of older women, it is important to remember that they will probably have worked for lower wages than men. This means that they are less likely to have an occupational pension than a man, and if they do, it will be lower. Married women or widows may be cushioned by the pensions of their partners, but the relationship between low income, poverty and ill health is a self-evident facet of life for some older people. The older man also may suffer from a degree of isolation and inappropriate health expectations. Phillipson (1986) recognized problems of older men networking, and increasing evidence relating to prostatic cancer indicates a rethink on older men's health.

Ethnicity

Coming into hospital as a patient is difficult for anyone who does not know what to expect, but it is even more difficult for people with different cultural backgrounds, who may find it difficult to communicate in English. If, as a nurse, you work on the basis of stereotypes you may make assumptions about people's backgrounds that are not correct and may cause offence. If you react to people according to skin colour alone, this does not give information about whether they are Muslim or Hindu, or whether they were born in Britain or in the Caribbean. The only way of finding out the information that you need to provide good care is to ask them.

Age

Older people do not always think of themselves as old. Nurses in the day hospital for older people often tell me that when they suggest to their clients who are coming up for discharge that they should attend day centres or luncheon clubs, the reaction they often get is 'I'm not going anywhere with all those old people'. So it is important to remember that the way someone appears to you may not reflect how they feel about themselves. There is no legislation to prevent employers advertizing jobs with age requirements, such as 18–25 or under 40. At present the government has resisted pressure to introduce legislation, though the Institute of Personnel Management encourages its members not to discriminate against job applicants on the ground of age. Before the recession of the early 1990s, when all the talk was about the demographic time bomb, some employers were very concerned about labour shortage and one DIY retailer experimented with recruiting staff who were over 50 years. They found it worked well and that older staff were more knowledgeable about the products and able to give better advice than younger employees.

The Realities

Most domiciliary services have been struggling to keep pace with demographic trends. For example, home help provision declined from 18.3 whole time equivalents per 1000 population aged 75 and over to 17.9, while meals served per year to each 1000 of population aged 75 and over also decreased from 143 000 to 142 000. Three fundamental problems with community care policy will have to be tackled if its aims are overall to be achieved. Emerging problems as a result of community care show that:

- *The organizational structures are fragmented and lack coherence; many different bodies with different sources of funding are required to work together to promote community care and are failing to do so effectively.*
- *Patterns of distribution of financial resources are incompatible with the aims of community care policies; local authorities attempting to expand provision in the community find themselves liable to financial penalties.*
- *Insufficient attention has been paid to the staffing implications of developing community-based provision; new forms of training need to be introduced and the redeployment of existing staff who works in institutional settings needs to be taken into account.*

A programme of radical change, on the basis of examples of innovative practice, should consist of these issues:

- *strong and committed local 'champions' of change;*
- *a focus on action, not bureaucratic machinery;*
- *locally integrated services;*
- *a focus on the local neighbourhood;*
- *a team approach;*
- *partnership between statutory services and voluntary organizations*

The need for radical change is now more urgent than ever, with the numbers of those aged 85 and over expected to increase. If a wider range and better quality of community care is to develop, it must receive a far larger proportion of resources than at present. If not, domiciliary care will be increasingly simple and the level of care provided will become increasingly inadequate.

THE COSTS OF CARING

The physical costs of looking after a frail older person are fairly obvious; lifting at frequent intervals during the day and possibly night; extra washing where incontinence is involved; special cooking; help with feeding and other personal care tasks; all of these add up to a considerable amount of additional work. These tasks are usually borne by one person. However, although the health of many informal carers is not good, it is difficult to demonstrate that the task of caring is itself to blame since so many of them are themselves in an older age group where health problems are more common.

The social and emotional costs of caring also seem to be fairly obvious. There is the restriction of social life, less time for friends, fewer opportunities to leave the house or have holidays, and a greater reluctance to invite friends home, especially where the older person's presence means that accommodation is more cramped and particularly where incontinence is a problem. Yet most carers do not find such difficulties overwhelming.

Ungerston (1987) has drawn attention to the ways in which some caring tasks in Western society are identified as 'female' and others as 'male' and has used the notion of taboo to explain this. If her argument holds, it may be extremely difficult to effect significant change in the sexual division of labour in caring. Other financial costs may be involved in caring: extra heating; and more expensive food for sensitive palates; wear and tear on furniture; the cost of special equipment; travel expenses where the cared for person lives in a separate household; and the cost of buying in services to ease the burden.

NEW ISSUES TO ADDRESS

Social and Economic Hardship

A survey by Townsend (1989) established that the continual fall of employment, low incomes and a number of short- and long-term policies has, within inner cities such as London, created material and social deprivation for older people.

The great majority of people aged 60 and over are no longer in paid employment and, although not exposed to poor working conditions, they fare badly with regard to housing and dietary deprivation. The poverty of a substantial minority is acknowledged in different ways by older people themselves. A larger proportion of older people, especially over the age of 80, have incomes on the margins of poverty. Townsend found that the overwhelming majority agreed that the gap between rich and poor is too wide. A clear majority agreed that the rich should be more highly taxed. The Joseph Rowntree Foundation has recently examined the financial wellbeing of older people. Their findings show that the level that divides the poorest and the richest has continued to increase. In 1989, the richest fifth enjoyed incomes nearly three times those of the poorest fifth (Hancock and Weir, 1994). The poverty of older people has three explanations according to Townsend:

- *long-standing cultural and class relationships within British society;*
- *loss of employment, status and income as an indirect, as well as direct, effect of market forces;*
- *weak and contradictory social policies of successive governments.*

Older people have had a prominent place in political debate over the last decade. There are three reasons for this. First, because of only partial comprehension about population changes, social policies display uncertainty towards radical adjustments to accommodate large numbers of older people. Second, political use may be made of certain gerontological facts, for example future ratios of the older population to that of working age. A good indicator of this political opportunism is use of the word 'burden' by economists and health service planners. A third reason is directly related to an ideological shift. A new challenge to the post-war collectivist welfare consensus has focused attention on the cost to the public exchequer of both income support and health and social services for older people.

At present, the political priority is to facilitate wealth generation rather than its distribution, thus reducing the role of the public sector in the community. Political debates frequently simplify issues related to age, commonly lacking clarity and consistency in the use of the term 'elderly'. It is important that we encourage precision in policy and service debate between those groups of the population. It is not the case, for example, that a 10% increase in the population aged 60 years or more will be accompanied by a 10% increase in specific health disorders in this group. This chapter recognizes the need to consider the age structure of the older population and the wide range of cohort differences in older people, life times, health care, nutrition habits, working and living conditions. Once digested, nurses need to consider these, in tandem with developments in medical technology and practice, and future changes in service provision.

CONCLUSIONS

This chapter has looked at the realities of older people's social worlds, addressing new horizons within which both nurses and older people operate. Older people have been seen as life-long risk takers who have fulfilling relationships at various levels. The familiar features of ageism in all its myriad forms have been addressed. The chapter has given guidance on using a biographical research method to enter the social world of older people. The positive aspects of growing old have been identified alongside some of the difficulties age brings. Knowledge in relation to community care, family care and the effect of social, political and health care policies has been highlighted. This chapter emphasizes the need to recognize older people's individual needs, understanding that gender, class and ethnicity impinge on growing old, no less than age.

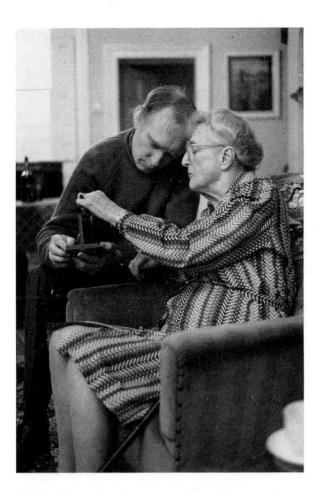

Fig. 2.2 *Joint ventures between the young and old benefit society*

Most older people want to stay in their own home and, if in hospital, to be cared for by nurses who recognize their individuality and needs. It is important that as we approach the twenty-first century, older people are recognized as having different traditions, different pasts and futures living within different cultures. This chapter has emphasized the continuing interplay between ageing and social change, identifying sources of misinterpretation and redefining the world of older people. The limited amount that is known about the social world of older people relies too much on stereotypes that can be wrongly used by nurses when giving care and advice. Older people value independence and social support. They need love, affection and affirmation and, on a practical basis, advice and help. A major feature in ensuring the social world is healthy for older people is to recognize the important role of the nurse in being a confidant within this world, having intimate knowledge of its needs. If as a profession nursing is to promote positive ageing, then initially the social world has to become our focus.

CLINICAL DISCUSSION POINTS

Try to apply your knowledge of the social world of older people to your specific area of nursing.

Acknowledge stereotypes and myths about older people, developing strategies to combat these within your practice.

Discuss the legislative events that have influenced the nursing of older people over the last 10 years. Use this knowledge to promote independence, preventing custodial care.

Evaluate a positive local national or international nursing initiative within gerontological care that would benefit the group of older people you care for.

How might you develop relationships with local schools and voluntary agencies involving the local community within your nursing strategies?

Discuss ways to network, cross boundaries, exchange and reciprocate and build alliances with other professionals.

SUGGESTIONS FOR FURTHER READING

Arber, S. and Ginn, J. (1991). **Gender and Later Life.** Sage, London.
This text has a large amount of data on the social world of older people.

Fennell, G., Phillipson, C. and Evers, E. (1988). **The Sociology of Ageing.** Open University Press, Milton Keynes.
This an easy to read enjoyable text that serves as an excellent introduction to the sociology of ageing.

Peace, S. (1990). **Researching Social Gerontology.** Sage, London.
This is an important text that offers the reader an introduction to various methods of research within gerontology. Nurses and health visitors benefit from the methods of research identified and applied.

Sidell, M. (1995). **Health in Old Age.** Open University Press, Milton Keynes. *Exploring the perspective of the older person, using case studies and official statistics, this work looks at the myths surrounding health in old age. It provides a positive framework for a healthy old age within its last chapter.*

REFERENCES

Arber, S. and Evandrous, M. (1993). **Ageing Independence and the Life Course.** Kingsley Publication, London.

Bernard, M. and Meads, K. (1993). **Women Come of Age.** Edward Arnold, London.

Bond, J. and Coleman, P. (1990). **Ageing in Society**. Sage, London.

Butler, R. N. (1969). Ageism: another form of bigotry. **The Gerontologist, 9,** 243–246.

Challis, D. and Davies, B. (1986). **Case Management in Community Care: An Evaluation Experiment in the Home Care of the Elderly.** Gower, Aldershot.

Coleman, P. (1986). **The Ageing Process and the Role of Reminiscence.** Wiley, London.

Cummings, E. and Henry, W. (1961). **Growing Old. The Process of Disengagement.** Basic Books, New York.

Department of Health (1992). **The Health of Elderly People: An Epidemiological Overview.** Vol 1. The Health of the Nation. HMSO, London.

Eisenhammer, J. (1994). Load silence on pensioners, as german election nears. **The Independent,** 21st September.

Ford, J. and Sinclair, R. (1987). **Sixty Years On—Women Talk About Old Age.** The Women's Press, London.

Gearing, B. and Dant, T. (1990). Doing Biographical Research. In: Peace, S. (Ed.), **Researching Social Gerontology,** pp. 143–159. Sage, London.

Grimley Evans, J. (1994). Can we live to be a healthy hundred? In: A Healthy Old Age. **Medical Research Council News** (Autumn), **64**, 1.

Hancock, R. and Weir, P. (1994). The financial well being of elderly people. **Social Policy Research, 57.** Joseph Rowntree Foundation.

Harris, D (1990). **Sociology of Ageing.** Harper & Row, New York.

Henwood, M. (1992). Through a glass darkly. **Kings Fund Research Report** 14, Kings Fund Institute, London.

Hepworth, M. (1993). Old age in crime fiction. In: Johnson, J. and Slater, R. (Eds) **Ageing and Later Life.** Sage, London.

Hockey, J. and James, A. (1993). **Growing Up and Growing Old.** Sage, London.

Iddedens, D. (1987). Sexuality during the menopause. **Medical Clinics Of North America, 71** (1).

Jerrome, D. (1990). Intimate Relationships. In: J. Bond and P. Coleman (Eds) **Ageing in Society,** pp. 74–81. Sage, London.

Kelly, J. (1977). The ageing male homosexual myth or reality. **Gerontologist, 17,** 328–332.

Khan, R. and Antonucci, T. (1987). Convoys over the life course: attachment role and social support. In: P. Balts and O. Brim, (Eds) **Life Span Developments and Behaviour.** Academic Press, New York.

Khun, M. (1976). Sexual myths surrounding the elderly. In: M. Oak and G. Melchorode (Eds) **Sex and Life Styles.** Grone & Statton, New York.

Masters, W. and Johnson, V. (1981). **Human Sexual Responses.** Little Brown, Boston.

Midwinter, E. (1991). **The British Gas Report on Attitudes to Ageing.** British Gas Publications.

Minosis, G. (1989). **History of Old Age: From Antiquity to the Renaissance,** pp. 303–307, Polity Press, Cambridge.

Newsome, J. (1994). Help the Aged: **Rwanda Appeal.** BBC Television, 25th August.

Nolan, M. (1994). Geriatric nursing: An idea whose time has gone? A polemic **Journal of Advanced Nursing, 20,** 989–996.

O'Connor, L. and Rodin, P. (1986). Never too late. **Psychology Today,** 66–69.

Pelling, M. and Smith, R. (Eds) (1991). **Life, Death and the Elderly.** Routledge, London.

Phillipson, C. (1982). **Capitalism and the Conduction of Old Age** Macmillan, London.

Phillipson, C., Fennell, G. A. and Evers, H. (1988). **The Sociology of Old Age.** Open University Press, Milton Keynes.

Phillipson, C. and Walker, A. (Eds) (1986). **Ageing and Social Policy: A Critical Assessment.** Gower, Aldershot.

Qureshi, H. and Walker, A. (1989). **The Caring Relationship.** Macmillan, London.

Sheppard, L. (1988). Intergeneration Equity or the New Ageism. **Ageing and Vision News, 1** (July), 6.

Starr, B. and Wiener, M. (1981). **The Star and Wiener Report on Sex and Sexuality in the Mature Years.** Hill, New York.

Stearns, P. (Ed.) (1985). **Old Age in Pre Industrial Society.** Holmes & Meirr, New York.

Thompson, P. and Perks, P. (1993). **An Introduction to the Use of Oral History.** National Sound Archives. The British Library Publications, London.

Tonnies, C. (1955). **Geminschaft and Gesellschaft Community and Associations.** Translation. C. S. Looms. Routledge, London.

Townsend, P. (1989). The social and economic hardship of elderly people in London. **Generations, Bulletin of British Gerontology, 9** (Spring).

Ungerston, C. (1987). **Policy is Personal: Sex Gender and Informal Care.** Tavistock, London.

White, R. (1982). **Human Sexuality and its Problems.** Churchill Livingstone, London.

Warnes, A. (1992). Elderly people driving cars: Issues and perspectives. In: K. Morgan (Ed.) **Gerontology Responding to an Ageing Society,** Jessica Kingsley, London.

Chapter Three

The Impact of Ageing

Helen Jones

Core Themes in Gerontological Nursing

Ageing Matters	New Social World	Lifespan Perspective	Health and Old People
Illness and Dependency	Quality Nursing Care	Therapeutic Intervention	Politicizing Gerontological Nursing

Key Words

Changes with Time • Theories • Primary Ageing • Social Construction • Political Ideology

INTRODUCTION

This chapter is concerned with ageing and its effects on people. But what do we mean by 'ageing' exactly? Ageing is a term generally associated with numbers and in this particular instance with chronological age, or increase in number of years since day of birth. Consider for a moment that a whole person is made up of, and influenced by, a range of component parts – their physical function; their personality and personal construct system; their ability to integrate and their social networks; and finally, the political and economic framework of their habitat. The effect of passage of time within and between each of these components will produce a range of effects and responses upon a person as wide and as varied as the numbers of individuals reaching old age. Thus, the passage of time will produce a rich source of individual older people, each one unique. The purpose of this chapter is to try and identify the patterns or trends that influence individuals as they increase in chronological age. Their influence may be from the micro-level of component part to the macro-level of whole person. Ageing effects all aspects but at different rates within and between components.

To help identify some of the threads in this intricate web of changes with age, the chapter has been divided into four parts. These are:

Theories of ageing

Ageing at microscopic and functional level

Ageing and social integration

Ageing and self image.

THEORIES OF AGEING

The theories and patterns described in this chapter should serve as a guide to assist the student in recognizing the ageing affects and effects on people, to assist in assessing need, help to plan the relevant care, and evaluate appropriately the care given prior to replanning and continuing the cycle of care or meeting need.

The cause for ageing itself is not well understood and no single cause is apparent. Theories of ageing suggest how, why and what happens to a person solely due to living through a passage of time, or the natural life cycle. They are not concerned with extraneous influences such as disease or natural disaster. Before proceeding further it is first necessary to define what is meant by theory. In this context, it is generally accepted that in order to be recognized as a theory, the following criteria modified from Spence (1989) must be met:

- *the change must generally be evident throughout mankind;*
- *the change must be progressive – i.e. more acute – as time passes;*
- *the change process must lead to some dysfunction.*

As previously suggested, the range of theories fall into one of three main categories: biological; psychological; and sociological.

Biological Theories of Ageing

There is no acceptable universal definition of ageing. Biological ageing studies are complex to undertake and interpret because effects occur at different rates and at different levels from the individual cell to the whole organism and at all levels – tissue, organ, system – in between. Since ageing effects vary in every individual, and because of the lack of an acceptable definition, it is perhaps more important to consider a person's functional age rather than their chronological age when looking at biological ageing. Some textbooks (e.g. Garrett, 1983; Spence, 1989) choose to list the theories. Alternatively, some choose to group the biological theories into, say, intrinsic theories and extrinsic theories (e.g. Christ and Hohloch, 1988). They define intrinsic theories as age changes that come from within and are due to a predetermined cause, while the causes of extrinsic theories are considered to be external to the body. The difficulty with this kind of categorization is where to place an external influence that has an internal effect. Its usefulness comes at the initial stages of learning and understanding when trying to make some kind of sense of the theories. Christ and Hohloch

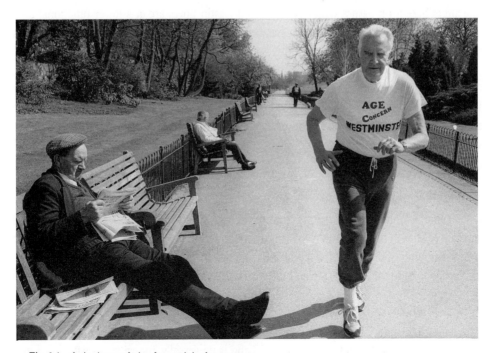

Fig. 3.1 Ageing is an exclusive characteristic of every person

(1988) further categorize theories into genetic, non-genetic and physiological theories. While this may be a useful tool to aid memory, it also serves to fuel the philosophical argument of the cause and effects of ageing.

Here, the theories appear simply in alphabetical order, to show no bias and to make the reader consider the characteristics of each. For further information, see Bromley (1974), Christ and Hohloch (1988) and Spence (1989).

In reading through the list, the reader should consider similarities and differences between theories since they develop around two main concepts. The first is the notion of genetic or programme-related changes. The second addresses the belief that all aspects of living, embracing environment, physiology, psychology and social influences, exert their effects and thereby affect ageing. Current thinking tends to favour theories that reflect the former concept.

Biological Clock Theory

The biological clock theory suggests there is a sequential biological process linked to the dimension of time. Thus, there would be a set period of growth followed by a longer period of decline. Writers vascillate on the actual siting of the clock, which is thought to be either in individual cells or in the hypothalamus. The debate has been long and complex. The biological clock is thought to set, run and monitor a genetic programme responsible for embryogenesis, growth and development. Thus this theory is sometimes called a Programmed Theory (q.v.).

Chemical Cross-link Theory

The affect here is on tissues where collagen and elastin fibres are at a lower functional level than earlier in life, due to knotting. It has been suggested that chemical changes may be a cause of the knotting. It is not clear if this is a cause or an effect of ageing.

Free-radical Theory

This theory describes where changes occur in chromosomes, pigments or collagen due to the presence of 'free radicals'. The free radicals are thought to be present due to environmental factors – such as radiation or air pollutants – external to the body and affecting biological systems.

Immunological Theory

With ageing, lymphocytes originating from the thymus gland fall in number leading to a T cell imbalance. This, in turn is thought to bring about an immune deficiency as well as an increase in autoimmunity. This is the theory of immunology. It is a combination of theories, more specifically the programme theory and the wear-and-tear theory.

Programme Theory

Another genetic theory is where it is thought that cells divide for a specific number of times only. This number is thought to be around 50 and is universally known as the Hayflick Limit

(Hayflick, 1977). This theory supports the notion of a species maximum lifespan and programmed destruction. Other programme theories address genetic disorders which are associated with premature ageing, for example Down's syndrome and progeria.

Somatic Mutation Theory

Clearly, this theory is genetic in origin. It embraces the failure of, or error in, DNA replication. However, this theory does raise the interesting question – is somatic mutation a cause or an effect of ageing?

Stress Adaptation Theory

Stressors both internal and external to the body trigger a biological response – they lead to stress activation. An accumulation of these responses through life is considered to bring about ageing. Stressors may present in any form such as wounding, disease, surgical procedure, losing your home or indeed, losing a loved one.

Waste Product Theory

As life continues, so there is a build up of waste products and toxins in the body. One example is lipofuscin, but there is no testimony in the literature that suggests this is harmful to body cells.

Wear-and-tear Theory

This theory is quite simple. Repeated use of, disease, or damage to anatomical structures and physiological functions leads to general wear-and-tear with the ultimate end result being wear-out.

Sociological Theories of Ageing

It is clear from the rhetoric that while social behaviour may be influenced by ageing, the reverse is not always true. As a consequence, sociological theories of ageing serve to explain why something is happening rather than to predict potential changes. More simply, these theories provide a form of order to social interactions and the socialization of elders that are observed in reality. Five main concepts are introduced here.

Continuity Theory

Continuity theory focuses on the individual's own responsibility and behaviour. It is based on the assumption that, in general, these two remain fairly stable and unchanged throughout life, despite advance in years and the changes that occur in a society at the macro-level, for example family structure or gender roles. In essence the theory purports that a person's pattern of living is the overriding factor. It reflects their life experiences and as such diminishes the affect of biological age.

Disengagement Theory

This was originally developed in the late 1950s/early 1960s by Elaine Cumming and William Henry (Cumming and Henry, 1961). The 'disengagement' concerns both the individual and society and is acceptable to both. It does not concern the social structure of society, for example social organization or the economy. The theory is based on observations of older people, influenced by personality and lifestyle. Personal finance, roles undertaken, and state of health have all been considered to influence patterns of activity and levels of disengagement. Further debate focuses around whether disengagement is imposed on, or desired by, an individual. The environment at the macro- or political level and its effect at micro- or individual level is also important.

Exchange Theory

This theory is based on the assumption that socialization involves giving and receiving, on valuing and being valued. As individuals move through life, the roles that they take on and shed slowly change. Western societies have evolved such that, for the majority of the population, retirement is enforced at an age specified by government and supported by law. Societal roles change dramatically on reaching the age of retirement and many of these new roles are underutilized and not particularly valued. Added to this, there is a structured societal dependence on health, social and welfare support to further reinforce the notion of taking, without the balance of the older person being able to give. Up to this point, exchange theory is similar to the theory of disengagement. However, exchange theory moves this argument further on and attempts to address the imbalance by suggesting that social policy could evolve to utilize and benefit from the skills and knowledge of retired older people. It is judged that the outcome of such policy changes would generate a population of older people who could truly take on roles valued by the rest of society, as well as continuing to receive the necessary medical, social and welfare support.

Political Economic Perspective

This hypothesis was not described until the early 1980s. It details how the national policies and their implementation actually promote dependency for older people. The mechanics of this perspective are rooted in lifestyles, roles and opportunities for the person when they were younger and strongly reflect issues of class, gender and race. A classic example of this is the national retirement age. Most people, whether they wish to or not, are forced to retire in the seventh decade of life. At present, this means that retired people are no longer eligible for paid work. They have to live on the state pension and a private pension, if they took one out. There may be an employer's pension which may or may not be index-linked. Total income from pensions cannot equal more than two-thirds final employment salary. Thus, these policies mean that income falls upon retirement (unless interest on investments can make up the shortfall, but this is not the usual case). Older people become dependent on the state. A lower income usually means that services can be obtained at concessionary rates. This system can feel like charity or hand-outs and, if it is perceived as such, may lead to lower self esteem. Enforced retirement is biased: females retire at 60 while men retire at 65 (currently under review – but to benefit whom?), while those in higher social class professions can and are encouraged to work well into their ninth decade of life or later. Examples of these roles include judges, politicians and doctors.

Role Theory

The concept of role theory came about in the 1940s. It is based on the notion that retirement is a critical event in life. The post-retirement phase provides a minimal number of, or no, significant roles for the individual. This theory has recently received much support with the development of pre-retirement programmes in large work environments. There is also a small but increasing recognition of the need for continued support for an employee as they move through this phase of their life. While the time of retirement is the actual pivot for change in role, a social framework of roles needs to be developed in society that continues to support the older person as they move through the whole of the post-retirement phase. Thus this theory requires policy support.

Psychological Theories of Ageing

Psychological theories of ageing concern lifespan development. For this reason, it can be difficult for the beginner to determine which age-related changes are due to natural biological evolution or changes in social circumstances or a maturing of a person's perspective of and approach to life. Thus, psychological theories tend to express changes with age in terms of cognitive functions, namely: intelligence and personality; learning and ability to solve problems; and memory. These changes are described in the next section. To list the theories here would not do them justice and therefore they are described in more detail later in the chapter. Lifespan development and its various protagonists are considered in the section on ageing and self image.

AGEING AT MICROSCOPIC AND FUNCTIONAL LEVELS

Primary ageing is the biological progression of becoming old, regardless of increase in years from birth. The cause of age-related changes is still unclear; however, current rhetoric favours genetic theories while not ignoring other influences external to the body. Age-related changes are seen to occur from the subcellular level, through tissues and organs, organ systems and, ultimately, through to the functional level of the whole organism. Though interesting, it is outside the scope of this book to describe the effects of ageing in this format and in such detail. This section lists the major changes observed, system by system. For more exhaustive information, the reader is recommended to peruse *The Ageing Body* by Whitebourne (1985).

While documenting age-related changes, this section is of most value if read in its entirety. This is so that the reader can become more than just conversant with the facts presented, but can start to inter-relate them and understand the true meaning of primary ageing.

The Ageing Cardiovascular System

The ageing process does not begin at any specific time but the whole body develops to maturity and then begins to decline slowly. Between the ages of 25 and 65 there is a reduction in stroke volume of the heart and cardiac output drops by around 40%. This approximates to 1% per year. There is calcification of blood vessels which become less elastic and consequently have an increased peripheral resistance. Thus, it is logical that pulse and systolic pressure increase. Overall then, cardiac output falls and there is a fall in blood circulation. Both arteriosclerosis and atherosclerosis occur. Thrombi, emboli and atheroma lead to peripheral vascular disease. In practical terms this means:

- *the heart is sensitive to the fall in oxygen and potassium thereby causing heart dysrhythmias and cardiac disease;*
- *a fall in circulating oxygen causes both anaemia and confusion;*
- *a fall in circulating blood volume leads to a reduction in waste removal which in turn can lead to confusion;*
- *poor blood circulation causes hypothermia;*
- *most amputees are older people and the main cause of this is peripheral vascular disease. The ratio of amputees is 2 males to 1 female. The second leg is usually removed within 2 years of the first and there is usually death within 5 years.*

The Ageing Endocrine System

Overall, with age hormones are less effective. It is thought that endocrine gland synthesis of a hormone remains unchanged or insignificant with ageing. However, the hormone receptor sites may be affected in some way to limit uptake of the hormone with age. Table 3.1 outlines overall changes. For greater detail consult Spence (1989) and Whitebourne (1985).

General observed effects include the following. The adrenal response to stress such as injury or anxiety, is reduced. The adrenals influence glucose store and utilization, reduce protein synthesis and increase urea in the urine. They also influence sodium ions and therefore water loss causing a fall in blood volume. This leads to a fall in blood pressure. Ultimately death can occur. There is an insulin deficiency. TSH is unchanged; T3 in the plasma is reduced; T4 secretion falls; T4 in blood plasma is unchanged, thus the hormone is less effective and there is thought to be a possible deficiency in the negative feedback mechanism for thyroxine control.

In practical terms this means:

- *the range of thyroxine functions will also be affected. This includes its control of red blood cell and eosinophil numbers and its influence on blood pressure;*
- *Addison's disease is common in older people – due to an underactive thyroid gland, while overactivity (Cushing's disease) is rare;*
- *mature-onset diabetes mellitus occurs;*
- *hypothyroidism leads to myxoedema.*

Table 3.1 *Hormonal changes in main glands, thought to be due to primary ageing. Modified from Spence (1989)*

	Circulating blood level		
	Rises	Falls	Unchanged/insignificant
Nature of change			
(Refer to text)			
Hormone synthesis			★
Hypothalamus releasing factor			★
Hormone receptor sites		★	
Main Glands			
Pituitary gland			
TSH			★
ACTH			★
GH			★
FSH	★ } females		
LH	★ } only		
Thyroid gland			★
T4		(★ possibly)	
Parathyroid gland			★
Adrenal glands			
glucocorticoids		★	
aldosterone		★	
Pancreas			
insulin		★	

The Ageing Excretory System

As previously noted, blood flow is reduced – by some 53% with ageing. Glomerular filtration reduces by 50% between the ages of 20 and 90. There is also a fall in the ability of the renal tubules to concentrate the urine. Bladder capacity is reduced by 50% from 500 ml to 250 ml. and the muscular bladder walls weaken. These effects are more evident at night. The prostate gland increases in size thereby narrowing the urethral passage. Bladder emptying may revert to reflex contractions. Nearly one-third of people over the age of 70 have gall stones (information gained from post mortems). A reduced liver mass leads to a consequent fall in liver function. In practical terms this means:

- *an increased risk of dehydration;*
- *likelihood of prostatism in men;*
- *risk of insufficient fat metabolism;*
- *such changes in the liver will bring about an increased effect for drugs, so smaller doses may be sufficient. Polypharmacy will be more risky. Further to this, alcohol intake will carry increased risks.*

The Ageing Gastrointestinal Tract

At present, around 60% of people aged 60 years are edentulous. Teeth become less white and more yellow due to dentine thickening. There is a loss of collagen and gums recede causing inefficient mastication. A change in taste occurs with altered sensitivity to sweet and salt. There may also be a change in sensitivity to bitter and sour. At the same time, older people are less sensitive to smells. Gastrointestinal tract secretions such as saliva, enzymes and gastric juices decrease and may even dry up. Vitamin B_{12} deficiency is common in older people. There is reduced muscle motility. In practical terms this means:

- *dentures may no longer fit and become uncomfortable;*
- *there may be an increase in the use of condiments on meals which can be unhealthy, e.g. salt;*
- *following an anaesthetic or cerebrovascular incident, dulled oral sensitivity may increase the risk of further damage;*
- *vitamin B_{12} deficiency leads to poor red blood cell maturation and pernicious anaemia in particular;*
- *reduction in secretions is likely to lead to blockages and incomplete metabolization of necessary foods.*

The Ageing Immune System

The thymus atrophies with age. There is an increase in diffuse lymphoid tissue and a reduction in organized lymphoid tissue. These changes in effect reduce the mechanism of defence causing a build-up of waste in the body, thereby adding to the problems previously described due to an ageing cardiovascular system. Furthermore, the spleen has less white pulp and follicular tissue and more red pulp, effectively reducing the body's protection by defence. There are cell defects in differentiation and in function affecting T cells. T cells provide immunity to viruses, fungi and mycobacteria as well as delay hypersensitivity. The levels of some immunoglobulins in the blood alter, increasing the risk of disease. Finally, toxin sensitivity is increased.

In practical terms this means that older people are generally more prone to disease and less able to fight the disease. As stated earlier, the body is less able to cope with stress and so the disease process is an even greater threat. The symptoms of toxin overload, for example confusion, will occur more readily due to an increased sensitivity and the body's reduced ability to filter out waste.

The Ageing Musculoskeletal System

There is less protein in ageing muscles. A fall in serum potassium and vitamin C causes muscle weakening. The skeleton has less support then and there is an average height loss of 5 cm between the age of 20 and 70. Calcium is lost from the bones and redeposited on the costal cartilages, trachea, bronchi, thyroid and wall of the aorta. The cause of this is unclear. Bones become less dense and brittle. Involuntary muscles thicken. Fibrous tissue in voluntary muscles increases, their speed of contraction falls and there is a reduction in activity. In practical terms this means:

- *there is an increased risk of pathological fractures;*
- *respiration movements become restricted thereby increasing the risk of infection;*
- *peristalsis slows, possibly affecting elimination;*
- *the voice alters due to changes in the laryngeal muscles.*

The Ageing Nervous System

The weight of the brain reduces by around 10% between the ages of 25 and 75. Co-ordination is less precise due to reduced cell activity and possibly reduced cell numbers. Atrophy of the brain and spinal cord depends on biological ageing elsewhere in the body, thus the maintainence of excercise into later life is important. Response and reaction time slows and the threshold for the special senses is raised. In the eye, the lens becomes opaque and less elastic, the cornea thickens and the iris fades. Cataract formation is a likely outcome. In practical terms this means:

- *there is increased susceptibility to hazards;*
- *there is less awareness of pain;*
- *there is less awareness of thirst, which leads to an increased risk of dehydration. There is also less awareness when the bladder is full and walking to toilet takes longer, therefore increasing the risk of voiding urine in inappropriate place. Consequently, older people drink less to reduce incontinence, and the complications of dehydration are a risk. The spiral continues;*
- *there is less awareness of cold, reduced ability to regenerate heat, thus increased risk of hypothermia;*
- *presbyopia.*

The Ageing Reproductive System

At age 60, 7 in 10 couples are still sexually active and over the age of 75, there are still 1 in 4 healthy couples still sexually active. A detailed overview of statistics and further references is available in Gibson (1992).

In females the following changes occur:

- *there is less elastic tissue;*
- *fat replaces vaginal muscle;*
- *glandular breast tissue is replaced by fat (from age 35);*

- *breasts, vulva and vagina are less sensitive;*
- *vaginal mucosa are drier, thinner, less elastic;*
- *rate of arousal and number of orgasms falls;*
- *quality and actual number of oocytes falls.*

In males the following changes occur:

- *there is a fall in the alkaline seminal fluid produced in the prostrate;*
- *the penis is less sensitive and arousal time increases;*
- *the angle of penile erection lowers;*
- *post-ejaculation recovery phase takes longer;*
- *testosterone levels fall. Testosterone promotes secondary male characteristics and helps regulate metabolism.*

Many of these changes reflect those described under previous headings, for example reduction in secretions; inelastic muscles; raised threshold for sensitivity. In practical terms this means that the sex act becomes more than just impregnation. The process is longer if this is desired, but alternative options of sharing and giving sexual arousal and pleasure become more important. The risk of unwanted pregnancy is no longer an issue. Gentle lubrication and finding alternative comfortable positions for coitus are perhaps the greatest need. It provides a useful and interesting challenge to the reader to take each of the above biological changes and consider how each might be viewed as an advantage rather than a disadvantage. For instance, the penis erection at a lower angle may encourage new inventive positions for sexual intercourse.

How do you think a nurse might prepare for or conduct such a discussion with an older person? It needs to be planned carefully and to help in this process, first consider the following aspects: should anyone else be present besides the client and the nurse? His or her partner perhaps? Where should the discussion take place? How do you plan to approach the subject and direct the discussion? What information are you looking for? and why? If the situation arises spontaneously during the course of some other aspect of care, is there sufficient privacy? What manner and approach does the nurse need to adopt? Are there any other communication skills that will be needed? Does the nurse know of any other sources of information or practical help that may be of value to the client? (or indeed, his or her partner?) How is the nurse going to (a) record, and (b) follow-up this conversation?

The Ageing Respiratory System

There is a reduced efficiency of coughing and fewer cilia. Bronchioles and alveoli increase in size and reduce in number. The alveolar elastic collapses due to thinning. Cardiopulmonary reserves are reduced. Respiration is less easily controlled due to a fall in CNS sensitivity. In practical terms this means:

- *there is an increased risk of chest infection;*
- *these are limited oxygen reserves for an increase in demand, such as strenuous excercise or shock; this increases risk.*

The Ageing Skin

Reduction of collagen and elasticity causes minor skin trauma and capillary rupture known as 'senile purpura'. Skin becomes more transparent. There is a loss of subcutaneous fat and a reduction in stored water, thus causing wrinkles. The numbers of sweat glands fall. Nails become hard and brittle. Hair becomes thin, sparse, coarse and turns grey. Warts – particularly on the trunk – are common. Temperature regulation is less efficient. In practical terms this means:

- *owing to changes in fat, elasticity and a fall in vascularity, skin wounds suffer from delayed healing and are at increased risk of infection;*
- *there is an intolerance to change in local conditions, for example going from a warm house to the outside on a cold day, or sitting in a draught;*
- *there is an increased susceptibility to trauma;*
- *owing to sweat gland changes, there is an increased risk of hyperthermia;*
- *fevers are more severe and less obvious, making it essential to record both pulse and respirations.*

Cognitive Changes

Learning and Memory

With age, the ability to remember recent events is poorer, while recollections of situations in the distant past can be quite vivid. In practical terms, reminiscence serves to assist in reviewing of life which helps construct personal meaning and worth.

Older people are able to learn. Evidence for this, for example, lies in the large numbers who commence Open University courses upon retirement. However, because short-term memory is poorer, alternative learning styles to those adopted earlier in life need to be developed. Primary memory is unimpaired. Secondary memory is affected with age, particularly concerning tasks of increasing complexity. So, for learning, the nature of the situation is not simple. As previously stated, response time is slower and there is a raised threshold for sensitivity. Responses err on the side of caution, possibly because of a fear of failure rather than a need to succeed. To learn we need motivation. To have motivation we need relevance and relevance may be less obvious when the 'student' is older.

Intelligence and Cognitive Development

Methods to determine intelligence may be quantitative – e.g. psychometric tests – or qualitative. The former measure various abilities by the use of standardized tests while the latter focus on the conceptualization or way of attending to the problem. It is now recognized that the results of such tests cannot be linked with age, partly because of the way they are administered and partly because of the changed responses to learning, response and reaction times described above. The tests are tailored more towards younger people and they do not take account of different experiences in life. Generally, it is thought that intelligence is not affected by age. Cognitive development may follow the biological model of growth, through maintenance and on to decline, or it may follow the path of growth, maintenance and then plateau or even rise. These possibilities are described in more detail in the section on ageing and self image.

Personality

Personality does not change with advance in years. Still evident are the four types of personality: integrated: disorganized; defended; and passive dependent (Neugarten, 1971). What may be seen by the voyeur, or experienced by the family or friend, is the individual older person becoming more themself. As a person moves through life's course they encounter and confront situations which initiate thought and reasoning. Their resolution helps the individual find out who they really are and what their life is all about. With age may come a kind of understanding of self which may give rise to reinforcement of some character traits. It is thought that emotional capacity does not change as age increases.

AGEING AND SOCIAL INTEGRATION

The fundamental thrust of this whole chapter is that ageing is a sociological construct. Justification for stating this is that biological age is the general marker used to help determine the effects of ageing. Age is frequently used by society to establish a whole scenario about an individual. For instance, think of a 16-year-old and a 70-year-old living on the streets of London. The picture drawn and preconceptions made as to why and how they live under these circumstances are likely to be very different. The young person may generate feelings of sadness and perhaps sympathy – they are more likely to be viewed as victims. On the other hand, the older person is more likely to be considered as master of his own destiny, and having only themselves to blame. Thus, there is a dimension of conforming to social norms that is age-related. Such age-specific social patterns of behaviour that are considered 'normal' are one way of separating out and examining a group of people in terms that have meaning to our everyday life. Ageing is merely a framework or vehicle through which that study can be conveniently explored. In this context, ageing is about one person's changes with time – both physically and psychologically – and their interaction/s and behaviour/s with other person/s.

In terms of social integration there are four main contributory factors. These are:

- *functional abilities;*
- *awareness of self;*
- *socialization abilities;*
- *external influences.*

All four are heavily interdependent which is why as a nurse, we can only consider the client as a whole or in total. Functional abilities have already been described in the preceding section. In summary, the level of functional ability is totally unique to each individual and different systems may be able to function at different levels but will always be, at best, functioning at the lowest level of function within the system. Awareness of self relies on preservation of personality and internal resources to maintain self esteem. This is explored further in the section on ageing and self image. It is offset by social images and stereotyping which influence socialization abilities. External factors such as social trends and political ideology also have a profound effect. Each of these needs to be explored in more detail.

Social Images and Ageing

The way of thinking and values placed on a subgroup of people within any given society are clearly evidenced by the visual documentation of the day. Thus, in developed Western societies, current visual evidence depicting older people is available on television, newspapers, books, journals and art studies. Different bodies within society – such as journalists, politicians, pressure groups, reporters, script writers – all utilize these various media forms in different ways to either portray or to characterize their image of age.

If age is a sociological construct, then in order to begin to understand these images we have to consider the context from which they are drawn. The life course based on a social structure begins at birth with total dependency of the newborn infant. In the social life course, this infant matures to develop an awareness and appreciation of self and of others. Components of that development are control of the body itself and its interreactions with other bodies, recognizing the influence of power and emotion. Social maturity moves the dependent infant to become an independent person with identity; that is, to become an individual. Continuing through this social life course and regardless of chronological age, old age brings a gradual loss of bodily control. At a critical stage, this in itself elicits redependence, thereby beginning to break down the whole, mature person. The concepts of individual and identity begin to crumble and are replaced by group concepts of infantilization and marginalization.

With this information in mind, what is the image of age that we currently experience? It is easier to start by looking at images that represent our aspirations of health and beauty. In Britain, in the mid 1990s, the 'in look' is elfin features and a waif-like body of youth. The look is virtuous. It is also evident that the mature model and the larger sized model are beginning to become popular. The argument in support of the former is that older women are beautiful too but in a different way – their beauty is in their maturity. Concerning the latter, larger sized models are more in evidence quite simply to acknowledge that a significant proportion of the female population – estimates suggest around 47% – is not waif-like, yet they are still beautiful. So, at present, older people are beginning to be accepted as beautiful.

Moving on to drama and fiction, the last few years have seen a proliferation of comedy programmes concerning the characteristics of older people or the dilemmas and situations around them. They serve to highlight different facets of the experience of old age at the present time. These include the fact that newly retired people are still very fit and able to enjoy and contribute to life. Here, the theory of reciprocity is sometimes clearly evident. Another facet is that older people may move into a home. Script-writers attempt to describe the current dichotomy that while the older person is supposed to be in control and have the final say – within the available market appropriate to their needs – in practice, those choices may be removed, thus eliciting infantilization of the older person.

Current trends in journalistic reporting tend to evoke feelings of sympathy and empathy for the older person. While this may be a compassionate view of society, is it not also degrading and demoralizing because it evokes pity and thus dependence?

There are many aspects to the social images of ageing and only a few have been raised here. At present, more positive images of ageing are appearing. Examples of positive role models for ageing include Joan Collins for her looks; Margaret Thatcher for her political activities; and the Queen Mother for her sheer warmth and stamina. Moreover, it would seem that the whole concept of ageing is currently being explored, debated and challenged. Only time and observation will inform us of the outcome.

It would be pertinent to digress slightly here and address the notion of sexual health promotion in later life. One image of ageing is that older people are not interested in sex. Older people and sexuality are perceived to sit together uneasily in the same sentence and yet the sexual needs of older people are just as important for a professional nurse to consider as if the patient were younger. In general, health care professionals seem reluctant to acknowledge, yet alone address, the sexual needs of their older clients. Occasional papers in the literature (e.g. Jones, 1994) serve to generate an interest in the subject. They help to highlight the notion that older people do have sex – there is no specific time in the life cycle when sex must, should or does stop.

Thus, if people are sexually active, it follows logically that their sexual practices and behaviour may put them at risk of becoming HIV positive. This, in turn, may lead to HIV-related disease, for example AIDS. Risky behaviour, the human immunodeficiency virus (HIV) and older people are discussed at length in Jones (1992) along with many other issues surrounding this subject. Concerning HIV, health promotion has a very positive role to play on at least four fronts. First, by encouraging older people to practice safer sex through the continued use of condoms despite a lesser risk of unwanted pregnancy in heterosexual relationships. Safer sexual practices must also target the significant numbers of older homosexuals. Gibson (1992) estimates there are 400 000 gay men in England and Wales. Second, health promotion also has a strong part to play on those caring for older people who may be HIV positive. It is important that anyone participating in care for someone who is HIV positive adopts universal precautions (CDC, 1988) to help limit spread. Third, a report by Age Concern (1993) made public the fact that carers of people who are HIV positive are often older people – they may be parents, siblings or loved ones. The effects of caring can be quite devastating – emotionally draining, socially isolating, to name but two significant effects. Thus supporting and advising a carer of universal precautions is a health promotion task. Fourth, and finally, in the light of increasing demographic numbers of older people with HIV infection, health promoters can inform and influence the debate for future planning of health care needs in communities (Jones, 1993).

Social Trends and Ageing

Examination of the social images of ageing can be developed further, based on the premise that 'actions speak louder than words'. In other words, what is happening within the actual structure of present-day society that has a marked influence on the lives of older people? Two major examples will be raised here – large retail parks and old people villages. Both of these have evolved in Britain in the last decade.

Large retail parks have evolved to provide better value for money in a traffic-free environment. They are generally situated on the perimeter of urban areas, easily accessible by major roads. While the aspirations of these ventures is commendable, the ripple-effect of their lower prices threatens the small, local shopkeeper. So how do the older, frailer, less mobile older people either access these parks or, alternatively, how do they afford to pay the higher prices at the local shops that have managed to survive such competition? If the continuity theory is about sustaining and maintaining life patterns, then how can this be achieved in these circumstances?

The evolution of 'villages' for older people is again a double-edged sword. These villages are small designated areas that have developed within existing towns. They offer all the basic amenities that older people may require. In Coventry, for instance, there is a range of housing available from small flats to a more intense nursing unit. Accommodation is located around a 'village green' along with a health centre where both health and social service staff are located. There is also a hairdresser, pharmacy and social club. While access to all essential items is within walking distance and some older people may enjoy mixing exclusively with others of their own age, there is also the feeling that 'the burden of the ageing population has been dealt with'. The trend seems to have been to see ageing as a burden when surely it is a challenge? How can we, as a community, ensure that the experiences and wisdom of our older people are not lost to future generations because they are unable to mix with each other and share their life stories? A more disturbing aspect of 'villages for older people' is the example of Sun City in Arizona, USA, which is a fine purpose-built village in the desert and serviced by younger people. The hospital is in the centre of the town. Financial resources separate out those who can afford to live there, therefore it is truly a ghetto for only the grand geriatrics. Those local older people unable to afford to live in Sun City are further marginalized by becoming a smaller minority and yet because of their financial status their health and welfare needs may be even greater.

These examples help to demonstrate how at the end of the twentieth century, ageing and social integration are not two easily compatible terms. It is for you to take all these questions further, to consider the difficulties of social integration for older people, and begin to try to formulate some practical solutions.

Stereotyping and Ageing

When asked, I tell people that my specialist interest is in older people. Frequently, the next question is 'What do you mean by older people?', to which I always reply 'Precisely!'. This reply serves two purposes – the first is that often the question is asked indignantly, as if to say,

'How can older people be interesting?' The second is to make the person who has actually asked the question stop and think.

Taking the second reason first, it is in the nature of being human that we wish to understand the conversations in which we find ourselves. Asking what is meant by 'older people' helps to put the topic into a little box, and helps to conjure up pictures and situations with which we can readily identify. Yes, we can begin to participate in this conversation now and perhaps even make some sensible contribution. But the contribution is only meaningful if it is based on truth.

In order to demonstrate this point, stop and think of the pictures that come into your mind when you read the words *older people*. Perhaps you picture an older man or woman, quite possibly with grey or white hair, and more than likely bent forward a little – certainly not tall and straight, facing the world head on. And what of their personality? Are they friendly or fierce, grumpy or happy, accepting or challenging? Perhaps they appear physically frail to some degree. Do they comply/harmonize with the unwritten rules in the sphere in which you socialize? Now, think of how many older people that you have met in your work and in your personal life who actually come anywhere near to this mythical person. Not one of them is likely to conform to all the characteristics you have imposed on them. How many of these characteristics have you ascribed to your character purely because of the word *older*? This is stereotyping at its most basic level. When we take this concept and begin to make policies and practices based on these stereotypes, then we move into the realms of ageism.

This brings us back to the theory of a social and political structured dependency. On a more personal level, such stereotyping may cloud the clinical practice of a professional nurse by assuming all too readily that the older person is incapable of participating in decisions about their own care. This comes about because the physical frailty may imply psychological incapacity and so the older person is marginalized and infantilized as decisions about their care are made for them. This may be further reinforced by the older person her/himself acting out the part of the stereotypes in which they themselves believe. The important issue is to see the person as the individual they are and not the little box or category in which they are placed because of their chronological age.

Going back then to the first reason for my reply is now simple. If we chose to come into nursing because we have a genuine interest in and care for our fellow man, then here is just another individual to whom we can offer our professional services. Like all the other people to whom we offer our services, their case is unique, and our interest is genuine.

Political Ideology and Ageing

Older people are affected by political ideologies both directly and indirectly. They are affected overtly and covertly. Direct political rhetoric concerning older people has been used in the national elections of the late 1980s and early 1990s. Political argument was used to target the very substantial vote of those people over the age of retirement – almost 20% of the total voting population. While it seemed the 'in thing' to try and gain the vote of older people, at the same time the political thinking was quietly counting the cost of health and welfare services received by this significant portion of the populace and looking at ways of reducing the costs. A good example is state pensions, which are a clear target for a change in administration. With the relative numbers of people in employment decreasing coupled with a relative increase in the numbers of retired persons, the finances to meet a full state pension for all are just not available. The policy is no longer valid, nor indeed appropriate for the current shape and form of the population. The portion of the population that is retired is such that the remedy has become a political nightmare.

Another development in political philosophy throughout the 1980s which, on first examination, would not seem to be targeting older people is the new-look free-market health service. The drives of a free-market are the business criteria of efficiency, effectiveness and a value for money service (HMSO, 1989). Under these conditions, older people who frequently require longer-term health, social and welfare support tend to reduce the efficiency and value for money dimensions of the service/s. This is because their needs are complex and protracted, and thus cannot be met and delivered quickly. Within this change of health service administration there has also been a move to transfer older people from long-stay and continuing care wards out into the community. Consequently nursing homes – both private and of Trust status – have proliferated. Monitoring standards and quality of care in such a fragmented system is hard to establish (see UKCC, 1994) and, without government or professional policy guidance, is even harder to enforce. It would seem that in a free-market economy in the health services, the case of older people is pushed to the margins.

AGEING AND SELF IMAGE

Regardless of whether the chronological age of a person is an appropriate marker against which to record changes, in developed Western societies this is a major criterion. People use the age of themselves and others as an indicator not only as to how they should or could live their lives, but also as a reference to how they believe they should feel or behave. Examples of people whose image has been retained or improved with age without medical assistance include Sean Connery, Felicity Kendal, Joanna Lumley and Roger Moore. It is also used as a guide for the image that they wish to project.

Self image is a broad and complex topic. This section can only highlight some of the principal concepts and issues involved. Salter (1988) suggests that body image is made up of three distinct concepts. These are:

- *body ideal – what we would like our body to look like, what we aspire towards achieving;*
- *body reality – what our biological body actually is inside, what it looks like on the outside and how it functions;*
- *body presentation – how we dress and adorn our body – or not – to show to other people.*

Body presentation is about making a statement which may in turn be about what we are, who we identify with, or about who we are not. Through body presentation we express our ideas and beliefs of conformity or non-conformity. Self image can draw from and utilize this perspective. Thus our ideal self image will be how we would like to be. It builds up our strengths and minimizes our weaknesses. The reality of self image would then be personal perceptions of what a person believes they really are.

How we present ourselves to others is the image we wish to project, and this may differ depending upon the situation in which we find ourselves and the role which we wish to undertake. We can advance this analogy further by revisiting the notion of personal perceptions. Consider that personal perceptions may or may not be accurate. They may only be accurate in part and they may change when other people's perceptions are made known to us. Thus it becomes an iterative process. From this viewpoint then, self image becomes an ever-evolving concept that relies on self awareness and feeds on information gained from experience and from other people.

In order to be self aware a person must be introspective at times. Theories of lifespan development examine and attempt to describe in qualitiative terms how such examination of self in relation to experience help to develop a person. Sugarman (1986) describes these theories in more detail and provides references to original articles. The reference frame from which these theories hang is chronological age. Three of the more popular ones are described below.

Erikson

No text on psychological development would be complete without reference to Erik Erikson (1963). His theory of psychosocial development was first described in the 1950s and 1960s. He proposes that development is influenced by, and therefore is a function of, each individual person and their sociocultural situation. The stage of development reached can therefore be recognized by psychosocial tasks. Erikson suggests that there are eight stages of development and links each to an approximate span of biological age. At each stage there is personal development and a concomitant social institution. An individual can only move through these stages in a specific order. Each stage places a demand in the form of an emotional crisis on the individual which must be resolved, the outcome emerging at any point on a continuum. As life progresses, earlier demands may be reconsidered and the person may re-exit at a different point on that continuum.

The stage for consideration here is the eighth stage. Erikson suggests this may occur around 65 years or over. The emotional crisis creating a demand for resolution is ego integrity versus despair and disgust. The two lie at either end of the continuum. Ego integrity resolves upon the notion of accepting your previous life course, accepting responsibility for your life. At the same time, it is acknowledging there were like-minded others from different social and cultural backgrounds. It also concedes the very small part an individual holds in the grand fabric of the universe. The converse of this is the despair and disgust, epitomized by a profound compunction that the life of the individual was not something different. A degree of despair will be evident if ego integration has not occurred throughout the seven earlier stages of development. It is thought that out of successful ego integration comes the virtue of wisdom. Major cultural institutions are seen as the social celebration of such a virtue.

Havighurst

Robert J. Havighurst also began describing his theory of developmental tasks in the 1950s (Havighurst, 1973) Developmental tasks occur at specific instances in life. If they are achieved successfully then the person moves on positively through life towards their next task. If they fail then future life is viewed more negatively. Developmental tasks arise from one of three fronts and these are: biological evolution; personal ambitions and beliefs; and the pressures that come from within the society in which the person perceives they belong. Developmental task demands will vary when they present according to the society and culture within which a person exists. There is no clear biological age to which the tasks are linked. Thus, this theory clearly demonstrates the complex nature of the whole process of ageing.

At present, the stage of concern for older people is mainly that of 'late maturity'. Havighurst's developmental tasks associated with this stage concern the changes in physical abilities, paid employment, income level, and social roles. The nature of these changes may in turn affect lifestyle and even a person's home. Near-future cohorts of older people will also be concerned with some developmental tasks linked with Havighurst's 'middle age' stage. These include, for-example, changes in their older parents, biological form and function, realizing social responsibility, and facilitating the growth of children into adulthood.

Buhler

Charlotte Buhler described development through a life course in the early 1930s (Buhler and Massarik, 1968). She uses phasic biological development/s as the basis for psychological development/s which occur in three areas. These are (a) the part a person plays achieving their individual goals in life; (b) the range of experiences available to a person throughout their lifespan; and (c) the way a person attends to change in or sustaining their life. She proposes five stages, each losely linked to biological age. The fourth stage, c. 50 years to c. 70 years reflects, in Buhler's biological phase, the beginnings of decline. Psychological development involves assessing the personal life course to date and identifying achievement or failure. Resolution here will provide a new foundation for the next stage in the life course. The fifth stage, c. 70 years until death, reflects continued biological decline. This may confer the final period of fulfilment or failure, but also it may be that old targets, as yet unachieved, are re-attempted.

How does all this relate to the older people who require our nursing services? First, It is important to remember that we all have our own self image which we project and which others will try to recognize and identify. It is essential that a nurse respects and values (but does not necessarily have to agree with) the self image that a person presents. To recognize, acknowledge and, most of all, respect that image will help in the assessment and planning process of relevant care. It will also help in defining appropriate evaluation. If care is planned, delivered and evaluated on our own personal beliefs rather than that of our client, then care is less likely to be (a) appropriate, and (b) evaluated effectively.

Lifespan development theories may be relevant to real clinical practice. For example, an understanding of Erikson's theory can perhaps assist in accepting the older woman at home who has her leg ulcer dressed daily. She continually complains to the nurse about her family who do not visit and the other nurse who comes and says she must walk more. 'I thought nurses were paid to help me, not make me do the work myself. They always used to be so kind. Not anymore.' Is this perhaps a case of life's regrets? Is she perhaps disgusted at herself because the ulcer increases her perceived dependence on others? From Buhler's perspective the older woman may be attempting to come to terms with what she perceives as her failures – that her children do not wish to visit her as frequently as she believes they should.

In general, our self image concerns how we think and feel about ourselves and how we choose to project that image. It concerns how others perceive us. If the older woman in the above scenario believes she has few visits from the members of her family, then she may feel that they believe she is not worth visiting. The negative image that she has of herself could make her less inclined to comply with treatment, that is, becoming more mobile. Consider how and what kind of care may be appropriate in this situation.

CONCLUSIONS

The aim of this chapter has been to look at ageing and its effects on people. The effects of an increase in biological age have been observed and described from various perspectives, namely: biological; sociological; and psychological. Each perspective has evolved its own theories of change, which are linked with concepts from other perspectives. In short, no single unified approach to the theory of the process of ageing is currently available.

This chapter has addressed the more popular theories of biological ageing. Theories that favour aspects of programme-related change or genetics at present enjoy more credence, for example those involving a biological timing device, such as a specified limit to the number of times a cell replicates. Sociological theories include an overview of the prevailing disengagement theory whereby disengagement of older people from society and society from older people is mutually acceptable. The political economic perspective has more recently contributed a well-documented argument for the more reasoned situation of older people in the 1990s.

The second section provided detail on biological ageing anatomically and physically. Close attention has been placed on this section not only because there is a dearth of sound information available, but because of what a person's functional abilities actually are and how the person believes they are seem to play a fundamental role in a person's ability to express themselves. This was clearly evident in the third and fourth sections. The third section on social integration examined the images we hold and cling on to of the role our culture believes that an older person should play. It showed how we stereotype older people and strip them of their individuality by so doing. We also looked briefly at the very structure of our government policy framework and the direct effect this has on older people.

The final section attempted to demonstrate that every older person is just ourselves in a few years' time. They are individuals in their own right, with emotions, needs, goals and concerns about how they live their lives. Their lifespan is nearer completion and they have evolved and perhaps become more wise, less exuberant, less cautious, but still in need. They have survived the convoluted process of living and evolving. The developments of age from each perspective are complex and interwoven. They produce this wise older person before you – your client. Value their needs and they will value you.

CLINICAL DISCUSSION POINTS

Identify some ways in which your knowledge of the physiological impact of ageing will inform your nursing practice.

Brainstorm with colleagues your own stereotypes of the impact of ageing. Remember, there are both positive and negative stereotypes. Discuss how these can be challenged in your practice.

Try to draw mental picture of yourself at 60 years, 70 years and 80 years, imagining both the biological impact of your age and its sociological construction. Use these reflections to develop positive strategies and responses to clients you care for.

SUGGESTIONS FOR FURTHER READING

Bromley, D. (1974) **Human Ageing,** 2nd edn. Penguin Books, London.
This book covers many of the concepts addressed in this chapter only in some more detail. It provides many references for further reading.

Whitebourne, S. K. (1985). **The Ageing Body.** Springer, New York.
This is more expensive but provides great detail on the process of primary ageing. Many examples of relevant research are also described and cited.

Sugarman, L. (1986) **Life-Span Development. Concepts, Theories and Interventions.** Routledge, London.
A small pocket-sized text that provides plenty of background knowledge to help the 'learner' not only understand the psychological theories of ageing but also to appreciate the concept of the lifespan development.

Warnes, A. M. (1989) **Human Ageing and Later Life. Multidisciplinary Perspectives.** Age Concern Institute of Gerontology, London.
This book is chosen for its simple yet detailed approach to the sociology of ageing. It contains many relevant statistics, studies and references.

REFERENCES

Age Concern (1993). **A Crisis of Silence: HIV, AIDS and Older People.** Age Concern, London.

Bromley, D. (1974). **Human Ageing,** 2nd edn. Penguin Books, London.

Buhler, C. and Massarik, F. (Eds) (1968). **The Course of Human Life: A Study of Goals in the Humanistic Perspective.** Springer, New York.

CDC (1988). **Perspectives in Disease Prevention and Health Promotion. MMWR 37; 24; 377–382; 387–388.** (Available through the National AIDS Information Clearinghouse, PO Box 6003, Rockville, MD20850, USA.)

Christ, M. A. and Hohloch, F. J. (1988). **Gerontological Nursing**. Springhouse Notes, Pennsylvania.

Cumming, E. and Henry, W. (1961). **Growing Old: The Process of Disengagement.** Basic Books, New York.

Erikson, E. H. (1963). **Childhood and Society.** W. W. Norton, New York. (Penguin, Hardmondsworth, 1965).

Garrett, G. (1983). **Health Needs of the Elderly.** Macmillan Education, Basingstoke.

Gibson, H. B. (1992). **The Emotional and Sexual Lives of Older People.** Chapman & Hall, London.

Havighurst, R. J. (1973). History of developmental psychology: socialization and personality development through the life span. In: P. B. Balles and K. W. Schaie (Eds) **Life-Span Developmental Psychology: Personality and Socialization.** Academic Press, New York.

Hayflick, L. (1977). The cellular basis for biological aging. In: C. E. Finch and L. Hayflick (Eds) **Handbook of the Biology of Aging,** pp. 159–188. Van Nostrand, New York.

HMSO (1989). **Education and Training.** Working Paper 10. HMSO, London.

Jones, H. M. (1992). **The Human Immuno Deficiency Virus and Older People.** MA Dissertation, Keele University. (Reference only copy available in University library.)

Jones, H. M. (1993). HIV mistreatment: policy, resources and practice. **Senior Nurse 13**(6), 19.

Jones, H. M. (1994). Mores and morals. **Nursing Times 90**, 47, 54.

Neugarten, B. (1971). Grow old along with me! The best is yet to be. **Psychology Today 5**, 7.

Office of Population Censuses and Surveys (1993). **Ethnic Group and Country of Birth in Great Britain.** (Census 1991). HMSO, London.

Salter, M. (1988). **Altered Body Image. The Nurse's Role.** Wiley, Chichester.

Spence, A. P. (1989). **Biology of Human Aging.** Prentice-Hall, London.

Sugarman, L. (1986). **Life-span Development. Concepts, Theories and Interventions.** Routledge, London.

UKCC (1994). **Professional Conduct. Occasional Report on Standards of Nursing in Nursing Homes.** UKCC, London.

Whitebourne, S. K. (1985). **The Ageing Body.** Springer, New York.

Chapter Four

Promoting Health in
Older People

Gillian Granville

Core Themes in Gerontological Nursing

Ageing Matters	*New Social World*	*Lifespan Perspective*	*Health and Old People*
Illness and Dependency	*Quality Nursing Care*	*Therapeutic Intervention*	*Politicizing Gerontological Nursing*

Key Words

*Healthism • Health Promotion • Communication •
Empowerment • Evaluation*

INTRODUCTION

Old age has been universally associated with ill health, decline and dependence. The focus has been on maintaining or treating medical conditions and coping with the burden of disease and disability. Very little attention has been devoted to health and the prevention of ill health in later years. In this chapter we aim to move away from that medical model and look at health in older people as a positive and dynamic process.

This Chapter is divided into three sections with the following aims:

To examine what we understand by health and health promotion and the attitudes of older people to their own health

---

To look at the theoretical background to health promotion and different methods of delivering the service

---

To provide practical examples of promoting health in old age.

UNDERSTANDING HEALTH AND HEALTH PROMOTION

Initially, it is necessary to understand what is meant by health. Are we talking about an absence of disease or are we considering a much wider concept? In 1948, the World Health Organization (WHO) described health as 'A complete state of physical, mental and social well being'. This moved away from describing health in terms of mortality and morbidity, but could be considered rather ambitious in terms of realistic aims and expectations.

McClymont *et al.* (1991) suggested five concepts of health, each leading to different models of delivering practice. These five conceptual ideas are:

- *health as the absence of disease;*
- *health as a positive state;*
- *health as a fluctuant experience;*
- *health as independence for living;*
- *health as adaptation.*

All five concepts could apply to health in old age and demonstrate the importance of older people not passively accepting ill health *because* they are old, but also allowing them to be realistic in achieving healthy goals. The role of the health educator is to assist people to reach their goals.

We have established, therefore, that health is not simple to define, but it needs to include social and emotional wellbeing as well as an acceptable level of physical ability and and absence of disease.

A word of warning here. It is important that health is seen as a *resource* for everyday living and not the *reason* for living. *Healthism* is the ideology that believes health is more important than rewards or satisfaction and that the achievement of health is the prime object of living. This puts the responsibility for health on the individual and can obscure social and economic factors. It can lead to the situation of '*victim blaming*' when a person blames themself if they become unhealthy because they believe it must be their fault for living an unhealthy life. The challenge for the health educator is to empower their clients to be responsible for their health but not to lead them to victim blaming.

Older People's Attitude to Health

We all develop our attitudes through a multiple range of experiences and responses throughout our lives. These experiences extend from our families and peer groups to cultural, religious and political influences as well as employment, our environment and major life events. We are all influenced by the views and trends of the society we live in and our behaviour reflects those views.

Older people, as part of the wider society, internalize the view that the ageing process leads inevitably to a time of ill health, disability and dependence and are often too willing to accept that a certain health problem is due to their age. The saying 'What can you expect at my age?' is only too familiar.

Listening to Older People

It is the responsibility of the health educator to listen to older people in order to understand their attitudes and assist them to reflect and examine their views. Through this reflection, the health professional can effect change in attitude and expectation and move to a more positive approach to health. Without this change, any attempts at promoting health in old age will fail.

A wider responsibility for promoters of health in later life is to challenge attitudes in other areas of society by fighting to combat ageism.

Research Findings on Health Beliefs in Old Age

The Health and Lifestyle Survey carried out in 1984/85 is a random sample of the British population and gives us some insight into the health beliefs across the generations. The survey asked the question 'Are more people healthy now than in their parents' time?'. The majority of people over 65 years of age (78% of men and 75% of women) thought that people were healthier now than in their parents' time. However, the proportion who thought people were healthier now decreased with age from 78% of those aged 65–74 years, to 67% in people aged over 85 years (Victor, 1991). This could indicate that people accept that ill health is part of the ageing process.

Table 4.1 *Why are people healthier now than in your parents' time? Percentage, in Great Britain, 1984. From Victor (1991), with permission from the Open University Press*

	18–59	65–74	75+
Medical advances and improved availability	37	38	36
Health education	20	11	8
Improved living standards	21	31	33
Better environment	4	1	4
Better hygiene	4	4	4
Better working conditions	9	10	11
Better diet	40	38	36
More exercise	10	8	8
N	5554	1040	575

The survey also asked why people are healthier now than in their parents' time. Results are shown in Table 4.1. Improved health services, better nutrition and improved living conditions were considered to be the most significant factors by all the generations, but older people put much less value on health education than younger people. This could be explained by the fact that older people have had less opportunity to be part of health education programmes and consider health more in the context of outside influences. The younger generations are made aware of the value of health education through the school curriculum and the emphasis on healthy lifestyles. Victor (1991) interprets the data as follows:

> *From the data, older people seem to be identifying the importance of structural variables (e.g. income, living standards, etc.) in improving health status. In contrast, the younger members of the population appear to be offering more individual, behavioural dimensions to explain improved health status.*
> (Victor, 1991; p. 96)

She continues:

> *If there are important differences in how varying generations perceive and conceptualise health, then this has important implications for the development of health promotion and education strategies.*
> (Victor, 1991; p. 96)

Research tells us that older people today need to understand what health education is all about before they can benefit from it. However, the next generation of older people will probably not need the same approach because they will have grown up with the concept and value of health education.

What Health Promotion Is And Is Not

Health promotion is not to be confused with health education or prevention of ill health, although these form part of it. Health promotion is a dynamic process which seeks to convince people of the value of health and the need to improve health throughout the lifespan. It is a way of enabling people to increase the control over their lives and the role of the health promoter is to sell health, much in the way that other products are sold. It is a commodity and people are the consumers.

Consumerism

Consumerism in health promotion is concerned with extending the control that people have over their lives and the choices they make. Nutbeam (1986) interprets this as meaning:

> *... the public should demand and receive the information with which to develop a more critical awareness of the impact of different goods, services, personal activities and environmental conditions on health. Subsequently effective consumer choice or behaviour implies the ability to use the information and the availability of selected services or other services.*
> **(Nutbeam, 1986; p. 117)**

In other words it is the role of the health promoter to give information in a way that can be used by the people. Consumerism is a very powerful concept and can be very challenging to professionals in the way they promote health in the population.

The Ottawa Charter 1986

Important recognition for health promotion came at the First International Conference on Health Promotion held in Ottawa in November 1986. A Charter for Action was presented in order to achieve health for all by the year 2000 and beyond. The Charter defined health promotion as:

> *The process of enabling people to increase control over and improve their health by empowering them... to identify and realise their needs... and change or cope with their environment.*
> **(McClymont *et al.* 1991; p. 149)**

The Charter claimed that health promotion went beyond health care and it should be put on the agenda of policy makers in all sectors and at all levels, directing them to be aware of the health consequences of any decisions they make and to accept responsibility for health. The Charter required policy makers in all sectors of public life to:

- *build healthy public policies;*
- *create health-supportive environments;*

- *strengthen community action;*
- *develop personal skills in individuals;*
- *re-orientate health services.*

Figure 4.1 shows this in diagramatic form.

Essential concepts underpinning health promotion policies were seen to be caring, holism and ecology. There was a need for all those concerned to be committed to a strong public health alliance (The Ottawa Charter for Health Promotion, in Kalache *et al.*, 1986).

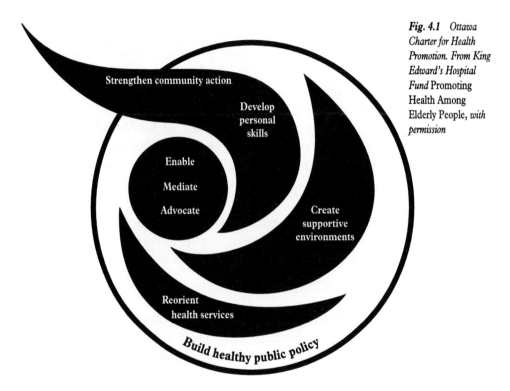

Fig. 4.1 *Ottawa Charter for Health Promotion. From King Edward's Hospital Fund* Promoting Health Among Elderly People, *with permission*

The Importance of the Charter

McClymont *et al.* (1991) remind us to be cautious of the dangers of rhetoric and to be aware that action speaks louder than words. However, the Charter did make significant advances. It shifted the emphasis from professional-directed goals to people-directed ones. It implied that future health promotion activities would be more effective if they became client-centred and focused more on group and community work. Table 4.2 shows how this shift in emphasis could occur. Clearly, this change could not happen suddenly; gradually some groups of people are challenging established medical views and are seeking alternative therapies or ecological and environmental answers to health (McClymont *et al.*, 1991).

Table 4.2 *Health promotion – shifting the emphasis. From McClymont et al. (1991) with permission*

From	⟶	To
Illness	⟶	Health
Health as an objective of living	⟶	Health as a resource for living
Concepts of cure of disease	⟶	Concepts of wellbeing, holism, care ecology
Reliance on professional direction and responsibility for health	⟶	Less reliance on professionals and more self-responsibility and self-directed action and goals
Passive reliance on professional decision-making	⟶	Active client, group and community decision-making
Passive acceptance of situations and services	⟶	Active involvement by individuals, groups and, communities in creating change
Health sector activity only	⟶	Multisector co-operation

Health Education

Health education forms part of an overall strategy in health promotion where there is an interchange of information between people and professionals. Opportunities for learning are consciously arranged in order to improve knowledge and develop understanding and skills conducive to health.

An example would be a series of talks on healthy lifestyles given to a seniors' group. The purpose of health education is to pass on knowledge from the professional to the people, in order that they can make choices about their health. People cannot make choices about their lives if they do not have enough information. Ultimately, people may choose not to adopt the healthy options and many would consider this the right of every individual.

Disease Prevention or Preventing Ill Health

This refers to strategies which aim to conserve health rather than actively improve it and is very evident in the medical model of health care. It is commonly divided into primary, secondary and tertiary prevention of disease. The different stages are illustrated here with reference to osteoporosis, a condition that affects older women after the menopause.

Primary prevention is any activity that seeks to prevent a disease occurring. A view is often put forward that it is impossible to have primary prevention in old age because patterns of healthy living have to start in childhood to prevent problems in later life. This rather simplistic attitude fails to take into account that, at certain phases in the life course, individuals are more receptive to health messages. It is known to be difficult to promote good health habits in school children as they are unable to visualize life as an older person and tend to be more conscious of the present. They are receptive to health hazards that would affect them as young people but not when they are older. However, as people age, they become more aware of the value of preventing ill health.

Primary prevention of osteoporosis would be promoting a good dietary intake of calcium and taking plenty of exercise throughout life, in order to build up a strong bone mass. Even in postmenopausal women, a healthy diet, regular exercise and no smoking would reduce risks. A medical way of primary prevention would be using hormone replacement therapy (HRT) after the menopause to slow down the rate of bone loss caused by lower oestrogen levels.

Secondary prevention is screening for a condition in its early stages when treatment can be effective. In older people, screening for certain conditions may have some relevance to preventing a disease from developing and enables the older person to become more conscious of their health. To illustrate with our example of osteoporosis, women with known risk factors could be screened for bone mass and alerted to potential problems. They could then choose a treatment to slow down the process.

Tertiary prevention refers to reducing occurrences or effects of an illness. In osteoporosis, this would involve rehabilitating a woman who has suffered from an osteoporotic fracture to enable her to live a safe and independent life.

All forms of disease prevention could form part of a health promotion strategy.

Who Delivers Health Promotion?

I do not intend to be specific about who should deliver health promotion. Everyone has a responsibility to promote health from policy-makers to individuals.

All nurses, as health professionals, will actively promote health. Certain types of nurses, such as health visitors, are specialists in health promotion and take a lead in the community to improve health, but we all need to be involved both as role models of good health and by enabling our clients to choose healthy options.

DELIVERING A HEALTH PROMOTION STRATEGY TO OLDER PEOPLE

In order to deliver an effective health promotion strategy we need to consider the action on three different, but integral, levels:

- *national policies;*
- *local communities;*
- *individuals.*

National Policy Level

It is the responsibility of every government to produce policies that are conducive to healthy lifestyles, and to reduce the inequalities in health caused by social disadvantage. This can be achieved by focusing on *planning* and *financing* at a national level. The Black Report (Townsend, 1982) clearly showed that poverty and poor housing caused ill health. An updated response to this is given by Benzeval *et al.* (1995). Any health promotion plan that ignored the issue reflected in the work quoted would fail.

An attempt to educate older people in healthy eating by discussing the most nutritious food available would be hopelessly ineffectual if the professionals involved did not seek to reduce the poverty in old age which prevents people buying more healthy food. It would be inappropriate to discuss the value of regular exercise with an older person living in damp, inadequate housing if the housing department was not also involved in rehousing or improvements.

In order to tackle these central political issues, powerful lobbying is required to bring about changes in legislation which promote healthy living. Health professionals have a responsibility to ensure that their professional bodies have these political issues high on their health agendas.

The working party from the King Edward's Hospital Fund (Kalache *et al.*, 1988), which examined promoting health in older people, felt there was a need to strengthen links between central government departments. This would provide an opportunity to consider policy concerns which went beyond the boundaries of any single department and show recognition of an holistic approach to health in old age.

> *The Department of Health (DoH) cannot be held solely responsible for initiatives designed to promote health but it might consider making it its business to put health promotion and ageing onto the agendas of other departments and agencies in the fields of transport, education, environment and housing to ensure that policy initiatives do not run counter to the notion of positive health. Perhaps the concept of health impact statements, akin to environmental impact statements, merits attention.*
> (Kalache *et al.*, 1988; p. 35)

Local Community Level

It is necessary to ensure that health promotional activities are appropriate to the local needs of a defined community. At this level the focus is on *practice* and is divided between local authorities, including housing, education, social services and transport, and health authorities, general practitioner services and voluntary organizations. Close liaison with all these departments enables effective health strategies to be delivered to meet the needs identified by the community.

Health professionals also need to form *partnerships* with local older people so they are part of identifying, planning and implementing activities. The perceived needs of professionals may be quite different from the needs expressed by the local people. Without this partnership it would be difficult to improve health and change attitudes.

McClymont *et al.* (1991) discuss the importance of 'tuning-in' to a community before engaging fully in health promotional activities through knowledge of informal *community networks*. She says:

> *They (community networks) help to maintain their (older people's) sense of belonging, provide outlets for older clients to voice their concerns, act as channels for information and can offer practical help. Their representatives include hairdressers, post office staff, pharmacists, milkmen, church workers, small shopkeepers and policemen.*
> **(McClymont *et al.*, 1991; p. 174)**

It is through these informal links in the community that the health professional can seek the most appropriate way to deliver the health messages which can influence health behaviour.

Individual Level

Health promotion at an individual level acknowledges the positive contribution that a person can make to their own health. This may require a change of attitude and the professional strives to *empower* the individual through knowledge and the skills of self care. Older people can be encouraged to exercise healthy choices and to seek out alternatives for themselves. The danger of individual action is that it can remove responsibility from the state and hide the wider social and environmental issues that cause ill health, discussed previously, at National level but are outside the control of the individual.

McClymont *et al.* (1991) remind us that individuals may actually choose to accept less healthy options:

> *Those faced with empowerment may choose to relinquish control in favour of greater dependency! When such is the case, these individuals must be allowed to exercise their rights without fear of recrimination.*
> **(McClymont *et al.*, 1991; p. 150)**

However, we must not forget that the choice to become dependent may affect the life of another individual who would also have the same right of choice. This applies to carers of older people. In these cases, compromise may have to be reached.

Communicating with Older People

We cannot hope to promote health among our older clients if we do not understand how to communicate effectively with them. We need to recognize certain communication skills in order to give effective health messages that people will act on.

Ewles and Simnett (1988) identify certain barriers to communication which need to be overcome before learning can take place:

- *social and cultural gap between educator and client;*
- *limited receptiveness of client;*
- *negative attitude to the health educator;*
- *limited understanding and memory;*
- *insufficient emphasis on education by health professional;*
- *contradictory messages;*
- *overcoming language barriers.*

Social and Cultural Gap

Communication can be ineffective if there are ethnic, cultural and religious belief differences between educator and client which are unacknowledged. It would be pointless to discuss a healthy diet with an ethnic older person without knowledge of religious demands regarding food. Social class, as well as gender, can also create barriers. To this list, for the purposes of our study, we could add age or generational gaps. An older client may resent a young nurse telling them what is good for their health if that young nurse does not acknowledge the depth of experience from the older person.

Limited Receptiveness of Client

Communication is a two-way process and the client may not be able to communicate with the health professional for several reasons. These could include illness, tiredness and pain, or being too busy and distracted by other events.

Another incidence when communication may break down is if the person does not value his or herself and their health. An older person who has recently suffered bereavement would have low self esteem and may find it difficult to value their own health at that time.

Negative Attitude to the Health Educator

A client may already have preconceived ideas of what health promotion is and be against any involvement. They may have had previous negative experiences with health educators failing to communicate appropriately, or they may not want to know about taking more exercise or eating healthier food if it means giving up a lifestyle they are used to. This is perhaps one of the most difficult barriers for the health educator to overcome.

Limited Understanding and Memory

A client may have limited intelligence or may be illiterate. A knowledge of the level of understanding is vital in order to adopt the most appropriate method of delivering a health promotion message. It would be totally ineffectual to give a person with limited understanding a series of handouts, or work sheets. The messages would be better given through pictures or sounds. Conversely, it could be inappropriate to give simple diagrams and cartoons to a person who was a recently retired headteacher.

Assessing understanding and memory in an individual presents the health professional with a personal and professional challenge.

Insufficient Emphasis on Education by the Health Professional

Health professionals may fail to recognize the value of health promotion in all aspects of their work. This may be due to lack of training or low priority in practice. He or she may lack the confidence in skills and knowledge through a lack of basic awareness or they may feel too busy and give health promotion a lower priority.

This particularly applies to work with older people, when the sickness model has been so dominant and the advantage of promoting health in old age has been grossly undervalued.

Contradictory Messages

Ewles and Simnet (1988) remind us that 'Communication barriers are erected when the client gets different messages from different people' (Ewles and Simnet, 1988; p. 100). For example, different health professionals may say different things; family, friends and neighbours can contradict what is being said by health professionals and give inaccurate messages. However, medical science is not without its criticism of giving contradictory messages as often new research disproves previous theories. It is the responsibility of the health professional to be as up-to-date as possible and to give clear information.

Overcoming Language Barriers

This applies especially to people who do not have a good command of the English language. However, Ewles and Simnett (1988) emphasize that language is only one of the barriers to communicating with people from other races. The health professional needs to be aware of his or her own *communication style* in order to deliver the most appropriate method of health promotion. 'The health professional's core attitudes to her clients are likely to be reflected in her style of communication' (Ewles and Simnett, 1988; p. 88). They identify four communication styles:

- *authoritarian*
- *paternalistic*
- *permissive*
- *democratic*.

Authoritarian Style In this approach, communication is one-sided, with the professional giving out information and advice and not encouraging the client to question or express feelings. This can lead to a failure of acceptance of the health message because the person is unable to reflect and discuss the relevance of the information for themselves. We would all recognize, I am sure, that this is an easy method to adopt by the professional as they cannot be challenged or their level of knowledge questioned.

Paternalistic Style The aim of the paternalistic health educator is to promote the good of the clients and protect them from harm. This can lead to a failure to appreciate the older person's needs and what may seem the best thing by the health educator may not be the best approach for the older person.

> ### Case Study: The independent older person
>
> *Mrs M is 92 years old with moderate arthritis and suffers from occasional falls. Her physical health would be maintained if she allowed a neighbour to do her shopping for her. By going out every day she risks falling but maintains her own self esteem. She feels independent and reduces her social isolation.*

The paternalistic health educator would aim to keep the woman at home with other people doing her shopping and failing to recognize her emotional needs.

Permissive Style In this approach, the health professional allows the client to reach their own conclusions and avoids any difficulties or confrontations. The clients are required to find their own solutions to promoting health but, unfortunately, this can lead to avoidance of difficult problems and no solutions being found. This is the opposite approach to the authoritarian style and equally ineffectual.

Democratic Style In this method, the communication is a two-way process with the experiences and resources of both client and health professional being used to find the right solution for the right client. Through listening to each other and discussing differences of opinion openly, disagreement and unacceptance are avoided.

Ewles and Simnett (1988) believe that:

> *... the democratic style is most in harmony with the health education philosophy of encouraging and enabling people to take responsibility – both individually and collectively – for health.*
> **(Ewles and Simnett, 1988; p. 90)**

For many of us this democratic style may be a difficult approach to adopt. It is safer to dictate and tell people, rather than to share and reflect. However, it is the only way to truly empower our older clients to value and improve their health and, in the methods that follow, it is the democractic philosophy that is used.

First, however, it may be helpful to examine your own style of communication so you are aware of any changes in your approach which may be required (Table 4.3).

Empowering the Local Community

The way to empower the local community is for the health professional to go to where people live, work, shop and have their leisure time and to deliver the health messages there. Identification with the community and its needs are essential. Here are some examples of possible approaches.

Table 4.3 *Looking at your communication style. From Ewles and Simnett (1988) with permission*

The following questions aim to help you to examine your own communication style. Put a tick in the appropriate box

	Never	Sometimes	Usually	Always
1 Do your clients say what they feel?	☐	☐	☐	☐
2 Do clients finish what they are saving before you respond?	☐	☐	☐	☐
3 Do you think you are able to see things from your client's point of view?	☐	☐	☐	☐
4 Do clients disagree with you?	☐	☐	☐	☐
5 Do you explore with your clients the consequences of alternative actions?	☐	☐	☐	☐
6 Do you help clients to discuss painful memories or sensitive issues?	☐	☐	☐	☐
7 Do you share all the information at your disposal?	☐	☐	☐	☐
8 Do you help clients to discover their own strengths?	☐	☐	☐	☐
9 Do you respect your clients' right to reject your advice?	☐	☐	☐	☐

Which communication style – authoritarian, paternalistic, permissive or democratic – do you think you usually use?
What were the influences which led you to develop this style?
Can you identify any advantages in using alternative communication styles in your work?
Can you identify any aspects of your communication style that you would like to change?

The Health Shop

A health shop for people of age 55 and over could be established in the middle of a shopping area. It would need to be near the transport system and could be staffed by a health professional and a group of volunteers. Its aim would be to provide information and resources in the form of posters, notices and leaflets. The professional could be available as a resource to discuss any individual fitness plans and to promote a healthier lifestyle in older age.

The Beth Johnson Foundation established a Senior Health Shop as part of its Self Health Care in Old Age Project (1986) and claims that 'Everyone over fifty is welcome and will find something of interest that could help them towards a new healthy and happy life'.

The Market Stall

The majority of communities have local markets and the health professional could establish a regular monthly market stall focusing on relevant health topics and supporting any national campaigns. For example, in the winter the theme could be on ways of keeping warm and information on heating allowances. In warmer weather, the focus could be on outdoor pursuits and the value of exercise in later life. A dynamic worker should have no problem in finding different themes that would attract interest. The stall could give information in the form of leaflets, or be a way of exchanging information about groups and activities in the area. It could become part of the local network.

The same approach could be used in other areas where older people congregate. The post office on pension day could be one example, or a cafe or restaurant known to favour older clients. Mobile displays could be used, promoting such things as influenza injections in the autumn.

Word of Warning Sometimes there is a conflict between health messages and the self interest of other people in the community. We were recently involved in an initiative to promote healthy eating to protect against heart disease. Our market stall was allocated next to the local hamburger stall and we had to cope with conflict and severe animosity from the stall owner. He did as much as he could to obstruct our stall and greatly influenced the effectiveness of our health messages. Careful planning could perhaps have avoided this but it is important to be aware that selling health is not always in everyone's interest.

The Community Groups

All communities have established local groups for older people where the pro-active health promoter can offer information on health. The examples are numerous and knowledge of the local community would identify where these groups are. Some examples could be:

- *women's groups – Women's Institute, Townswomen's Guild;*
- *men's groups – Rotary Clubs, Probus;*
- *luncheon clubs;*
- *day centres;*
- *sheltered housing areas.*

Talks could be given on chosen topics, or health courses, covering several weeks and tailored to the needs of each group, could be offered.

The Local Media

Local radio, television and newspapers are excellent ways of raising awareness of health concerns and supporting other activities, such as a market stall, in which you may be involved. They are an ideal medium for health campaigns and issues, as long as the professional is aware of the limitations of this approach for changing health attitudes and behaviour.

An effective way of trying to influence policies affecting health is to write a letter to the editor of the local newspaper. This can keep a topic in the public eye for some time and facilitate debate on controversial issues. It is recommended that letters should be short and to the point in order to capture interest.

The Community Action

It is the responsibility of the health professional to support or initiate community action against situations hazardous to health. Campaigns such as poor lighting, which could cause an older person to fall, or convincing the local leisure centre to hold sessions for people over 55 years of age, all merit the attention of the health professional seeking to empower their local community to a healthier old age.

Empowering the Individual in a Group Setting

We can empower individuals to change their attitudes and behaviour through small group work. It is a demanding and time-consuming approach which is not suitable for all clients, and requires the development of certain skills which need to be learnt and understood by the

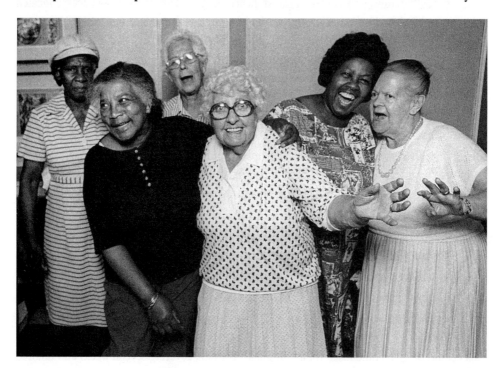

Fig. 4.2 *A group of older women getting together to improve their health*

professional. However, with experience and confidence, it can become a most rewarding and successful way of delivering health promotion.

The role of the professional in group work is one of *facilitator*. Facilitate means 'to enable' people to share and reflect upon their experiences and reach their own decisions. It is very much to do with valuing the person's own thoughts and resources and, in a group of older people, the wealth of experiences throughout the life course would be vast! It is dependent upon the democratic style of communication. The authoritarian approach would be disastrous but the professional also needs to be aware of the permissive style and be prepared to allow difficulties and confrontations to occur in a group when it is appropriate.

Informal and Formal Groups

McClymont *et al.* (1991) discuss informal and formal groups within a community: natural or *informal* groups arise spontaneously, tend to have fewer goals and operate with fewer restrictions. They give, as examples, small groups of 'regulars' who meet in the parks, cafes or shopping areas. These informal groups can provide valuable insight into the health needs and wishes of the older people and help in the planning of appropriate interventions.

A *formal* or formed group is brought together for a deliberate purpose and has a more structured membership with clearly defined goals. These types of groups can be *closed* groups, when the same people meet for a specific period of time with a clearly defined purpose. An example of this could be a structured course on older women's health running for 8 weeks. No new members would join the group during the course. This allows a closeness and security to develop so that individuals feel safe to exchange confidences. A *rolling* or *open* group would be one which may have been established by a professional, meeting a defined need, such as loneliness in a sheltered housing complex. This type of group has a much looser structure and people come in and out the group as the need arises.

We now examine more closely the structure, process and outcomes of closed groups as these are the ones the health professional is most likely to be involved in.

The Structure

Size The ideal size for small group work is 8–12 people. Too few will limit the exchange of experiences and some people may feel very threatened and exposed. Too big a group will prevent everyone participating and may cause subgroups to form.

Where Ideally, meetings should be held on neutral territory to prevent any feelings of ownership within the group. It does not always follow that the newest, smartest health centre is the best venue as this may indicate that the professional knows best and members may feel intimidated. The best location is the one where the community feels most comfortable, for example a community centre, village hall or library.

How The group will only run smoothly if the lighting, heating and ventilation are correct. A group of menopausal women may wish to have plenty of windows open to enable those suffering from hot flushes to feel more comfortable. A group of older people meeting together for reminiscence therapy may wish for a warmer environment.

A crucial factor is the arrangement of the chairs. Each group member, and this includes the professional facilitator, needs to be able to see everyone and everyone should appear equal. For this reason the circle is ideal, with sufficient space allowed between the chairs enabling emotional space as well as physical space (Fig. 4.3).

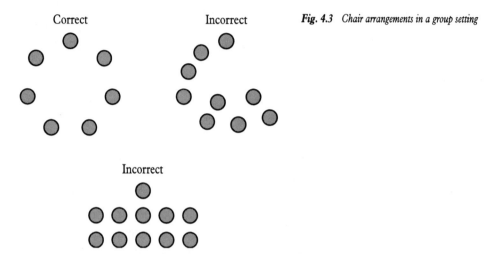

Fig. 4.3 *Chair arrangements in a group setting*

Similarly, the types of chair should all be the same so there is no indication of hierarchy and everyone feels they have an equal part in the group. Ideally the chairs should suit the client group. Very soft, low-slung chairs for a group of older people may prevent them from getting up without assistance, thus putting them at a disadvantage.

When The correct timing for groups is vital to their success. The professional should not be surprised if a preretirement course held in the local community centre during the daytime fails from lack of support. It would be equally inappropriate to run a health and fitness course for older people during dark winter evenings.

The facilitator should ensure that time is closely adhered to with the sessions beginning punctually and, equally important, finishing on time. Between 1 and 2 hours is usually long enough for a session.

The Process

Ice-breakers It is important that each person's name and a little bit about them is known so group members can relate to each other and feel they all belong to the group. It would be the role of the facilitator to ensure the process takes place either through introductions in pairs or name games. Name games can be used at the beginning of each session.

Confidentiality At the start of any group the issue of confidentiality must be addressed. Groups helping people with personal problems need to have high levels of confidentiality so that people feel safe to disclose private thoughts. A rule of confidentiality may be made from the start and possibly reinforced later in the sessions.

Exchanging Information If the function of health promotion in the group situation is to empower people to change attitudes and behaviour conducive to health, the experiences of the group need to be used and valued. The way to use the group's experiences as well as influencing health is through active participation.

'Brain storming' is an excellent method of exploring a certain area and collecting ideas from the group. A flip chart and pens are used and the group throws out relevant ideas as they occur to them. It enables the facilitator to know the range of knowledge and attitudes present and to develop certain areas if appropriate.

'Buzz groups' means dividing the group into smaller groups of two or three where they are given a point to discuss or a task, such as a questionnaire, to complete. This enables full participation of group members as the quieter ones feel able to talk more freely in a small group. The groups then all return to the larger group and exchange information.

'Gaming methods' is using games, such as quizzes or specially designed board games, to test or reinforce information.

'Role play' is only successful if the group members are well integrated and feel safe and comfortable with each other. Its purpose is to enable people to see another's point of view. For example, in a carers' group, the role of a dementia sufferer, the carer and the professional may be acted out in order to lead to a greater understanding of each other's position.

Facilitator's Role Facilitating a group needs skill and experience if it is to be effective. No group member must be allowed to dominate and it is the facilitator's role to ensure the group focuses on the topic in hand, whilst still allowing participation; a difficult balance to achieve if one group member is determined to tell everyone about his or her prize chrysanthemums, when the group is discussing ways of eating more nutritious food! If the discussion is irrelevant, some of the group members will feel let down by the group and probably stop coming. Another dilemma is when the health professional wants to discuss a particular health matter but the group continually reject the suggestion. If the educator tries to impose their view, it will not be taken on by the group and their health status will not change.

Outcomes

Group Endings It is important that small groups have endings, to prevent people becoming too dependent on them. The aim of the groups is to empower members not to develop dependency on the professional. A very cohesive group may choose to maintain a self-help function by meeting informally to exchange and share experiences. In this case, the facilitator's role will have finished and he or she will withdraw.

Discussion of outcomes of the group will enable the individuals to reflect on their learning and development and to realize what they have gained from the course. It also allows consideration of future requirements.

Evaluation is discussed in more detail at the end of this section.

Empowering the Individual in a One-To-One Setting

Health promotion can be carried out on a one-to-one level for those individuals who are unable, or do not wish, to join groups. A professional can still empower an individual by assisting them to make health choices. Choice is only possible with knowledge and this knowledge can be used to develop healthy lifestyles.

One-to-one situations can be created at any time a health professional has contact with an individual, whether in the home, in the surgery or clinic or out in the community. The educator needs to be aware of all the opportunities available to promote health.

Evaluating Health Promotional Activities

We cannot be effective at promoting health unless time is spent monitoring and evaluating our work. This process allows us to enhance and improve our practice and plan effectively for the future. Evaluation should form a continuous and automatic part of all our activities and the results acted upon, enabling changes to be made if necessary. Evaluation methods should also allow for short-, medium- and long-term goal planning.

Evaluation can be effective at all three stages of the structure, process and outcomes of a procedure, with self evaluation occurring at all three levels.

Evaluating the Structure

This entails questioning when and where certain activities were performed:

- *Were the posters displayed in the right place to attract the target group?*
- *Was the market stall situated in the best place and on the correct day?*
- *Was the preretirement course held at the right time of day?*
- *Was the best use made of the media facilities?*
- *Was I effective in enabling an older person, visited at home, to make some choice about their health?*
- *Was the group held in the most appropriate room at the health centre and should I have ensured the chairs were comfortable?*

Evaluating the Process

This applies to the way information is given:

- *Was the use of questionnaires the best way of finding out how much knowledge the group had on dementia?*
- *Did I allow too much irrelevant discussion during the session?*
- *Were some of the questions in the health survey at the market too personal and did not allow confidentiality?*
- *Would that health message have reached a wider audience if I had used the local paper rather than the doctor's surgery?*

Formal groups can evaluate each stage of the course by asking people verbally to score sessions as good, fair, poor, or by using number ratings. This will given an overall impression of the group's reactions. More detailed information on the process can be obtained using sentence stem completion (see Fig. 4.4) and can be performed on a sample of the group.

Right now I feel _____

Next session I hope _____

The best thing about this session was _____

I would change _____

Fig. 4.4 *Example of sentence stem evaluation method*

Evaluating the Outcome

Evaluating outcomes depends on the original objective of the service. Sometimes the outcomes are easy to measure:

- *At a smoking cessation group how many of the members stopped smoking?*
- *In a healthy lifestyle group for older people, how many of the people took up a regular form of exercise?*

Often the outcomes are less easy to measure because the results are not so clear cut.

- *Was the self esteem of a group of isolated residents in sheltered housing enhanced through their attendance at a reminiscence group?*
- *Did a group of carers gain emotional support through belonging to the group?*

Outcomes also need to be set against realistic objectives. Perhaps a more realistic outcome for some members of a smoking cessation group would be to reduce the number of cigarettes they smoked each day. Or, in the healthy lifestyle group, did all the members attempt some sort of exercise, even if it was not on a regular basis?

Evaluating is an on-going activity of questioning and examining each stage of the structure, process and outcomes of an intervention. It should be done with a positive approach, recognizing when success has been achieved and where improvements can be made. Most importantly, it should become an automatic part of good practice in health promotion.

PUTTING IT INTO PRACTICE

In this section we look at practical examples of putting the theories we have discussed into practice. We examine health promotional activities at strategic times in the life cycle of older people, the times when people may be more receptive to changing their health and lifestyle. The areas we cover are:

- *promoting health in retirement;*
- *promoting health in women at the time of the menopause;*
- *promoting mental health in a sheltered housing complex;*
- *promoting health in a carer of an older person suffering from dementia;*
- *promoting health in an older person following a bereavement;*
- *promoting health in an active, recently retired couple.*

Promoting Health in Retirement

Case Study: The working man at retirement

Mr E is a skilled workman in one of the small local factories in the town and is due to retire in 10 years' time. He has worked hard all his life, doing overtime and shift work when required. His wife has had a part-time job since the children have grown up and left home and she is responsible for the domestic running of the home. Mr E has had very little time to develop any leisure activities, except watching the television and going to the local pub. He is apprehensive about retirement.

Aims of Health Promotion in Preretirement

- *To plan for increased leisure time.*
- *To have financial security.*
- *To develop a healthy lifestyle.*
- *To maintain close relationships.*
- *To be a valued member of the community.*

Structure

1 *To arrange a meeting with the factory management (the factory is too small to have its own occupational health department).*
2 *To raise the awareness of the management for the need for employees to have some preparation for retirement.*
3 *To plan to hold an 8–10 week course for approximately 10 employees who have 10 years to retirement.*
4 *To plan a suitable time and venue within the factory through negotiation with the management staff.*
5 *To advertize the course in the factory with suggested plan for programme.*

Process

Suggested programme for a preretirement course which should be flexible, depending on the needs of the group:

- *what retirement means to you;*
- *reviewing income;*
- *healthy lifestyle – exercise, food and drink, smoking;*
- *ways to relax and relieve stress;*
- *preparing for leisure;*
- *what retirement means to you and your partner (possible combined session with partners);*
- *review of the course and further support.*

Outcome

The group could be reconvened annually, or more often if required, to monitor progress and maintain momentum. The aims of the course can be evaluated and further courses planned.

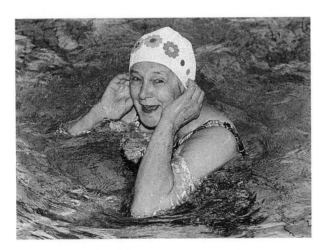

Fig. 4.5 Swimming for health

Promoting Health in Women at the Time of the Menopause

Case Study: The older woman at the change

Mrs M is having irregular periods and hot flushes. At times she feels tired and weepy. Her son has recently married and her daughter has gone away to college. Her husband is very preoccupied with a demanding job. She has read a lot about hormone replacement therapy (HRT) but feels uncertain whether she wants to take tablets or not. She made an appointment to discuss her feelings with the GP. Unfortunately, the doctor was rather busy that day but suggested she had a blood test for oestrogen levels and then come back to have a prescription for HRT if that was what she wanted.

Aims of Promoting Health in the Menopause

- *To help women to understand the changes occurring at the menopause.*
- *To enable women to adapt to these changes with a positive attitude.*

- *To have sufficient knowledge about HRT in order to make an informed choice.*
- *To have appropriate support and advice as required.*

Structure

- *Menopause clinics – held weekly at the general practitioners' surgery or health centre during the late afternoon. Women could refer themselves and either make an appointment or 'drop in.' The facility could provide a close monitoring system for women on HRT or for those who want to discuss its use on a one-to-one basis in a relaxed atmosphere.*
- *Self-help group – the health professional could facilitate a small closed group of women who wish to share information about the menopause. This could be held at the most appropriate venue within the community.*

Process

This is a suggested programme, depending on the needs of the group, for running a course with a small group. Some of the sessions could be facilitated by other professionals, such as a trained counsellor discussing relationships, or a GP giving information on HRT, but these people must be acceptable to the group.

- *Attitudes towards the menopause.*
- *Understanding our bodies and the changes that occur.*
- *The value of diet and exercise.*
- *Stress and relaxation.*
- *HRT and osteoporosis.*
- *Relationships in later life.*
- *How to be assertive.*
- *Where do we go from here?*

Outcomes

The outcomes should be measured against the aims. This could be done in writing, using the sentence stem evaluation or by verbal feedback from the group. The self-help outcome can be assessed by the relationships that have developed within the group and whether the group forms a network of support.

Promoting Mental Health in a Sheltered Housing Complex

Case Study: The older woman with memory loss

Mrs C moved from her home in the town 5 miles away after her husband died and now lives near her daughter in a group of sheltered flats attached to an older persons' home. The individual flats are in long corridors with communal sitting areas on each floor which are rarely used. Mrs C only knows her next door neighbour. Her daughter works at the local hospital and visits occasionally. Mrs C is aware that she has early signs of dementia with recent memory loss but she is coping well by using 'aide memoirs'. However, she remembers very clearly when she was a weaver in the Lancashire cotton mills. She misses her family and is tearful at times.

Aims of Promoting Mental Health

- *To promote self esteem.*
- *To facilitate friendships and social contacts.*
- *To enable maximum potential of mental health functions.*

Structure

To facilitate a reminiscence group once a week in the communal sitting room. Visit residents of the sheltered housing area, explaining what the group is and inviting them to attend.

Process

- *Initiate a 9-week course.*
- *Divide the course into three parts to reflect the lifespan of the older people, for example childhood/school days/First World War; young adulthood/work; Second World War and today.*
- *At each session, old photographs, slides or music can be used to facilitate discussion.*
- *The older people can be encouraged to bring along their own memorabilia to the sessions.*
- *A visit could be arranged to the local museum or the museum attendant invited to attend a session.*

Outcome

The success of the group, and whether the aims have been met, can be assessed by the attendance at the group and whether the group wish to become an open group, meeting regularly and supporting themselves.

It is important in reminiscence work that the facilitator is sensitive to any unpleasant memories which may be brought out and to be prepared to deal with any difficult situations on a one-to-one basis after the session has finished. The excellent research by Fieldon (1990) showing the value of this type of intervention for improving the mental health of residents is recommended.

Promoting Health in a Carer

Case Study: The caring older person

Mrs S is an active, intelligent, older woman living in a bungalow on the edge of the town with her husband who is a retired architect. Over a number of years Mr S's memory has faded and he is now not safe to be left alone. He sometimes has difficulty in getting to the toilet on time and has occasionally wandered outside, becoming angry and aggressive if his wife tries to restrain him. Mrs S is devoted to her husband and wishes to care for him as long as possible. They have one daughter who has home, family and job commitments. The local Social Services Department has recently become involved.

Aims of Promoting Health in a Carer

- *To focus on the health of carers.*
- *To develop a support network for carers.*
- *To allow information on available services to be disseminated.*

Structure

- *Group of local health professionals and carers to meet and plan a health workshop for carers.*
- *The venue would depend on what is available in the community but it would need to be of sufficient size for a large group.*
- *Consideration must be given for care of the older person at home to allow the carer to come to the workshop. Organizers would need to arrange a voluntary sitting service in the home, or hold the meeting in a venue where the older person can come too and be cared for, for example home for older people.*
- *Transport for carers would need to be available.*
- *A suitable day, probably a weekend, would need to be decided, when the maximum benefit for carers can be ensured.*
- *The event would need to be advertized widely using all available sources such as local media, posters, leaflet drops and personal contact with known carers.*

Process

The programme for a health workshop for carers held from 10.00 am to 4.00 pm on a Saturday at the local older persons' home may be:

10.00 am   *Coffee and welcome*
                     Plan of the day (facilitator)

10.30 am	*What is a carer? (facilitator and a carer)*
11.00 am	*Leading a healthy lifestyle*
	Nutrition (community dietician)
	Exercise (community physiotherapist)
11.45 am	*Lifting – practical demonstration (district nurse)*
12.30 pm	*Light Lunch (provided by the WRVS)*
1.30 pm	*Entitlement to benefits (local DSS officer)*
2.00 pm	*Trying to cope with aggression (community psychiatric nurse)*
2.45 pm	*Stress and relaxation (counsellor)*
3.30 pm	*Forming support networks and carer groups (facilitator)*
4.00 pm	*Close.*

Outcomes

The outcomes will depend on whether a support network is established.

Promoting Health in the Bereaved

Case Study: The bereaved older person

Mr E is a fit, retired council worker whose wife died 6 months ago after a short illness. He has two children, a son and a daughter, who live within 10 miles and visit him from time to time. Since his wife's death he has not felt like going out and has stopped going to the local bowling club. Neighbours have expressed their concerns to the health visitor that Mr E is not eating properly.

Aims of Promoting Health in the Recently Bereaved

- *To assist the client to pass through the stages of grieving towards acceptance of loss.*
- *To raise their self esteem.*
- *To keep physically and mentally fit.*

Structure

- *One-to-one approach in the client's home to establish level of grief and counselling.*
- *Alternatively, facilitate a small closed group for bereaved older people. The suitability for this group may depend on one-to-one interviews and personal invitation.*
- *The venue would need to be carefully chosen, possibly within primary health care facilities.*

Process

Within a small group, the weekly discussions would need to focus on the needs of the group. The facilitator would require skill and sensitivity to establish the group so each member would obtain benefit. Suggested topics for discussion are:

- *looking at bereavement;*
- *financial concerns;*
- *examining other losses in life;*
- *establishing networks;*
- *ways to have a healthy lifestyle;*
- *stress and relaxation methods;*
- *developing new hobbies;*
- *practical skills of daily living.*

Outcomes

Did the group members establish new ways of coping and are no longer dependent on the group? Do they have informal support networks to maintain their wellbeing? These would be the main outcomes you would hope to achieve when promoting health in bereavement.

You might spend some time thinking about loss and older people and whether this approach would be appropriate for other losses in old age.

Fig. 4.6   *Keeping active together*

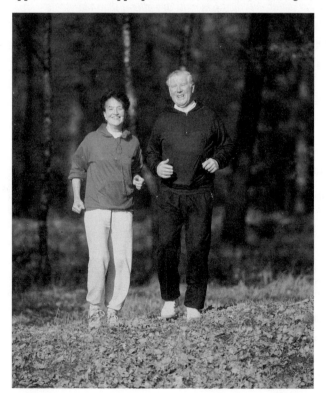

Promoting Health in an Active, Older Couple

> **Case Study: The active older couple**
>
> *Mr and Mrs G are both retired school teachers. They have one child who lives abroad and another who lives about 30 miles away. They wish to be active and healthy and to retain their independence throughout their lifespan. They also want to remain in contact with their peer group and play a useful part in the life of the community.*

Having worked through the previous examples, try planning a health promotion strategy for this couple. You may decide on more than one approach. Use your knowledge to establish clear aims and devise structure, process and outcomes for the methods.

Summary

We have looked at six examples of promoting health in older people at strategic times in the life cycle. You will have noticed that certain themes follow through each scenario. It is important to always include a healthy lifestyle as the basis of all good health. Money concerns are also of importance because we know that poverty leads to ill health. We have aimed to empower clients to make informed choices on their health through the sharing of knowledge and development of self esteem. We have aimed to support clients in order that they can lead as happy and healthy an old age as possible.

CONCLUSIONS

In this chapter we have examined the value of promoting health in old age. In the first section we looked at the meaning of health and the way that older people perceive their own health. This was important information to establish if we are seeking to alter attitudes to health.

In the next section we examined the scope of health promotion and the importance of recognizing the influences of policy on health. We realized that to promote health effectively it had to be considered on several levels which were national, local communities and individuals. We then moved on to consider communicating with older people and the importance of recognizing our own style of communication. Finally, in this section, we looked at ways of empowering the local community to improve health as well as methods of empowering individuals, either in the group setting or on a one-to-one approach. We ended with ways of evaluating our activities by examining the structure, process and outcomes.

In the final section, we concentrated on case studies to illustrate some of the times in the life cycle of an older person when health promotional strategies could be effective. This approach was considered the most appropriate in a gerontology textbook, rather than defining the needs by chronological ages.

It is to be hoped that this chapter will inspire nurses to actively promote health in our older generation in whatever setting they are working. In this way attitudes can be changed and society can begin to value the contribution of older people.

ACKNOWLEDGEMENTS

I thank Joy Tricklebank for patiently interpreting my writing and producing the typed copies, Ruth McGrath for her enthusiasm in producing positive images of older people, and, not least, to all the older people who have given me inspiration and brought this chapter alive.

CLINICAL DISCUSSION POINTS

These link specifically to the practical examples in the final section of the chapter.

Discuss other ways to promote health at this stage of the life cycle apart from through the work place. What sources could you use to identify the client group and what different venues would be appropriate?

Consider whether it is appropriate to discriminate positively for older women and to hold women-only courses. Discuss other ways of promoting health in older women.

Discuss other approaches to improving the mental health of clients in residential settings. Consider the value of school children becoming involved with older people as part of a project in intergenerational activity.

Discuss how you might set up a support group for carers. Should separate workshops be set up for people looking after dementia sufferers or should they be combined with other disabilities?

SUGGESTIONS FOR FURTHER READING

Carnegie Inquiry into the 3rd Age (1992). **Health: Abilities and Well being in the Third Age.** Research Paper **9**. The Carnegie UK Trust.
The Carnegie Inquiry was set up to consider issues affecting the life, work and livelihood of people who have finished their main job or career or bringing up children but may have 20 or more healthy, active and independent life ahead. This 9th paper in the series gives a comprehensive and up-to-date review of the issues relating to health and well being in later life.

Sidell, M. (1994). **Health in Old Age Myth, Mystery and Management.** Open University Press, Buckingham.
This book explores the myths which surround the subject of health in later life. It looks at the resources and social support available as well as implications for public policy provision and explores the problems and possibilities for ensuring a healthy future of old age.

Shapiro, J. (1989). **Ourselves Growing Older. Women Ageing with Knowledge and Power.** Fontana/Collins, Great Britain.
A complete health and living handbook for mid-life and older women. A practical, useful reference book which discusses women's health and ageing issues. It draws on the work of experts, but also listens to the voices of women themselves.

REFERENCES

Benzeval, M., Judge, K. and Whitehead, M. (Eds) (1995). **Tackling Inequalities in Health.** King's Fund, London.

A Beth Johnson Foundation Project (1986). **Self Health Care in Old Age Project.** Beth Johnson Foundation, Stoke-on-Trent.

Ewles, L. and Simnett, I. (1988). **Promoting Health: A Practical Guide to Health Education,** 2nd edn. John Wiley, Chichester.

Fieldon, M. (1990). Reminiscence as a therapeutic intervention with sheltered housing residents. A comparative study. **British Journal of Social Work 20,** 21–44.

Kalache, A., Warnes, T. and Hunter, D. (1988). **Promoting Health Among Elderly People**. King Edward's Hospital Fund, London.

McClymont, M., Thomas, S., Denham, M. (1991). **Health Visiting and Elderly People. A Health Promotion Challenge,** 2nd edn. Longman, Singapore.

Nutbeam, D. (1986). Health promotion glossary. **Health Promotion** 1(1), 113–127.

Townsend, P. (1982). **Inequalities in Health: The Black Report.** Penguin, London.

Victor, C. R. (1991). **Health and Health Care in Later Life.** Open University Press, Milton Keynes.

Section 2

Individual Perspectives

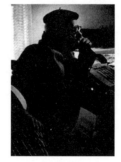

Gender, Race and Social Responses to an Ageing Client
Helen Jones

Loss and Bereavement in Later Life
Margaret Foulkes

Individual Responses
John Dean, Glenys Dean and Mary Savage

"With the Ancient is wisdom; and in length of days, understanding."

Job 12:12

The second section of this text recognizes the insider's view of ageing – the older person as a central voice within gerontological nursing. Helen Jones' chapter on gender, race and its impact on ageing immerses the reader immediately in an experiential exercise. As the reader is asked to consider the experience of becoming an older émigré faced with accessing health in a foreign country, many of the key issues faced by older people in ethnic minority groups come to life. Issues on the effect of gender offer a balanced picture of older women and older men's issues and the effect these issues have on health. Margaret Foulkes' chapter on loss and bereavement similarly focuses on the very individual response to loss. This chapter extends nursing's image on loss, highlighting the fact that loss relates just as much to animate as well as inanimate objects. The chapter offers very tangible advice, which is both sensitive and research based, on helping older people cope with grief and loss.

The final chapter within this section on individual responses is a powerful and unique account of two different experiences of caring for older people. As a result of themselves being less than one generation away from being the recipients of care, each writer demonstrates diversity and insight into care provision. A central tenet that runs through this chapter is the ambivalence of choice within the scenario of the carer and cared for. Outlined by John Dean, Mary Savage and Glenys Dean poignantly discuss the issues of providing care and the specific life biographies that make this care so complicated.

Chapter Five

Gender Race and Social Responses to an Ageing Client

Helen Jones

Core Themes in Gerontological Nursing

Ageing Matters	*New Social World*	*Lifespan Perspective*	*Health and Old People*
Illness and Dependency	*Quality Nursing Care*	*Therapeutic Intervention*	*Politicizing Gerontological Nursing*

Key Words

Racism • Jeopardy • Access • Status • Inequalities

INTRODUCTION

Why, you may ask, are two independent concepts being brought together in one chapter? Race and gender are two totally separate and distinct issues with relevance to ageing in Britain in the 1990s. However, there are some similarities to be noted between the two, and perhaps of greater concern to the nurse as an informal advocate to the patient – for a nurse can be no more than that – there are some cumulative effects of both race and gender, of which nursing needs to be aware.

This Chapter aims to explore the following issues:

How race influences the experiences of older people

How gender influences the experiences of older people

The comparable dimensions of both issues and their cumulative effect on health and care.

RACE AND RACISM

Imagine the situation – you qualified as a nurse a few years ago and now with little chance of promotion, under constant pressure from your manager to do more in the limited time available, and the prospect of further study because you have to continue to develop academically, it is no surprise that as a consequence of all this you thoroughly enjoyed your recent holiday to France. So, you decide to pack your bags and emigrate there. You live in a clean white apartment by the ocean where you swim in the sea almost every day. Days are warm, bright and sunny – work is in a local shop where they close for afternoon siestas. Politics and bureaucracy are no longer a part of your life. You live a reasonably healthy life – ensuring the necessary operation in your mid-forties conveniently coincided with a timely trip back to visit relatives in Britain. But now, you are 72-years-old, a little frail, and do not want to travel far for treatment. You drive to the nearest Health Centre and obtain the following written advice leaflet (Cancer Relief Macmillan Fund, 1995) (Full translation on p. 132):

Case Study: *Information de votre santé*

Il y a plusieurs organisations nationals qui sont capables d'aider de differentes façons. Il est souvent juste une question de savoir comment trouver la bonne pour vous. Dans cette brochure nous donnons une liste des organisations nationaux qui peuvent vous procurer tout information et conseil ainsi-que support moral et practique. Ils travaillent tous en collaboration avec les Service professionel de Sante, et offrent aussi bien de l'aide qu'un conseil medical où qu'un traitment.

A far-fetched tale or a possibility? And what do you think of the help available to you? We will return to this tale shortly.

Before proceeding, it is necessary to clarify what is meant by 'race'. The terms 'race' and 'ethnicity' are used interchangeably by many people. Historically, the main distinction between the two terms is that race tends to label a person according to their physical characteristics, most notably their skin colour, while ethnicity tends to label a person depending on their social circumstances – mainly characterized by language, culture or religion (Mares *et al.*, 1985). While the finer details of this debate are of great importance, they lie out of the scope of this chapter and for more detailed discussions see, for example, Fenton (1991). It is suffice to state here that there is an inherent belief throughout Great Britain that there is a difference between the white Anglo-Saxon indigenous population and all other members of the populace. This is true – there are some differences. However, the difficulties arise when a person from either the 'indigenous' category or the 'other' category believes that difference to cause one category to become superior or inferior to the other.

When considering race – that is, skin colour – it is often believed, or worse still, taken for granted that the 'other' category – that is, the non-white, non-indigenous population – is inferior. This hierarchy of social value belief systems is not only incorrect and immoral, in the context of health care it provides a strong negative barrier to communication and therefore rehabilitation. As a nurse whose primary aim is to meet the needs of the individual requiring your services it is necessary to explore your own attitudes and beliefs, the foundations of your barriers, so that they may crumble. This text is intended to provide some facts and further references so that you may explore issues concerning race and ethnicity in more detail. Examples are described to help you develop a critical awareness of your own professional practice.

Since the title of this section uses the word 'race' – this chapter will be mainly concerned with people in the NCWP category (New Commonwealth and Pakistan). Or, more simply, older people whose skin colour is not white. Furthermore, for the purposes of this chapter, racism can be defined as those who not only discriminate against a group of people characterized by their non-white skin colour, but also disempower those people by abusing their own power. For nurses working within an integrated structure of health and social services it is important to understand that racism exists at various levels: from the highly complex socio-politico-economic level, through the institutional level and right down to individual racism. Sometimes, perhaps unknowingly, one level may influence another.

Double Jeopardy

Whenever racism appears and at whatever level, the effects are more accentuated when a person is older. The presence of one deepens the influence of the other; that is, prejudice and disempowerment due to the bio-socio-economic deprivation associated with old age is further enhanced when race becomes a factor. Since social status is linked with type of employment, and older people – in most cases – are forced to retire from paid labour on reaching a specified age, then if they have no job they simply have no status. In some cases a status may be conferred on that person according to their preretirement employment. This places any older person at an immediate disadvantage – because of their age they are forced to retire from work and because they retire from work they are forced to survive on financial and service handouts that the community feels fit to bestow on them. It is only more recently that private pensions and savings have been encouraged throughout the general populace. As state pensions and benefits are often perceived as gifts or charity, the receiver is expected to be greatful and consequently meant to feel somehow inferior. The notion of being disadvantaged because of old age and suffering discrimination is known as 'double jeopardy'. Add to this the inaccessibility of these services because of say, racism, and this is 'triple jeopardy'. Norman (1985) explores these issues at great length.

The converse of this hypothesis is the notion of 'age as a leveller'. Here, when considered as a measure of wellbeing, both the indigenous population and peoples of other races are seen to come closer together with advance in years, so ageing serves to lessen the differences between races. The debate goes on.

So how does all this influence the nursing skills required? Well, nursing is about caring and meeting a person's needs, yet everyone's needs are different. There are different cultural norms, which in turn influence beliefs and expectations. People of different races have different perceptions, different expectations and use a different form of language to communicate these ideals. The fundamental principle here is that the best and only person to communicate their need/s is the person her/himself – even a best 'guesstimate' will be inaccurate somewhere. Being patient-centred is never more important than with a patient of a different race to the nurse's own race. This is quite simply because you start from a position of having less knowledge and understanding. Communication is the key to obtaining knowledge and developing insight. What complicates communication are the images of old age inherent in society and in the media portrayals. A typical example of how British society views ageing is the caricature of Victor Meldrew in the BBC television series 'One Foot in the Grave'. I use the word caricature deliberately since he represents a conglomerate of many negative stereotypes and beliefs concerning old age in the 1990s. He is portrayed as arrogant, aggressive and intolerant. Far more realistic are the characters in the BBC television series 'Waiting for God', yet this programme seems less popular in the viewing ratings. It is pertinent here, then, to look in more detail at images of old age, expectations and use of language.

First, the negative image of ageing is reinforced by a lack of resources. It is the social forces – of which the political system is just one part – that limit resources. In turn, they are further limited by the resource distribution systems. In practical terms this means that older people are not only forced to retire from paid labour at a specific age, but on doing so are eligible for limited pensions and incomes. Eligibility for such finances are biased towards the indigenous population since many older people of 'other' races have not worked in Britain for sufficient years to qualify for the full amount. This concept, coupled with access to resources affecting life chances, is described more fully in Fennell *et al.* (1988). The health advice document written in French earlier in the chapter provides a classic example of how access to services can be so easily limited. At a time of stress and in a less familiar language, the words mean nothing and limit the actual help that is or may be available (for full translation; see end of Chapter). It is easy to 'blame' the emigrée for not learning the language and this shifts the burden of responsibility to provide an adequate service. The social structure, policies and laws, are planned and prepared, based on the indigenous population. Clearly, this disregards the fact that Britain is multi-ethnic, and that so-classified 'ethnic minorities' make a significant contribution to the population numbers as a whole. Table 5.1 shows the population of older people by ethnic group for 1991.

Table 5.1 *The population of older people in Great Britain by ethnic group (country of birth) for 1991. Modified from OPCS (1993)*

	All those aged 60 and over (Numbers in thousands)
Country of birth	
UK	10 913
Eire	195
Old Commonwealth	33
New Commonwealth	214
European Community (excluded above)	103
Rest of Europe	88
Turkey	2
USSR	23
Africa (excluded above)	22
America (excluded above)	18
Asia (excluded above)	22
Rest of world	<1
Total	11 633

Moving on to expectations, nursing is part of the service provision for health and illness and each race enjoys cultural norms and beliefs that embrace a range of religions, values and customs. There are threads of feelings and views that run through populations. For example, incest is regarded as appalling in Britain, while in some North African tribes, such close family inbreeding is positively encouraged – for sound biological reasons. All people of all races have met with different life experiences, their choices being limited or increased because of the differing social circumstances in which they find themselves. Ethnic minorities in Britain consist of those who came here by choice, or as exiles, or as refugees, or because they were born here. For more detail refer to Fennell *et al.* (1988) and Patel (1990). Thus they may have lived in Britain from a very young age, right through to their old age. Indeed, others may have lived here all their lives and be second generation British. The reason for living in Britain and the age upon arrival will affect life experiences and expectations. As a consequence, the strength of belief in cultural norms and values will be as varied and unique to each person as there are people. Acknowledging and internalizing that all people are unique is a fundamental principle of good nursing care. Thus, the patient is the only person who can identify their own personal needs which automatically involves them in their nursing care plan.

What is also important to recognize in relation to expectations is that immigration has given rise to fluctuations in size of ethnic minority groups according to geographical location. This is largely due to the suitability and availability of work open to immigrants. Suitability here means that in some areas, some cultures believe that women cannot or should not perform certain jobs. The same applies to specific types of employment for men. Here, then, it is the cultural beliefs that limit the employment. So, we find that in the 1950s, people from the Caribbean tended to settle in London, Bristol, the Midlands, Leeds and Manchester. People from southern Asia also settled in London, but other areas include Leicester, Lancashire and Yorkshire. More specifically, Sikhs settled in Southall, Gujeratis in Leicester, and Muslims in Bradford (Fenton, 1991). Geographical variations have important implications for health service provision. The service providers have a responsibility not only to be aware of the extent of the multi-ethnic population they serve, but also to identify the needs of the different cultures in order to try and meet them.

The immigration rate is far less now than it was from 1950 to 1970 when people of different races were positively encouraged to come to Britain to undertake often low paid employment. This, in itself, raises two very practical issues. The first is that working in low paid jobs means that only lower quality housing and education are available to immigrants. With ageing, this not only means that ethnic minority older people may be in need of more services due to the conditions in which they are forced to live, but being less well educated they can neither improve their options nor be aware of the limited services that may be available. The second point here is that the proportion of ethnic minority groups is not likely to increase in the twenty-first century as immigration laws are now more restrictive. As a consequence, they will remain a minority group for a longer period of time with a correspondingly lower voice.

Finally, a note about use of language. Each culture may speak in the same tongue, such as English, but their use of the words may be very different. For example, British people do not like to admit to having pain – they attempt to dismiss their discomfort or put up with it for fear of being considered weak. Furthermore, if they do admit to being in pain, the nurse tries to encourage the patient to 'hold on a little longer' before administering the prescribed analgesia. South Asian people, on the other hand, seem to express their pain more freely through cries, but they do not necessarily mean a physical pain and the actual cause of the cry needs to be determined. This is the responsibility of the good and caring nurse to determine, for an analgesic may be inappropriate treatment.

Summarizing, I refer back to my fundamental principle – that every patient is a unique individual, and as such is the only person who can identify their own needs. The nurse's skills are in communicating with that individual to help determine the exact nature of care needs. Where the language and/or cultural needs of the client may affect communication with the nursing staff, then other help must be sought. This may be from an interpreter associated with the health care service, or from within the family, or from a friend, or teacher of the faith from the client's religious belief. Choice of help must be from someone who is sensitive to the client's needs and must be acceptable to them. However, they must also be able to take account of the professional help that is being offered. This must be closely followed by careful planning, full implementation and thorough evaluation of the solutions so that she/he provides real care that is meaningful to the client.

The Current Context

It would be most inappropriate to look at ethnic minority older people without considering the sweeping changes currently occurring through the framework of the social and political policies. There are three main themes to be addressed:

- *the community care legislation;*
- *the changing nature of the NHS;*
- *the approval of traditional therapies.*

Taking each in turn, I describe briefly the macro-trend and then try to relate that to the micro-setting to make this relevant to each individual nurse as a practitioner.

The Community Care Legislation

In the 1990s the shift in care is moving from more formal institutions out into the community. Definitions and debates concerning this topic are well documented elsewhere (e.g. Phillipson, 1988). Within the legislation, certain groups are specifically targeted including ethnic minorities and the elderly mentally ill (EMI). This is a positive move intended to help redress the imbalance of services to people in the particular 'groups' listed. However, in the light of the foregoing, caution must be exercised. For the nurse working in the field, consider for example the group labelled EMI. Where mental health is considered, population characteristics help to determine criteria for diagnoses. A nurse ignorant of cultural norms and cultural behaviours and not prepared to ask the client, may lead to misunderstanding, inaccurate diagnosis of the nursing need and consequent inappropriate treatment being planned and given. A nurse who truly practises client-centred care that is needs led, can more readily assess and plan appropriate rehabilitative treatment. Doku (1990) details this scenario most eloquently.

The Changing Nature of the NHS

The world-renowned British NHS was first established in 1948 to provide a quality health service available to the whole population. Improved technology and raised awareness has increased demand on the service dramatically so that the original aims are no longer realistic. Private health care has been introduced and some modification is required. The question here then is – should services for black older people be separate or mainstream? Segregation of services deals with the symptoms and not the cause. Patel describes 'black projects' for 'black elders' and suggests challenge to such exploitation and oppression. She suggests future service provision for black older people resist separation and be based on the following principles:

- *that there is a role change for care providers;*
- *projects relieve the pressure but provide only short-term solutions;*
- *general financial pressures limit services and further marginalize black older people;*
- *separate services assume there is already access to statutory mainstream provision;*
- *'ethnic' identity is not best maintained by pluralistic separation;*
- *maximize the freedom of choice of the individual.*

In her conclusion she states 'black elders are part of this society and hence entitled to mainstream services' (Patel, 1990; p. 58). For the nurse practitioner, treating every client as an individual regardless of race or ethnic identity should help improve the services on offer. It is the responsibility of the nurse practitioner to treat every patient as an individual regardless of race or ethnic identity. Nursing based on this principle, coupled with the function of informal advocate should bring to the fore the services that are needed and not currently available. This will include some of those services required by ethnic minority and black older people and should help to increase the range on offer. The Community Care Policy Guidance (HMSO, 1990) clearly describes how services should be needs-led. A significant portion of

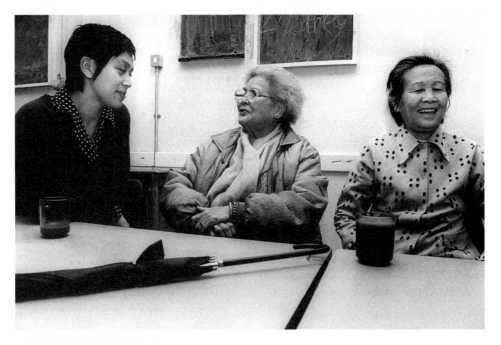

Fig. 5.1 *Sharing individual needs*

service-users are older people. Inappropriate services limit the use by ethnic minority and black older people. Identifying need could help develop apposite services.

The Approval of Traditional Therapies

The nature of health care and medicine falls into two natural categories – traditional or those modes essentially developed and practised in the Eastern world; and modern, more usually practised in the Western world. Older people from different cultures are familiar with and favour different therapies. To a certain extent, their compliance with a therapy reflects their strength of belief in its abilities. Compliance may strongly influence success or failure of a treatment. In order for nursing care to meet the client's needs it must embrace both modern and traditional therapies as necessary. Again, the successful nurse–client relationship relies on good communication skills that sustain the flow of information to and between both parties. Care must be taken to ensure complimentary treatments rather than dual treatments. Aslam and Healy (1986) describe the dangers of dual treatment in detail, citing as example the case of a Pakistani woman living in Bradford who was suffering from asthma. She was not only following her GP's advice but also that of the hakim back in their family village in Pakistan. Eventually the situation reached a climax resulting in hospitalization and careful monitoring of her physical signs and symptoms. This led eventually to an appropriate, single treatment.

In short, appropriate care of older people of ethnic minorities can only be offered within the context of the current social, political and economic framework *in situ*. This underlines the holistic approach advocated by expert nursing practice. The next section details the nurse's responsibilities towards older black people.

The Nurse's Responsibilities

'Service provision' is more than one dimensional (see Cameron *et al.*, 1989) – it is concerned with nurses and the nature of nursing; it is concerned with clients and their expectations; and it concerns racism at all levels, to name but three. The theory of nursing aims to be client focused, but in practice this rarely occurs. Generally, the clinical practice of nursing remains bureaucratic and inflexible, viewing the clients in subsections or parts, with their nursing care being largely determined by the medical model. Clients are rarely consulted directly as to what they perceive are their needs, particularly if they are older – thus ageism becomes yet another dimension of nursing. Ageism in nursing – the notion that clients are not valued simply because of their advanced years – is a major obstacle in providing and delivering a quality service to our older citizens. To help limit this hurdle, the practice of nursing needs to adopt a more client-led model (for all clients of any age) that draws on innovation and succeeds through flexibility. Unless nursing becomes person-focused in clinical practice in this way, then the needs of black older people are not even going to be identified, let alone met.

The nurse has a responsibility to *establish a healthy communication with each client*. 'Understanding the elderly ethnic minority client's name is part of the basis of a good professional relationship' (Duncan, 1991). Through lack of knowledge of the naming system it would be an insult to ask an already distressed wife at seeing her husband ill in strange clinical surroundings if she is Mrs Singh. Ignorance is an excuse, not a reason. In any race it is necessary to acknowledge that – with age – naming systems differ; with greetings – systems differ; status – may change according to sex, age, employment position; and that relevant questions may only be asked by the appropriate sex. Duncan also suggests liaison with the client's family to ensure:

- *the nature of the problem has been identified;*
- *the concept of the problem is clarified;*
- *the aims of rehabilitation are understood by all involved.*

Initially, this seems an easy and reasonable task. However, consider the scenario at the start of the chapter. You are back in France and can speak enough of the language to achieve general daily living tasks. Assuming your dysfunctional need is physical and further assuming that you understood the passage quoted and know where and how to get help – who do you want to interpret for you? In Britain, people available to interpret in such cases come from a variety of sources – larger hospitals hold lists of staff prepared to perform the task; a spouse may be willing; a grandchild may be able; an official interpreter may be employed. Each different source of interpreter brings with them a unique range of other problems. Would *you* like a complete stranger translating your very personal details into French? If a family member is translating – have they fully understood the health care terminlogy and explanation given by the nurse? If your physical malaise had any sexual or self esteem effects, would you wish someone of the opposite sex or two generations younger to be involved? Perhaps the important point here is *sensitivity and empathy towards a clearer understanding of the ethnic older person's needs*. The following case study, based on the author's own experience, gives an example of the practical issues raised.

Case Study

In the mid 1980s I was a Sister on an acute admission and assessment ward in the older person's care unit. Mr A, an Asian man, was admitted. He spoke little or no English and so any questions had to be asked through his 14-year-old grandson. The only real problem this raised for me was the fact that his grandson could not be there 24 hours per day. I was very concerned that the man may feel isolated, lonely and probably very frightened. For him it must have been very traumatic – in unfamiliar surroundings, unsure what was happening to him. Beyond these very personal issues I was also placed in a dilemma with regard to even simple routine tasks. Despite being a very large inner city hospital, the catering service could not cope and provide Mr A's meals. Consequently he had food brought in. However, another man, Mr B, was Polish. Communication within the Polish community was tremendous. A rota was set up and every day at every meal, traditional food prepared according to his beliefs was brought in and thoroughly enjoyed. Unfortunately, for both Mr A. and Mr B., there had recently been a change in the hospital policy regarding food, and the reheating of food brought in from outside the hospital was no longer allowed. How does a nurse meet the cultural needs of a client in these circumstances? What would be your professional responsibility today?

Thus, *obtaining access to the services* must be one of the nurse's key responsibilities for black older people in their care. In the community it is often reported that the GP acts as 'gate-keeper' to the district nursing service, yet while black older people are just as likely to require this service, there is less GP referral – see for example Cameron *et al.* (1989) To make things more complex, cultural gerontological studies suggest that disease patterns of ethnic minority people must be viewed in relation to their social economic position. Bowling *et al.* (1992) state 'These results raise the question of what is "real" need as opposed to "perceived" or "reported" need.' I would like to suggest that if a need has been identified by a client then regardless of whether it is 'real', 'perceived' or 'reported', it is the nurse's responsibility to help determine the cause because it is disabling to the person as long as the 'need' – as described by the client – is present.

As a nurse, we have a responsibility to *limit our preconceptions*. One of the many sweeping generalizations concerning black older people and their care is the classic belief that they are 'cared for by their own'. This is refuted by Fennell *et al.* (1988), Patel (1990) and many others. This misbelief masks the actual situation where perhaps an older person is housed by their family but not looked after and so their isolation is magnified in reality. This may further distance the black older person from access to help. The nurse cannot blindly assume that a visible family is a family who can and are providing practical help. A large home was opened in the early 1990s in Birmingham, specifically for oriental older people. It would be interesting to know why the project was initiated. Speculation throws up many issues. Was it because needs were not being met, or cultures respected? Or was it because as people age they wish to mix socially with those whom they feel they can identify more closely? Perhaps it was because it is Eastern culture to house people at a certain age in a certain way, that is a 'cultural norm'? There may of course be many other reasons and, whatever it was, we can only find out by asking.

The nurse's responsibility lies in *empowerment of the older non-white Anglo-Saxon citizen* in need of his or her caring skills. This is a skill to be learned and brought about by education, practice and experience. Until nurses empower their clients and allow them to identify their needs – regardless of skin colour, race, ethnic group, gender or age – the caring cannot be client focused but is merely service determined. If nurses themselves are not aware of their own racial or ethnic or cultural biases then they can only provide a less than adequate service to older people requiring their very special nursing care skills.

In summary the nurse's responsibilities in caring for any older citizens are:

■ *To establish a good professional relationship which is reciprocal in nature and sensitive to cultural norms and beliefs.*

- *Care must be none other than person focused, acknowledging the social network and structure in which the client exists.*
- *To keep all access to services open and an open mind to the nature of services required. Be self aware and recognize personal bias and prejudices.*
- *To scrutinize stereotypes and myths concerning older people and ethnic minorities closely – many have no foundation in reality.*
- *Most important of all, to empower each individual person. If empowerment is achieved fully, the other responsibilities will have already been met.*

The need for good communication cannot be over emphasized. The studies carried out in Coventry, Nottingham and Birmingham and described by Fennell *et al.* (1988; p.125) all show that older people in Great Britain of Asian or Afro-Caribbean origin would like more Day Centres. This is interesting because since these studies in the 1980s, and maybe as a result of these studies, more Day Centres have opened which target particular communities.

Case Study: The successful day centre?

In Birmingham, I have contact with one such social service day centre. It is situated in a densely populated multicultural inner city area. Its remit is to target all the local population of older people. Partly to encourage Asian older people to come, the centre manager himself is Asian. The centre is run such that different groups are targeted on different days. Wednesdays at the centre see older Asian women with mental ill health. Tuesdays are attended by older Asian men. A centre minibus collects those who cannot be brought and discussions, games, and activities (including Asian cooking) are well organized. The cook comes in and makes wonderful Asian menus. This all seems positive, successful and idyllic. However, in reality there is little integration of different cultures, and although they have agreed to come, when the bus turns up to collect some older people they may refuse to come because it is a religious feast or whatever. The point is the older people themselves seem unable to communicate this to the centre manager, even though he himself is Asian. This often infuriates the manager. How can these difficulties be circumvented?

The Ageing Client and Race – Summary

All people are unique in their belief systems because of their race, culture, life experiences and personal make up. As a nurse trying to meet the needs of ethnic older people requiring her/his care, it is therefore imperative to consult each individual in order to assess, determine and offer an appropriate plan of nursing care. Without consultation, such care is impossible. These needs may be easier to meet where the proportion of ethnic minority groups in any geographical location is greater. Nurses need to be sensitive to racial beliefs, for example where gender, of either the client or nurse, may become an issue.

The fact that immigration is no longer encouraged, but almost discouraged, means that the long-term trends will not continue as in previous years for which there are clear records. Thus, past experience may not always be relevant to present-day issues. To a certain extent, future numbers and percentages will be unpredictable so long-term service plans will be limited. With a minority, yet still significant, portion of ethnic older people in the foreseeable future, the nurse will be obliged to take on the role of informal advocate more frequently. The purpose of this will be to obtain the necessary services for her/his clients, particularly in areas where the population numbers of black older people are very low. The current national changes in social and health care policies will influence both the services that are available and affordable, and the abilities of nurses to meet the needs of ethnic older people. Nurses have a wider professional responsibility to make themselves aware of these changes and to consider the implications of them for their practice. Nurse are accountable and therefore have very specific responsibilities in relation to their professional practice when caring for this particular client group.

Finally, *open and honest communication that flows in both directions* is the key to achieving a high standard of professional competence and practice.

GENDER

In Britain today, do we view older people the same as younger people or do we consider them differently? Do we think of older men in the same way that we think of older women? Are the same services and opportunities available to older women that are available to older men? Should the services be exactly equal anyway? – is this fair?

In order to begin to look at some of the answers to these questions, and many more, it is intended that the information shall be presented logically, progressively and, hopefully, without a bias, favourable or otherwise towards females or males. It is not the purpose of this section to explore women's issues, but to provide a description of what is known and then perhaps raise relevant questions. This section looks initially at the images and stereotypes associated with ageing, particularly those that are gender specific. Relevant demographic statistics and trends are then described. Following this, there is a more detailed exploration of the social, health and psychosocial aspects regarding age and gender. Finally, all aspects are drawn together to try and draw some kind of 'mind-sketch' to illustrate the present situation and factors that should be considered.

The Images and Stereotypes Associated with Age and Gender Issues

Think back to when you first started to read this section on gender issues. Think about the pictures that began to appear in your mind – perhaps it was pictures of older people that you know or have come across in your life to date, but more likely it was a picture of no-one in particular, more a model or representative of what you were reading about. It is to this model or representative that I draw your attention. This picture will be the final outcome of your life experience to date. It will be drawn from years of information gathering from many experiences – family attitudes, friends' comments, social role models from school teachers to members of parliament among many other influences. Probably the most important and most influential of all these today is the effect of the media. While this includes the effects of books, radio, advertisements, newspapers and magazines, the most powerful of these is the influence of television. It is the myths and stereotypes that assist in labelling and thereby produce a popular image that evoke a negative or positive attitude in the voyeur. The initial impact and result of this stereotyping and imagery may be either beneficial or deleterious.

What is the Present-day Image of the Older Woman and the Older Man?

It is generally considered that all older people are alike. They are perceived to be one homogenous mass. In Britain today, 'they' are commonly thought to be a burden. Other stereotypical reviews include the following:

- *They are generally perceived to be in poor health and draining the limited employment, health and welfare services. It is often said in casual conversation that paid employment should belong to the younger population because they still have their life to lead.*
- *Older women are thought to be more emotional than men. They cry at funerals, they cry at weddings, they get upset if family do not visit or meet their 'great expectations'.*
- *They are not interested in, yet alone capable of, an active sex life. People do not like to think that their parents are still having an intimate, personal and active sexual relationship, simply because they are too old / lost their marital partner / have arthritis, or some other excuse.*
- *Retirement for a man who has worked all his life will provide a major source of problems.*
- *Media portrayals suggest that older men are far less tolerant – consider the popular character of Victor Meldrew in 'One Foot in the Grave' (BBC, 1993).*
- *Similarly, older women are seen to be physically large and powerful characters who dominate the whole family infrastructure, for example the ageing Pauline Fowler as her role replaces that of her dead mother Lou Beale in 'EastEnders' (BBC, 1993).*
- *Older women are most at risk of crime and violence.*
- *Women use their age and frailties to their advantage, for example to jump queues and ensure they have the last seat on the bus. They cry poverty to get things cheaper such as holidays; bus-passes; cinema tickets. They also use these failings to get family to visit, even move house and care for them.*

We can pick up a thread running through many of these 'images', and that is the negative adjectives and nouns ascribed to each characteristic, for example burden; problems; intolerant; dominate; frailties; and poverty.

Does life come from the images, or, images from the perceived view of life? This philosophical discussion is not for elaboration or debate here, save to note that people form impressions by drawing on a range of evidence available to them. Images and stereotypes of ageing are drawn from observation – of a person's age, their gender, their skin colour, their clothing. These things form a major first impression and lead to a range of assumptions. Observation is also made of social behaviour from, towards and about issues that concern a particular person. This may be what is actually said to or concerning the individual, or how the words are actually spoken. These observations may reinforce and/or change the original observation. A final important aspect is the unique judgement of the individual person who is carrying out the observation.

Thus, the fears and fantasies of gender-related attitudes are filtered through the social structures (Stevenson, 1989). A very clear example of this is society's attitude towards attractiveness and sex already mentioned earlier. Attractiveness in women is more closely associated with youth, and sex is similarly related to attractiveness. An older man can be considered attractive regardless of a few grey hairs – in fact this becomes a positive attribute since he looks 'distinguished' – or a small increase in weight. On the other hand, in order to remain attractive a woman must not gain weight, wrinkles or change hair colour. This message is woven into the fabric of society in that it is deemed acceptable for older men to marry younger women but the reverse is totally abhorrent.

Another example is how social policy places the 'burden' of family care quite clearly on to women. The role of informal carer clearly affects economic comfort and security, particularly since domestic tasks are not finanacially remunerated. It has to be remembered here that many carers of older people are in fact older people themselves, since the group 'older people' spans such a range of years. As Stevenson also notes, the social world of older people is deemed to be 'abnormal' with male residents in homes being 'spoilt' since their domestic dependence is deemed to be acceptable. Again, the choice of negative adjectives reinforces the stereotype. In reality, all situations are unique and therefore there is no such thing as abnormal in the truest sense of the word.

It is important to recognize that subsequent cohorts of older people will provide a constantly changing picture of previous life experiences. Further to that, each cohort will not be homogeneous, although some similarities may exist within the group experience, each individual will perceive this experience differently and thus make unique choices that will ensure a totally different life history for each person.

Statistics and Trends

The average life expectation on birth in 1985 was 71.5 years for males and 77.4 years for females. This compares with an expectation of 48 and 51.6 years respectively around the turn of the century (Victor, 1991; p.53). Clearly, life expectation of women is greater than for men. This characteristic is linked with mortality differences associated with gender differences which noticeably follow two main trends. These are:

■ *For people over the age of 65, with an increase in age, so too an increase in mortality is also recorded.*

- *In each category, this increase in mortality rate is greater in men than women.*

Compare:

> **At age 65–74**
> **Males = 41.2 per 1000**
> **Females = 22.8 per 1000**

with

> **At age 75–84**
> **Males = 96.3 per 1000**
> **Females = 60.1 per 1000**

and

> **At age 85+**
> **Males = 191.5 per 1000**
> **Females = 158.6 per 1000**
> **(modified from Victor, 1991; p. 45)**

These trends can be seen more clearly in Fig. 5.2.

There is an on-going debate in the literature attempting to explain these gender differences in rates of mortality. Essentially, they are based on three themes that focus around two main hypotheses. Some suggest the differences are linked with biological causes, for example that the female chromosomal make-up is XX while the male comprises of one X and

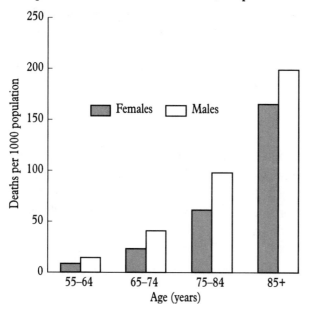

Fig. 5.2 *Death rate/1000 for females and males by age in England in 1989. Data source OPCS (1990)*

one Y chromosome. It is suggested that the female is afforded greater protection from genetic disease on the recessive genes because of this double-X factor. The second theme concerns social dimensions linking an increase in mortality with such things as the more physically dangerous and aggressive leisure activities of men such as rugby or 'bunji-jumping' as well as less healthy social habits such as smoking. The third theme suggests that both the previous themes have an effect but at different times in a person's life.

Regardless of cause, the overall situation that presents itself is that approximately two-thirds of the older population is female and one-third male. The proportion of males to females changes and the difference is greater as age increases from 65 years to 90 years and over.

Compare:

> *At age 65–69*
> *Males = 1155 000 in 1983*
> *Females = 1413 000 in 1983*

with

> *At age 85 and over*
> *Males = 148 000 in 1983*
> *Females = 489 000 in 1983*
> **(modified from Wells and Freer, 1988; p.100)**

Move recent figures and their corresponding ratios are shown in Fig. 5.3.

In short, the population over the age of retirement in Great Britain today is largely a

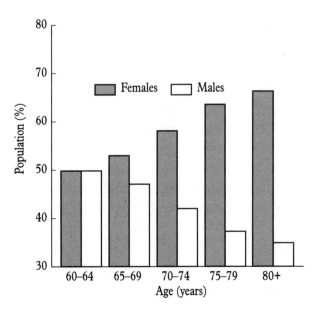

Fig. 5.3 *Changes in population gender composition by age in Britain in 1988. Data source, ACIOG (1992)*

female population. However, the number of males is large enough to take account of them as a significant minority. To ignore older males would be ignoring one third of the total older population and this would be wholly inappropriate.

Status – Independence versus Dependence

A person's social status may be considered in two different ways. The first is personal, relating to marital status and family life. The second is more public and concerns the status afforded to a person because of their position in paid employment. The former could be argued to be less valuable in the eyes of society since people do not – currently at least – get paid for being married or not married; for having a certain amount of children or not having children. Alternatively, it could also be argued that the political and social economy is heavily biased towards supporting those who come together as a couple to form and support a 'traditional' family unit. This is evidenced by, for example, single people having to pay supplements to have a hotel room to themselves when booking a holiday; or 'family' tickets at the theatre or leisure facilities providing a discount. These regulations in themselves ensure a dependence for one person upon another person. How does all this affect older people?

Already it has been noted that the increase in longevity is greater for women than for men. This has not altered despite a general increase in the population numbers as a whole (Bond and Coleman, 1990). It has also been noted that in the older population as a whole there are more women than men. The different effects of these trends are quite markedly different for both men and women. In 1990, the following percentages were recorded:

	Males	Females
Married	73	38
Widowed	17	49
Divorced/separated	3	3
Single	7	10

(taken from Arber and Ginn, 1991; p.13)

In turn, this means that older women live alone or have the potential to live alone more than older men. This in itself is a morphous situation that changes with times and attitudes. At present, the numbers of older people living with others is currently falling. This is associated with a range of factors:

- *Parents are having fewer children. A major influence on this trend is that infant mortality has fallen rapidly with the advent of certain vaccines and the introduction of child immunization programmes. Also, the evolution of the Poor Laws throughout the nineteenth century led to the introduction of a modified state pension around the turn of the century. To a limited extent, this no longer meant that parents needed several sons in paid employment to provide financial assistance to support them in old age.*

- *Marriages were occurring at a younger age and more frequently, thus children were moving out of the parental home.*

- *There is an increase in geographical mobility as adult children move to areas where paid employment is available. Also, some older people choose to move away from urban dwellings towards coastal and rural areas for their retirement (Jones and Armitage, 1990). This, however, only affects around 10% of the population, older people preferring to remain in their lifelong family home.*

- *Employment opportunities for women have increased. Not only do women choose to go out to work more, there are facilities – albeit limited – to help support that choice. These facilities cover a range of measures from work-based creches to equal opportunities/ discrimination policies.*

- *There is an increase in availability of housing suitable for younger families.*

Each of these factors bring with them their own gender-associated issues. An increase in reliance on the state pension and less on offspring earnings, while encouraging independence from the family, increases dependence on the state. Furthermore, until recently the pension was closely linked with years of service in full-time paid employment. This applies to many of the current cohort of older people, when many women did not work at all, and the few who did tended to work part-time only. This immediately highlights a financial difference between older women and men. In fact 'Elderly women are substantially more likely to live in poverty than elderly men in… Britain' where poverty is defined as 'having an income at or below the level of eligibility for means-tested benefits' (Arber and Ginn, 1991; p. 79). When comparisons are made between personal income of older men and women aged either 65–74 or 75+, consistently the most affluent group are those men aged 65–74, while the least affluent group are women aged 65–74 (Arber and Ginn, 1991).

This leads to consideration of an alternative aspect to this issue. Retirement from full-time paid employment is in itself a major life event. Therefore, there must be adequate planning and preparation. The effects of a husband retiring will influence both partners. On the one hand, the male will be moving from his domain of a highly structured and formal 'work' environment where he was respected and valued for his skills and knowledge, to a less structured and less formal environment of more 'domestic' skills in which he may have little or no knowledge and experience. The wife, on the other hand, perceives the home to be her domain and will soon have an intruder in the form of the person who has paid for her food, clothing and shelter most of her life.

An increase in geographic mobility and employment of women means that there are less women available at home to provide care for parents and parents-in-law. These trends particularly challenge the concepts of traditional patterns of caring. Since the majority of older people are female, this may add further stress to an already intolerable situation. Consider a woman who has never gone out to work since having children and who makes her domain the domestic arena. This is in part by choice, but in part it is thrust upon her by the 'norms' of the society in which she lives. On reaching pensionable age, and losing her partner, she now turns to her daughter or daughter-in-law for help and support as she once helped her mother and mother-in-law. But that person is no longer available – she does not live close by and if she did, she is not at home during the daytime to help with shopping and washing and the other household chores that need attention. To ask for help is perceived to be the equivalent of asking for charity.

Despite changes in lifestyle that are occurring on a grand scale, it can be said that the present group of ageing and older women have experienced a very different life history and lifestyle to ageing and older men. Thus nurses cannot consider all older people as one homogeneous whole. There will be more women requiring their services. Their needs may not currently be being met adequately by the services on offer. Equally, older males may have some of their needs ignored and so too be at a disadvantage.

Health

In a broad context, there are clear links between housing, education and health status. The person who is less well educated and in low quality housing is more likely to suffer from ill health. Alternatively, the educated person in the higher social class is more likely to be in better health. This has clear implications for people over the age of retirement who will automatically be limited by their social status – house and pension in particular – at the point of retirement. Furthermore, unless these are index-linked, with time, they will devalue in relative terms and buying power, so further limiting their access to a healthy lifestyle.

From the individual's perspective, an older person's perceptions of their own biological and functional state of health may not marry with the objective measures of the same things. In other words, older people seem to be over-optimistic about their health status. Victor (1991, p.97) identifies three different perspectives that respondents use to define health. These are:

- *health as a state of positive fitness;*
- *health as a state of not being ill;*
- *health as being functionally active.*

She says that older people tend to describe health in terms of the third definition, relating it to their ability to maintain social contact and activities. So, although a 'healthy state' would historically infer and be directly related to the medical model, it clearly involves a social dimension. Added to this is a psychological dimension, demonstrated by the fact that older people tend to compare their health state with that of their acquaintainces of a similar age rather than with younger people who are nearer their physical peak. This may explain, in part, the discrepencies between perceptions and objective measures. However, overall, both women and men over the age of 65 seem to hold the same views about what constitutes health.

With regard to the perception of health status, women appear to be more pessimistic than men, for example while 44% of men aged 65+ rate their health as good, only 38% of women aged 65+ apply the same rating. Over the age of 80 years, there is little difference in perceptions of health status between the sexes. A more detailed description of the intricate nature of these trends can be found in Victor (1991). Women tend to report more symptoms than men, older women visiting their GP for symptom relief rather than a cure. A question of interest here is – does the present system of health care deal with the health needs of older women? The wealth of literature available on the subject tends to show that women ask more questions, but obtain less answers; they do not or cannot articulate the need to see a female GP; there is a dissatisfaction with GPs in the way they give and receive information – they lack a 'personal' approach and may have both an ageist and a sexist approach; and finally, prescriptions are handed out but older women are reluctant to take medication. This last trend not only raises the question of compliance but also the question of whether appropriate treatment is being offered to older people, and older women in particular?

Primary and Secondary Ageing

It is rarely acknowledged but of fundamental importance when considering an older person, that in the biological context changes are occurring on two fronts. These are called primary and secondary ageing and are outside the scope of this chapter. In essence, primary ageing is the changes taking place within the cells, systems, organs and whole body due to the passage of time and natural processes of chronological ageing. Secondary ageing concerns the effect of infection and disease processes that affect the biological status and functioning of the body. For further and more detailed information on primary and secondary ageing, see Whitebourne (1985).

Primary ageing is generally described for males and females together; however, it is bound to affect gender differences simply because there are anatomical and physiological differences between males and females. A typical example here is that until the age of 40 the blood level of oestrogen in females remains fairly constant. From around 40 to 60 there is a steady decline that then stabilizes. A 'knock-on' effect of this is that more calcium is released from the bones resulting in a higher incidence of osteoporosis in older women. Recently there has been a rapid increase in the use of hormone replacement therapy which is considered to help alleviate these and other symptoms caused by the menopause.

Concerning secondary ageing, scan any of the OPCS tables showing UK mortality rates and it is soon evident that while, for example, more women die of circulatory disorders and more men die of neoplasms, the main mortality trends within the sexes of the main cause of death remain the same. These observed statistics demonstrate gender differences in what an older person is likely to actually present with to her/his GP or doctor. For instance, 70% of all cancers occur in people over 75 years of age (Faithfull, 1993) and the commonest form of malignant disease in the West is primary lung cancer. However, while it is the most common cancer in men in England, breast cancer is the most common in women (DoH, 1993). Millions of pounds are currently being spent on breast screening programmes. In view of the discontent with GPs voiced by older women, this positive strategy would tend to conflict with the view that the health needs of older women are not being met.

Nurses must challenge the view of older women as sickly with inferior needs. They must also ensure an understanding of the process of primary ageing as distinct from secondary ageing. By improving nursing knowledge in these two main areas a more informed assessment and plan of care can help provide more appropriate treatment for older female and male clients.

Psychological Wellbeing

Psychological wellbeing is intrinsically linked with a person's sexuality. Social attitudes and expectations are important to the behaviour, including sexual activity, of the individual. Older people are often seen as asexual beings (Jones, 1993), and yet 'Sexual expression affirms the older woman's sense of herself as feminine, a sense undermined by the media and popular stereotypes' (Huyck 1977, in Bond and Coleman, 1990).

Women are only allowed one standard of attractiveness and beauty which rapidly declines as age increases. Ageing is said to be a thief. Not only that, ageing women are subject to negative stereotyping which includes the belief of a lowered interest in sex and thus obsolescence. The historical view is that ageing, for women at least, is a negative experience, and that because of the physical changes, the psychological and social factors are ignored.

In the case of widows, they do not have a confirmation of their femininity. It is only perceived to be legitimate in marriage. Without a partner they lose companionship; material support; a partner in a world that is orientated to couples; and their link in a society that is male dominated. The advantages to being an older woman with no male partner include a personal freedom, the potential for personal development, and the opportunity to build more relationships with peers.

For widowers, the potential loss is even greater. They now exist largely in the domestic environment which is often quite alien to them, especially if they have worked all of their life. Also, men are less likely, even less able, to build meaningful peer relationships. There are fewer widowers because of the decrease in longevity in men and because men generally marry younger women. The remarriage rate is less for women than men in all age groups, further increasing the numbers of lone older women.

Enjoying a lifelong relationship with a single partner gives immense satisfaction. Many older homosexuals have enjoyed such kinship – their relationships are often long-lasting, very strong and very supportive. The loss of a lifelong partner – heterosexual or homosexual – leads to pain and grief as well as organization or disorganization depending upon the involvement with each other's life. A lack of understanding of this on the part of the health care professional can easily lead to a deterioration in the mental health and wellbeing of the older person. A few years ago, one lesbian older person described on the radio how when her partner was in hospital she had to pretend to be the patient's sister for fear of non-acceptance by staff. I often remember this interview and as a result try to be more sensitive in meeting client's needs.

Depression itself covers a continuum from a low mood in the average person through moderate to severe states of depression and mental ill health (Lodge, 1988). The suicide rate increases with age, particularly in the age group 65–74. After this age, the rate for males increases while the female rate falls. In trying to explain these statistics, the role change for men upon retirement, and their involvement in friendships and networking, cannot be ruled out of the equation. For women, the friendships made throughout life persist to old age – they are more extensive and more meaningful. The female capacity for intensity and responsiveness is not only greater but brings an increased vulnerability. Death of loved ones in old age brings inaccessibility and stress but an increased capacity for new friendships perhaps means that women are better off. Men tend to rely on their wives for intimacy and their death leads to disruption. Men tend to be less intimate in their social relationships, the sharing of the activity being the focus. In contrast, the relationships of women tend to have an emotional intensity that incorporates a lot of self disclosure.

However, the picture overall is not quite so precise and distinct, studies that examine the different classes (described in Bond and Coleman, 1990) show that middle-class men and women form ties outside of the family through their different associations, such as shared activities and voluntary work. Often the nature of the relationship allows reciprocal visits. Working-class men form ties with similar groups, whereas working-class women only join clubs and groups upon bereavement or retirement. Furthermore, these links are more age-specific. Their family achievements and commitments remain a priority.

The nursing implications of psychological wellbeing are great. The focus of care has to start from the individual client and their own perceived needs. Society's beliefs and expectations about older men and women will have an influence on that person, as well as the sex of the person.

Case Study

To give a simple example, when I was a Ward Sister, one woman came in with a severe stroke. She did not die but took many months to recover sufficiently to be able to be discharged home. During her rehabilitation on the ward, she suffered many setbacks and it was not always clear that she would ever be discharged. Her husband visited every day and often came in the mornings to assist with her care and just be with her. As time passed, it became clear to ward staff that he had developed a close relationship with a family friend. Eventually the wife, requiring home services was discharged home. Many staff were upset by the husband's friendship, and yet, in all these very sad and traumatic months of worry and changes for him, where could he go for help? What kind of help did he need? The hospital services were sufficient only to meet the needs of the client, his wife. Were his anxieties ever shared and considered? This scenario raises many issues for wider discussion.

Communication skills must be carefully used to pick up and explore possible areas of a more hidden need. It is immoral to say 'What else do you expect at your age?' This is evasive of the real cause for concern and inappropriate.

The Ageing Client and Gender – Summary

The images of ageing men and ageing women differ. Perhaps as a consequence of this stereotyping the expectations of each also differ. Women live longer than men. Above pensionable age there is a higher proportion of women than men. More women reside in residential and nursing homes. Traditionally, the state pensions and benefits have been based on the life style of the male; that is, if a person is able to work full time for 40 years or more, and has paid their National Insurance contributions, then they qualify for a full pension. This places the current cohort of older women at a disadvantage, particularly since it was not until the 1960s and 1970s that women were encouraged to join the paid workforce. Older women, therefore, are more likely to live in poverty. In parallel to this, it is a myth that retirement from paid labour affects only the partner who is retiring – it affects both parties.

Concerning their physical health status, women seem to suffer more chronic illnesses, while men suffer more acute illnesses. The health services available are more sensitive to acute illnesses, at a disadvantage to older females.

The evidence suggests that ageing is less harmful psychologically to men than women; that is, ageing is less deleterious and may be even beneficial to men while the converse seems to be true for women. Age is more likely to bring extreme loneliness and depression for older females and nurses have a responsibility to be aware of this, particularly when assessing. When assessing older men, their responsibiltiy is to be aware that these clients may feel that they have no confidant and do not readily wish to share their anxieties. However, it is recognized that women do have a greater ability to network, and so improve their socialization, than men. Thus not only are the needs of older men and women different, they both have real needs that are currently not being met by the nursing and health care services.

CONCLUSIONS

There is a current dichotomy. At one end there is the structured dependence of old age whereby the older person, and in particular ageing women – since statistically there simply are more of them – do have greater expectations of their family, friends and society as a whole. On the other hand, society is moving largely towards accepting any older person as an equally valued and independent member of society. With this move towards independence there has to be a clear responsibility for self. As the two situations lie at opposite ends of one continuum, then there will be confusion while the changes are being made and many older people will fall into the grey area in the middle. In fact, this is likely to be the case for the foreseeable future as the process of change is political and therefore unlikely to be completed to its end point.

Inequalities in old age are a function of access to resources in earlier life (Bond and Coleman, 1990). The occupational status held prior to retirement influences the salary received, and this in turn affects the opportunity to save or invest for future reserves. The presence or absence of an occupational pension depends on employment status. In the past, the labour market has discriminated against women, ethnic minorities, older people and those with disabilities. While these issues are beginning to be addressed, for the present population of older people, the effects continue to have their effect. Older women are discriminated against because of their sex – a form of 'double jeopardy'. Older black people have largely unmet needs because of their race. Sadly, older women of ethnic minorities are not only disadvantaged because of their age and sex, but also because of their race too – a 'triple jeopardy'. The length of survival in retirement is a further disadvantage since resources diminish with advance in age. As women live longer, they are thus more deeply affected, and particularly black older women.

The bio-psycho-socio dimensions are heavily interwoven and cannot be seperated from each other. They are different for both men and women as well as for people of different races, and, to a different extent depending on each situation. The similarities between race and gender issues and older people are that every older client should be treated as a unique individual. Relevant and appropriate care cannot be offered unless the individual is consulted and two-way communication maintained throughout the caring process. In the new climate of needs-led services the nurse is in an ideal position to highlight the unmet needs of black older people, older women and men. Further than that, they have a professional responsibility to do so.

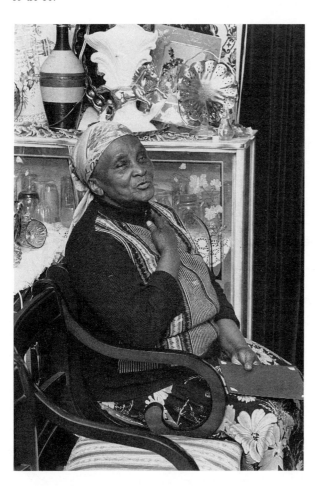

Fig. 5.4 The needs of the client are paramount in the health services of the future

Translation of paragraph on p. 108 (CRMF, 1995):

... there are many national organizations who are able to help in many different ways. It is often just a question of knowing how to find the right one for you. In this leaflet we list national groups which can provide you with information and advice as well as emotional and practical support. They all work alongside health service professionals, and offer help other than medical advice or treatment.

CLINICAL DISCUSSION POINTS

Identify ways in which you can find out more about the needs of the older people you work with.

Try and arrange a visit to a local day centre which caters for the needs of black and Asian older people. What kind of activities and services are on offer?

Discuss with a ward manager how homosexual relationships are accommodated (or not) within their care.

SUGGESTIONS FOR FURTHER READING

This chapter introduced the reader to various aspects of ageing. For a more detailed exploration of race-related issues and ageing, the reader is referred to *A 'Race' Against Time?* (Patel, 1990). The Age Concern conference proceedings *Recent Research on Services for Black and Minority Ethnic Elderly People* (Morton, 1993) is also recommended. For more information on gender-related issues and ageing, the reader is referred to such texts as Arber and Ginn (1991) *Gender and Later Life* and Bernard (1992) *Women Come of Age.*

The following are easy to read while providing valuable insight and further references for the interested student.

Arber, S. and Ginn, J. (1991). **Gender and Later Life.** Sage, London.

Patel, N. (1990). **A 'Race' Against Time?** The Runnymede Trust, London.

Squires, A. (Ed.) (1991). **Multicultural Health Care and Rehabilitation of Older People.** Edward Arnold and Age Concern, London.

REFERENCES

Age Concern Institute of Gerontology (ACIOG) (1992). **Life After 60. ACIOG,** Gerontology Data Service, London.

Arber, S. and Ginn, J. (1991). **Gender and Later Life** Sage, London.

Aslam, M. and Healy, M. (1986). Transcultural medicines: their impact on Western healthcare. **Pharmacy Update (September)**, 333.

Bond, J. and Coleman, P. (Eds) (1990). **Ageing in Society.** Sage, London.

Bowling, A., Farquhar, M. and Leaver, J. (1992). Jewish people and ageing: their emotional well-being, physical health status and use of services. **Nursing Practice 5** (4), 5–16.

Cameron, E., Badger, F. and Evers, H. (1989). District nursing, the disabled and the elderly: who are the black patients?. **Journal of Advanced Nursing 14**, 376.

Cancer Relief Macmillan Fund (CRMF) (1995). **Help is There.** Information leaflet, CRMF, London.

Department of Health (DoH) (1993). **The Health of the Nation. Key Area Handbook – Cancers.** HMSO London.

Doku, J. (1990). Approaches to cultural awareness. **Nursing Times 86** (39), 69–70.

Duncan, D. M. (1991). Communication. In: A. Squires (Ed.) **Multicultural Health Care and Rehabilitation of Older People.** Edward Arnold and Age Concern, London.

Faithfull, S. (1993). Age-related problems. **Nursing Times 89** (38), 66–68.

Fennell, G., Phillipson, C. and Evers, H. (1988). **The Sociology of Old Age.** Open University Press, Milton Keynes.

Fenton, S. (1991). Ethnic minority populations in the United Kingdom. In A. Squires (Ed.) **Multicultural Health Care and Rehabilitation of Older People.** Edward Arnold and Age Concern, London.

HMSO (1990). **Community Care in the Next Decade and Beyond.** HMSO, London.

Jones, C. and Armitage, R. (1990). Population change within area types: England and Wales, 1971–1988. **Population Trends Summer**, 25.

Jones, H. M. (1993). HIV mistreatment: Policy, resources and practice. **Senior Nurse 13** (6), 19–22.

Lodge, B. (with assistance from Grant, J.) (1988). Handbook of Mental Disorders in Old Age. In: **Mental Health Problems in Old Age, Pack P577.** Open University Press, Milton Keynes.

Mares, P., Henley, A. and Baxter, C. (1985). **Healthcare in Multicultural Britain** NECT and Health Education Council, Cambridge.

Morton, J. (1993). **Recent Research on Services for Black and Minority Ethnic Elderly People.** Age Concern Institue of Gerontology, London.

Norman, A. (1985). **Triple Jeopardy: Growing Old in a Second Homeland.** Centre for Policy on Ageing, London.

Office of Population Censuses and Surveys (OPCS) (1990). **Population Trends 61.** HMSO, London.

OPCS (1993). **1991 Census. Ethnic Group and Country of Birth. Great Britain,** Volume 1 of 2. HMSO, London.

Patel, N. (1990). **A 'Race' Against Time?** The Runnymede Trust, London.

Phillipson, C. (1988). **Planning for Community Care: Facts and Fallacies in the Griffiths Report.** Working Paper No.1, University of Keele.

Stevenson, O. (1989). **Age and Vulnerability.** Age Concern, London.

Victor, C. R. (1991). **Health and Health Care in Later Life.** Open University Press, Milton Keynes.

Wells, N. and Freer, C. (1988). **The Ageing Population.** Macmillan, Hampshire.

Whitebourne, S. K. (1985). **The Ageing Body.** Springer, New York.

Chapter Six

Loss and Bereavement
in Later Life

Margaret Foulkes

Core Themes in Gerontological Nursing

Ageing Matters	*New Social World*	*Lifespan Perspective*	*Health and Old People*
Illness and Dependency	*Quality Nursing Care*	*Therapeutic Intervention*	*Politicizing Gerontological Nursing*

Key Words

Grief Reaction • Emotional Needs • Cultural Needs • Relationships • Counselling

INTRODUCTION

Bereavement is normally associated with the death of a significant person, such as a close relative or friend, or perhaps even a much loved pet, but in fact it occurs in any state of loss. *Chambers's Dictionary* defines bereavement as 'to rob of anything valued; to deprive by death of some dear friend or relative; to snatch away'. With loss and bereavement come a grief reaction which, when understood, can be identified and responded to.

This Chapter aims to:

Consider some of the major losses in later life

Consider older people's reactions to losses

Examine the professionals' role in identifying the problem and helping clients come to terms with the loss.

LOSSES

Losses of one kind or another occur with increasing frequency as we get older. Friends and relatives die; children move away; diminishing mobility makes it difficult to maintain contact with previous interests; and other physical functions such as sight and hearing become impaired. Homes and familiar neighbourhoods are often left behind as older people move to be with family or move into more suitable types of accommodation or residential care. The emotional and social problems related to our complex modern society also create greater vulnerability for older people, who often feel that the security and familiarity of their youth has been lost. Consider some of the implications of the following losses for older people:

- *loss of physical health;*
- *loss of mental health;*
- *loss of friends/relatives/neighbours;*
- *loss of role (work; husband/wife; mother/father; etc.);*
- *loss of income;*
- *loss of home;*
- *loss of pets;*
- *loss of independence, status, security, familiarity, trust/emotional losses;*
- *loss of life;*
- *loss of spouse.*

The list can be endless and, when thought out in detail, many examples can be given. The older father of one nurse moved a distance to live with his daughter and kept asking for his local daily paper, which he had read for the past 50 years. Small losses can be as devastating as some major ones. Loss of a pet through death or when moving home or entering hospital can be a major concern. It is important to consider general loss with older people because the multiplicity of loss in later life may complicate the grief process when a significant death occurs. For example, when a spouse or carer dies, the bereaved person may need to move into some form of residential or hospital care because they were completely dependent on the other person and are unable to cope alone. Although many of these losses are unavoidable, the effects can sometimes be minimized by preparation and some losses in later life could be helped by education and changes in attitude to the ageing process.

Any kind of loss, and bereavement in particular, brings with it a grief reaction, which is often not recognized with general loss. This is dealt with later in the chapter, in relation to bereavement, but it is also important to remember the reactions of grief in relation to loss of health, loss of a part or function of the body (mastectomy, sight, hearing) and loss of home environment, when a patient is admitted to hospital.

Consider the losses that occur on admission to hospital or any form of residential care. These may include:

- *loss of privacy;*
- *loss of dignity;*
- *loss of control/self determination;*
- *loss of home;*
- *loss of family/friends/neighbours;*
- *loss of role/status;*
- *loss of familiarity;*
- *loss of pets;*
- *loss of independence/choice.*

Loss of Life

In the twentieth century, there has been a major shift in patterns of disease and treatment. Today, the leading causes of death are chronic diseases such as heart disease and cancer rather than acute infections. Many of the childhood infectious diseases have been eliminated and with improved standards of housing, nutrition and sanitation, there has been a great reduction in infant and childhood mortality. There is also a deep-rooted belief in society that medical technology can eradicate most disease and thus illness and disease are increasingly seen as the prerogatives of older people. This has implications for nurses and other caring professions, where young people starting on their career have not been exposed to death and dying. They also encounter curative orientated care and are less likely to be trained in effective nursing models of comfort oriented care.

Approximately 60% of deaths take place in hospital, 30% at home and 10% in other places, including nursing homes and hospices. Thus, care of the dying patient may be provided in a variety of settings. Parkes (1978) and Hinton (1979) compared the care of dying patients in hospital, at home and in a hospice. It was found that hospices were able to provide better symptom control, emotional care and meet the needs of relatives and carers more effectively. The work of the hospice movement, pioneered by Dame Cicely Saunders in the 1960s, and the subsequent setting up of the MacMillan nursing service in the 1970s, has greatly improved the care of dying patients in all settings. More recent studies (Hockley, 1983; Parkes and Parkes, 1984) have pointed out that although symptom control in hospital and home is improving, there is still a need to improve the emotional care for patients and relatives in these settings. Many families wish to nurse their loved ones at home, but fear and anxiety levels can remain high if adequate emotional support is not extended to relatives and carers. In some areas, carers groups have been formed, especially where long-term support is needed (e.g. Alzheimer's, stroke, MS, etc.).

Emotional Needs

For many people, death is still a taboo subject in Western society. Prior to the twentieth century, it was part of everyday life, usually experienced within the family and often within the wider community. In recent years, Aries (1983) has stated, we have 'removed death from society, eliminated its character of public ceremony, and made it a private act'. It can very often be a lonely event, as illustrated in Fig. 6.1.

This is a simplified diagram which illustrates how a person's view of the world may change during a terminal illness. Not all people will respond in this way, but many patients and also their relatives can find their world diminishing and contacts depleted when there is a long illness and particularly in later life where other losses are also involved. Compare this with Fig. 6.4 – rebuilding the world.

All of us live with the potential for death. There is a 100% chance that we will all face it one day, but many people plan their lives without any thought of death. Then, suddenly, when faced with a 'crisis of the knowledge of death', life is changed and it is essential to deal with this crisis appropriately and help the patient come to terms with the knowledge. There are still arguments revolving around telling or not telling a patient the bad news, but the issue is far wider than this. There are many levels of communication between people, and many degrees of awareness. There can be much denial or complete openness, but the most important issue is that there should be opportunity, availability and possibility for open communication. The dying person and their relatives should feel comfortable and secure in discussing what they want to discuss. This can present problems for the nurse, who must also feel comfortable in this type of emotional communication, so that the messages are not confused, ambiguous or contradictory.

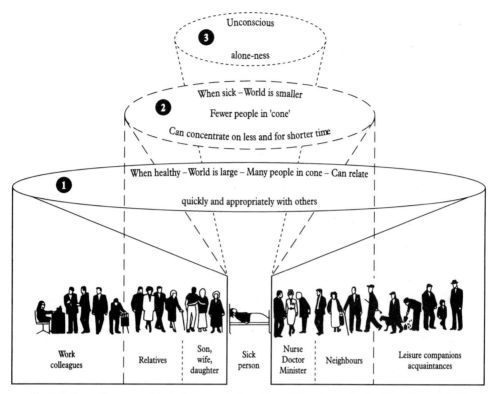

Fig. 6.1 *Cones of awareness. How the dying person's view of the world may change. Reprinted from Ainsworth-Smith and Speck (1982), with permission*

Many writers have argued that death is less of a problem for older people. Studies have shown that older people think and talk more about death than younger age groups (Cameron *et al.*, 1973; Kalish and Reynolds, 1976). Most speak about it calmly and with little fear. This has been linked with disengagement theory (Cumming and Henry, 1961), where the sense of loss diminishes as attachments diminish in later life and the individual and society prepare in advance for the final disengagement of death. A strong religious faith may also reduce fear of death. However, there are many individuals who are very involved in their lives and are anxious about giving life up or leaving loved ones. Sadly, many professionals have taken the view that older people are more accepting of loss of life and have failed to recognize the emotional needs of older people as they face death and also, those of their bereaved spouse, who may need considerable help in coming to terms with the changes that particular loss brings.

Kubler-Ross' (1970) study identified the sort of feelings that a dying person may experience. Her work has much in common with that of Parkes (1972) on bereavement, because it deals with the grief reaction to loss of life. The dying person will experience loss of family, home, and all the other losses which have been mentioned and a period of mourning can occur.

Case Study: Reactions to loss and impending loss	
The stages of dying (Kubler-Ross)	*The phases of mourning (Parkes)*
Denial	*Shock, numbness, disbelief*
Anger	*Feelings – anger, guilt, protest and resentment*
Bargaining	*Yearning, pining, searching*
Depression	*Disorganization, despair*
Acceptance	*Recovery, reorganization*

These stages must not be interpreted too literally, as all patients and bereaved people react differently, but they are useful as a guideline to some very common types of reaction.

Meeting these emotional needs presents a considerable challenge to the nurse. It is a time of great emotional strain and anxiety for all involved. Feelings of inadequacy may lead to avoidance of the situation. Therefore, it is important to assess where the patient is at, their awareness and the possible reactions (as indicated in the Case Study). A knowledge of the situation and understanding of the reactions will help staff deal with the situation. Having the time, space and privacy to communicate with patients and their relatives will help them express their feelings and voice fears and anxieties. These can often be dealt with by listening and helping the patient achieve simple, realistic goals. Valuing the person as an individual and acknowledging their specific fears can alleviate much emotional pain. Finally, perhaps the most important area is teamwork when dealing with dying patients because staff need support and opportunity to talk about some of the distressing personal experiences (see section on the needs of staff).

Social Needs

On admission to hospital, many patients are particularly distressed because of social problems such as finance, housing, benefits, family problems or perhaps being alone, with no-one to deal with everyday tasks. Some older people will be concerned about rent, bills, council tax, or who will care for their spouse or their pet. Claiming benefits to which they are entitled needs to be approached with sensitivity as many still find this a problem area. Reassuring them that the Attendance Allowance is not means-tested and they are entitled to claim, sometimes needs time and patience. The new claim for Attendance Allowance under the Special Rules, where a person is terminally ill, can be received within 2 weeks and is dated from the day the claim is received at the DSS office.

The social worker needs to be alerted if the person has been living alone and has no-one to deal with practical matters. If a patient has few or no visitors, they may need a little extra consideration. Do they need some personal items bringing in? Those with relatives may also have problems. In our complex society, with divorce and remarriage, or families living at a distance, the variety in relationships can be complicated. On occasions, the nurse may be involved in trying to balance the needs of the patient and the needs of various members of the family.

> ### Case Study: Recognising family stress
>
> *Mr A was in the hospice for terminal care. His first wife had died 20 years previously and his daughter had cared for him until 3 years ago. He had gone on holiday alone and met a woman, whom he had married on return from holiday. She had grown-up daughters, with whom she had a very close relationship. Mr A's daughter felt excluded, but coped until her father became very ill. Now she wanted to spend time with him alone, but found that her stepmother and family were always at the bedside. A nurse quickly became aware of the problem and alerted the social worker, who discussed the situation with the daughter and the stepmother. They both realized the needs of the other, though found it impossible to discuss it together. They agreed to separate visiting times, but on the day of Mr A's death, they sat together, each holding one hand.*

Families often need as much or more support than the patient and this can be time-consuming. However, if it is recognized and dealt with as soon as possible, it can alleviate much anxiety and distress for all concerned. Often small practical details, such as visiting arrangements, what can be brought in for patients, or what is available in the community can help relatives make decisions or organize their time more effectively.

Cultural Needs

In our multiracial society, it is important to consider patients' individual cultural, ethnic and spiritual needs. The nurse will need to identify any specific beliefs, wishes or traditions that are important to a patient. It is essential to listen to the wishes expressed by a patient and their family and also to give patients the opportunity to express their needs. Even patients who show no specific interest in any formal belief may wish to talk to someone about life and death. It is often the nurse to whom they turn, especially at quiet times when visitors have gone and they have time to think. For most staff, it is not possible to discuss these issues in depth, but a basic understanding of different beliefs and traditions can help staff communicate with their patients and respond to their anxieties. On many occasions, just to ask a patient to explain their culture or beliefs can be helpful in resolving a difficulty. The fact that someone has cared enough to listen is the first step. Basic information on a variety of ethnic groups should be available for nurses to consult – see the further reading list.

Facing death is also a time that can awaken past difficulties or old feelings of loss or anxiety about family or cultural heritage. In both death and bereavement, ethnicity is significant in many ways. Luborsky and Rubinstein (1990) have identified four ways in which ethnicity is significant to bereavement life reorganization, but which is also true for the dying patient.

Ethnicity:

- *provides a continuity in traditional values and practices;*
- *guides as to what to do in times of stress;*
- *gives a sense of rootedness in times of stress;*
- *draws on religion and family traditions. Often returning to reinvolvement with ways from earlier life.*

BEREAVEMENT

There are many losses in later life, but the one that stands out as the most disruptive and stressful is the death of a spouse. Other significant deaths will also be stressful, such as children, partner, close friend, relative or carer, depending on the nature of the relationship. Bowlby (1980) stated that the 'loss of a loved person is one of the most intensely painful experiences any human being can suffer. And not only is it painful to experience but it is also painful to witness, if only because we are so impotent to help'.

Why is it so Important to Look at Bereavement Today?

Death has become a taboo in our modern society. It is an embarrassment to people and is often something that is hidden behind closed doors. Almost gone are the days when everyone gathered in the parlour to pay their last respects; when all the community attended the funeral; and everyone talked about the person who had died. During the televising of the Gulf War, it was interesting to note the overt emotional grieving of the Arab world in contrast to the quiet, solemnity of public Western funerals (Fig. 6.2). There are several reasons why it is necessary to look at death and bereavement more carefully and bring the grieving process out into the open. Many bereaved people are unsupported in their grief for the following reasons:

- *silence and taboo surrounding death;*
- *many deaths occur in hospitals, nursing homes and residential homes, away from the community;*
- *the break-up of the extended family;*
- *lack of mourning ritual;*
- *fewer people attending funerals and being involved in the ceremonies;*
- *stiff upper lip and fear of expressing emotions openly;*
- *changes in modern society and medical technology;*
- *cultural differences and isolation from cultural traditions.*

With all these changes has come a denial of the painful grief that occurs with a bereavement and other losses. Society often fails to recognize the need to grieve, as can be seen in the

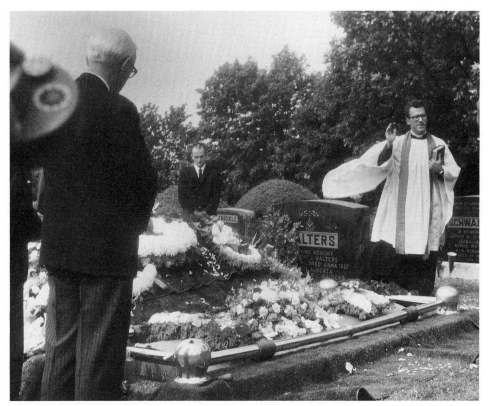

Fig. 6.2 *A traditional English funeral*

amount of compassionate leave allowed at such times and the fact that most people are expected to have got over their grief within a few days or weeks. Grief may be experienced less frequently in our modern society, but it is often experienced more intensely, because the emotional involvements are not diffused over an entire community or widely shared with others. Many cultures have had built in ritualistic conventions in the mourning period, which have been observed for hundreds of years, but some people have now relinquished these and serious problems in adjustment are being experienced. One example can be seen in Fig. 6.3. During the period from 2 to 12 months, all bereaved men also gather twice daily in the synagogue to pray together. This provides the support and self-help group, which professionals are now trying to set up as a form of modern therapy, but has been recognized for many centuries.

For many people, grieving will take its normal painful course, some may not grieve at all and for others, support will be needed. It is important to recognize that there are different ways of grieving, different lengths of time to readjust and different reactions to a similar loss. During a long illness, some older people may have experienced anticipatory grief and already worked through many of their feelings. In order to understand some of these differences, it is important to look at some of the theories surrounding relationships earlier in life.

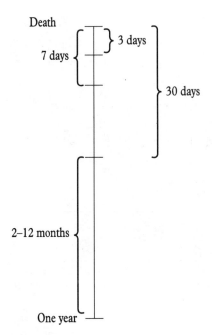

Fig. 6.3 *Jewish grieving schedule*

- 3 days – Deep grief
- Remainder of first 7 days – Condolences. Visitors listen and prepare food
- 30 days – Time of adjustment, when bereaved live restricted life
- 2–12 months – Period of remembrance and healing
- 1 year – Anniversary, Kaddish recited and memorial candle lit

Relationships

In order to experience loss, we need attachment. There are many theories why humans (and some animals) make strong emotional attachments with others. Bowlby's (1980) work on attachment is the third volume of a trilogy, which developed from his early work in 1951 on maternal deprivation. Bowlby believed that attachments come from the need for safety and security and that attachment behaviour is learnt from the time of birth. It is the goal of attachment behaviour to maintain the affectional bond and when this is endangered, very specific reactions occur. These reactions, as with children who cannot find their parent, are clinging, crying and anger. These reactions cease when the bond is restored, but when the bond cannot be restored, as in bereavement, the reactions may continue for some time.

Much work has also been done on adult pair bonds and how these grow and develop over time. There is mutual exploration, disclosure, acceptance and adaptation as couples share a life together, but also partners gain meaning and identity from each other in their lives. Thus, a woman may feel that her identity is very closely linked to her function as a mother or wife, and a man to his function as father, husband and provider. The image each person has, may be dependent on the other. The end of a relationship may involve not only the loss of intimacy and social interactions (both frustrating and rewarding), but also a loss of some meaning one partner gave to the other. With older people, they have usually spent a long time with a marital partner (or grown-up children or friend) and there is a comfortable relationship in which everyday interactions are regular and secure. Even in a difficult relationship, there is an element of security and familiarity and many couples may actually miss the arguments and bickering that characterize some relationships. In later life, paid work has ceased, socialization has often diminished and there is a focus on family life. Where there is ill health, there is a mutual dependence and a comfortable compromise might be reached where various tasks are redistributed and shared. This sharing can at times become exclusive and the outside world may be unaware of serious problems, until the stronger partner dies.

Case Study: Recognising the needs of dependent family members

Mr B was admitted to the hospice in the terminal stage of cancer. His wife had Alzheimer's disease and he had cared for her without any outside help. Even though Mr B had been seriously ill and struggled for many months, it was Mrs B who refused to have a home help, meals on wheels or to consider any form of residential care. When Mr B was admitted to the hospice their only son had to live in the house with his mother, as she was unable to care for herself. This caused strain within the son's family and eventually, following the death of Mr B, Mrs B was admitted to a nursing home. The grief, stress and guilt created many problems and considerable unhappiness for all involved, at a time of great emotional strain.

Relationships are characterized by many different needs that they meet. Weiss (1974) outlines a series of provisions or needs that are normally met in relationships:

- *attachment, which provides a sense of security and place;*
- *social integration and friendship. This is particularly important in our couple-orientated society;*
- *nurturing, which provides a sense of being needed and meeting needs;*
- *reassurance of worth;*
- *sense of reliable alliance in that the person provides dependable assistance and is always there;*
- *guidance. The person is always there at difficult or stressful times.*

Thus, relationships are made up of many interactions, which operate on different levels and with different intensity. They may not always be positive or rewarding, but even differences and frustrations may be valued, arousing and missed.

Many older couples have dependent or complimentary relationships. Specific roles are assigned over time such as gardener, driver, decorator, financial controller, holiday arranger, cook, washer-up, confidant, social host/ess, etc. Consider the following relationships and what each person provides for the other:

- *husband – wife (or partner);*
- *parent – child;*
- *friends and neighbours.*

When a death occurs, what other losses are involved?

The Process of Normal Grief

Simos (1979) compared grief to a physical illness stating that:

> *both may be self-limiting or require intervention by others. And in both, recovery can range from a complex return to the pre-existing state of health and wellbeing, to partial recovery, to improved growth and creativity, or both can inflict permanent damage, progressive decline and even death.*

Colin Murray Parkes, who has written extensively on bereavement in this country, speaks of grief as 'the only functional psychiatric disorder whose cause is known, whose features are distinctive and whose course is usually predictable' (Parkes, 1972).

One of the earliest attempts to look at grief in any systematic way was done by Erich Lindemann in 1944. A major tragedy occurred in Boston, USA, when a nightclub was burnt down and nearly 500 people were killed. Lindemann and his colleagues worked with the families who had been bereaved and discovered similar patterns of grief. He listed these as:

1 *somatic or bodily distress of some type;*
2 *preoccupation with the image of the deceased;*
3 *guilt relating to the deceased or circumstances of the death;*
4 *hostile reactions;*
5 *the inability to function as one had before the loss.*

Although there are limitations to this study, it does identify many reactions to grief that bereaved people experience. It is, however, the work by Parkes (1972) that has elaborated and further developed the concept of grief. Parkes (like Bowlby) suggests that bereavement constitutes a loss of security, which is perceived as threatening and which produces a state of stress and alarm. He suggests various stages which the bereaved person goes through until they finally begin to establish a modified identity and purpose. Unfortunately, sometimes these stages have been interpreted as distinct and in a specific order – that a person should progress from Stage 1 to Stage 4. If, however, these stages are seen as types of reaction to grief, which may occur at any time and in any order (or not at all), then they prove to have immense value in understanding some of the normal reactions to grief – see p. 140.

Shock, Numbness, Disbelief

Initially, a person may not be able to accept the death. The shock of the news can cause a temporary 'anaesthesia', which may last for several days, allowing the bereaved relatives and friends time to deal with the funeral and all the practical details.

Disbelief or denial can occur and the bereaved person may not be able to accept the death, believing that the person will return. This may be to avoid or delay the grief, but grieving needs to take place and it may be more severe or difficult to resolve, if not confronted at the time.

When this has worn off, the bereaved person begins to feel the 'pain' of grief. This can be an intense physical pain, which many have likened to the severing of a limb, being cut in half or mutilated. There is a great emptiness and life suddenly becomes meaningless. As one person expressed it, 'there was nothing, *nothing*, that made the future look anything but a dreary, meaningless trudge'. Thoughts of death and suicide are common because the world looks so bleak and there is a desire to join the deceased. This can be very frightening as most people have not experienced feelings like this before and may feel they are going mad.

Yearning, Pining and Searching

Many bereaved people have a preoccupation with thoughts of the deceased person. They scrutinize events to understand what has happened. They may need to repeat over and over again the events leading up to the death. It is as if the days, weeks or even minutes prior to the death are encapsulated in a time warp and every minute detail can be remembered. Looking for the deceased person may become a preoccupation, they may hear the voice, footsteps or noises connected with the person and even imagine they have seen them, or sense their presence. Dreams are often very vivid at this time and a particular event may recur in dreams. All this may be very frightening for the bereaved person and it is important to reassure them that these sort of events are quite normal.

This is also a time when the bereaved person may visit the grave regularly or may come back to the hospital. There is a need to return to the place where their loved one was last seen or to speak to people who shared those last days. Many bereaved people find it most helpful to see the GP, district nurse or staff in the hospital or hospice after the death. Sadly, many staff avoid these situations, sometimes from fear of anger or inability to cope with the emotions expressed, but for the majority of bereaved people it is one of the most helpful experiences for them.

Anger, Guilt, Protest and Resentment

These feelings occur at various times throughout the mourning period, but particularly after the numbness and denial have subsided and when the bereaved person is searching for an answer to the many questions of why did this happen... and *if only* I/they/anyone had done something differently. These feelings can sometimes be overwhelming and quite intense, and thus can be frightening and confusing.

Consider some of the situations in which people can feel anger and to whom it may be directed:

- *towards the person who has died;*
- *towards those believed responsible for the death;*
- *towards those who cared for the deceased;*
- *towards medical staff;*
- *towards relatives and friends;*
- *towards those who are not grieving;*
- *towards other couples/parents/children who have not suffered a loss;*
- *towards God, for allowing this;*
- *towards self, for not doing more.*

Anger is one of the most common reactions to bereavement and towards loss of life in dying patients and their relatives. The most difficult type of anger to resolve is where some blame may be attached, for example drunken driving. Where a court case or other legal action is involved, then resolution of grief may take much longer because the person will be unable to move forward until the hearing has taken place. It is important to be aware of these negative feelings because they are often directed at nursing staff or colleagues in other departments. Care must be taken not to be drawn into the criticisms or react angrily to personal attacks. Robert Buckman in his book, *I Don't Know What to Say*, gives some clear and useful guidelines in dealing with anger and other difficult situations.

When anger is turned inwards, it becomes guilt and many bereaved people feel that maybe they failed to do something. They may feel that the death could have been prevented if they had responded earlier. Maybe they could have got help sooner; encouraged a partner to see the doctor; not taken on some major work in the house; or not complained about various tasks. In marriages or relationships where there have been difficulties, the family might be confused because the bereaved person has such an intense grief reaction, often related to guilt.

Guilt

Case Study: Reactions in grief

Mr C was in his eighties and had always had a difficult and unhappy relationship with his wife. Mrs C was admitted to hospital and asked her daughter not to bring Mr C in to visit because she could not cope with the arguments. However, she deteriorated suddenly and died. Mr C was angry with his family for not taking him to the hospital and he started talking about all his wife's virtues, calling her, his `angel'. This alienated the family even further because they felt that he had not treated his wife properly during their marriage. Both children and husband were then unable to express and share their grief.

Another expression of guilt can be seen when a person is actually relieved by the death. Often, after a long illness and perhaps much suffering and pain, there can be relief that it is all over. If a relationship has been difficult, relief can be felt. However, this reaction can also bring with it guilt and feelings that there should be grieving. Guilt also occurs when a person has experienced intense grief and then starts to make a new life and actually has days when they are happy. Permission to stop grieving is as important as giving people permission to grieve.

The protest and resentment can be seen in other negative attitudes to situations that occur. One lady was angry because she was invited out for a meal and everyone was happy and laughing. Small incidents which would have been passed over before, now take on major proportions. Someone says the wrong thing or a mistake is made and the bereaved person may react quite out of character. This tension and resentment may cause friends and relatives to withdraw, just at the time when they are needed most.

Disorganization, Despair, Apathy, Depression

After the active anger and protest, it may appear that the bereaved person has given up the struggle to bring back the lost person. There is a restlessness, a search for activities to take up their time, but these remain unfinished. There is a lack of motivation or initiative and most commonly, a lack of concentration. Former hobbies, reading and television have lost their interest because the person cannot maintain their concentration for long periods. Things seem to go wrong, such as illness or accidents, and many normal everyday occurrences become magnified. Loss of confidence occurs and many bereaved people feel unable to cope alone or have dificulty even venturing out. They may feel cut-off from those around them and compound this by declining help or invitations out.

The bereaved older person may become very sad and lonely and this may be confused with depression. They may appear to withdraw from the world, which they see as hostile and changing. This is particularly true when a bereaved person is ill and has to enter hospital or perhaps permanent residential care. They no longer have a partner or soulmate to confide in. The work by Lowenthal and Haven (1968) shows clearly the importance of a 'confidant'. They studied 280 people, aged over 60 years, who were living in the community and found that a 'confidant' served as a buffer against loss. However, they found that having a 'confidant' was not a buffer against the psychological effects of physical illness. Many older people, of course, do suffer from illness or disability and this can be a particular difficulty when loss occurs.

It is important to comment on suicide at this point. Suicide rates rise steadily through life, with a noticeable rise between the ages of 65 and 74. With men, the figure continues to rise, but declines in women. Loss and depression were first linked together by Freud (1953) and it has been recognized that older people may take longer to get over their grief. There may be suicide attempts arising from clinically disturbed mental states or for other reasons, but for some older people, they may become stuck in their grief and unable to move on to recovery.

Physical reactions may also occur during the grief process and can be quite frightening:

- *sleep disturbances;*
- *nausea;*
- *difficulty digesting food;*
- *weight loss/gain;*
- *sighing;*
- *difficulty breathing;*
- *tightness in the throat;*
- *headaches;*
- *muscular aches and pains;*
- *rashes;*
- *dizziness;*
- *loss of energy;*
- *fatigue.*

Some bereaved people may experience similar physical problems to those associated with their loved one's illness.

Reorganization, Recovery, Redefining Roles

This is a time of restoration and readjustment, a letting go and relearning the world. There is a new identity, a new pattern of living, but also a renewed sense of hope integrated with memories of the past. New activities, interests, relationships gradually help the person regain their confidence and begin to enjoy life again. With this will come a realization that the past cannot be taken away but can actually be remembered without sadness and can be part of their total life. Recovery is not necessarily progressive and there will be 'minefields'. The bereaved person may feel fine one minute and then a memory will suddenly be reawakened and grief may return. Certain events and dates such as anniversaries, birthdays, holidays, Christmas and special times for that person, will cause renewed pain. However, eventually, new patterns of living will emerge after weeks, months and maybe years. Sometimes older people do not really seem to get over their grief and they have fewer opportunities to rebuild their lives, but most manage to cope with the loss to a greater or lesser extent. The question of when this becomes abnormal will be dealt with later in the section.

An alternative way of looking at the process of grief has been put forward by Worden (1983), who sees recovery being achieved via a series of four tasks. These tasks need to be worked through. The bereaved person is in control and must help themselves to adjust, although they may need some outside help to facilitate the process.

1. To Accept the Reality of the Loss　The person must accept that their loved one has died. For many people, it can take a long time before they can say the word 'dead' and euphemisms such as 'passed away', 'no longer here' or 'gone' are used regularly in our society.

2. To Experience the Pain of Grief Again, modern society does not encourage people to express their grief and many people are embarrassed by such expressions. Friends or outsiders say 'Don't cry' or 'You are upsetting yourself or others'. Grieving is as natural as eating when you are hungry or waving goodbye to a friend, it helps to heal the pain and crying is the most normal expression of this. It is hard to watch, but giving permission to cry and staying with the person is important for them.

3. To Adjust to an Environment in Which the Deceased is Missing Some of the other losses associated with relationships have been explored and it is during this task that the bereaved person becomes very much aware of all the roles the other person undertook. For older people, it is hard to begin to learn to cook, drive a car, change a plug or pay the bills. Often these are tasks which one partner preferred to do and the other partner may feel totally unable to take on. It also serves as a reminder of the loss.

Case Study: Other losses

Mrs D had never dealt with the household finances. When Mr D died, she was advised to open a bank account in her name and was given a cheque book. She was afraid of asking anything at the bank and only when she had no money and several bills were overdue, did someone realize she did not know how to write a cheque.

Mr E had been ill and unable to work for 20 years, but the one job he could do in the house was the washing-up. When he died, Mrs E found this the most difficult task because it was a constant reminder of her loss.

4. To Emotionally Relocate the Deceased and Move on With Life This is a difficult task because bereaved people may feel that they are being 'unfaithful' to their loved one. Some people feel that they can never love again and this restricts the new life that is opening up to them. It may not just be partners, but also friends or parents and children, who feel no-one can replace their lost love. Adult children may become very angry if their elderly parent becomes involved in another relationship and this can cause friction in families. Jealousies can be seen if new friends are made or new interests taken up and yet some changes are essential to build a new life. For some people, loss can mean gain and eventually their life might positively blossom with the new-found freedom and ability to engage in pursuits that were not considered previously.

This view of bereavement is useful because it gives a positive step by step guide to the movement of a bereaved person through the grieving process. However, it needs to be used in conjunction with Parkes' work because Parkes so clearly describes the feelings/reactions that bereaved people experience.

Finally, return to Fig. 6.1 and compare this with Fig. 6.4, which illustrates how an older person may have become isolated and withdrawn following the death of a spouse, especially if there has been a long terminal illness. They will, therefore, need considerable help in rebuilding their world.

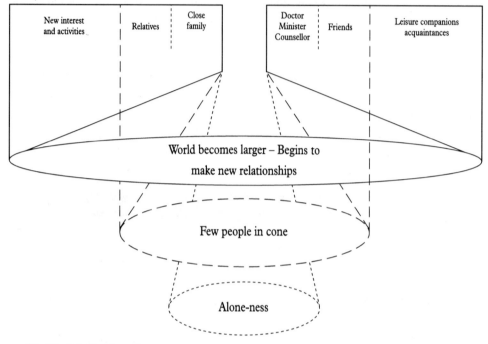

Fig. 6.4 *Rebuilding the world*

Factors that May Affect the Grieving Process

Each person will grieve in their own way and in their own time, but how long this takes and whether the person may need help or support during this time will be influenced by a number of factors (Fig. 6.5).

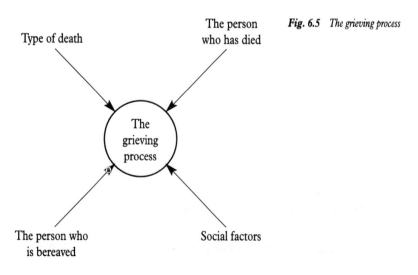

Fig. 6.5 *The grieving process*

The following are some of the factors that may create problems during the grieving process.

Type of Death:

- *sudden or unexpected;*
- *painful or horrifying;*
- *suicide or violent;*
- *preventable or avoidable;*
- *blame on survivor;*
- *not able to say goodbye;*
- *changed body image or personality prior to death;*
- *no body to bury.*

The Relationship with the Person who has Died:

- *dependency;*
- *closeness in relationship – perhaps to exclusion of others;*
- *guilt or ambivalence;*
- *age (very young or very old);*
- *last surviving relative/friend.*

The Person who is Bereaved:

- *guilt-prone personality or depressive;*
- *over-anxious or low self esteem;*
- *previous unresolved losses;*
- *physical disability or ill health;*
- *history of mental illness;*
- *unable to express feelings;*
- *angry or aggressive personality;*
- *loner or isolate;*
- *No time to grieve because of other responsibilities (e.g. dependent family).*

Social Factors:

- *financial problems;*
- *housing problems;*

- *family problems;*
- *unemployment/retirement/unhappy at work;*
- *lack of support – friends, community;*
- *family seen as unhelpful;*
- *other concurrent losses;*
- *detached from traditional culture or religious support system.*

Thus, the response to loss can vary in many ways, depending on the other circumstances involved. For a few people, the grief process can become complicated or unresolved and may lead to abnormal grief.

Abnormal Grief

Various types of abnormal grief have been identified. Lindemann (1944) felt that most pathological grief was caused by repressing thoughts and feelings surrounding the loss. Parkes (1990) identified three types of syndromes:

- *Unexpected grief syndrome, where profound, sudden shock caused high levels of anxiety. This has also been likened to post-traumatic stress disorder, seen in those involved with major tragedies such as Hillsborough and Zeebrugger.*
- *Ambivalent grief syndrome, where a negative or ambivalent relationship led to conflict in grief, for example relief mixed with guilt or denial and little grief, followed by anger, guilt and long-term pining.*
- *Chronic grief syndrome, characteristic of a clinging, dependent relationship. Grief remains acute and mention of the deceased is forbidden or a shrine is made. Queen Victoria was the perfect example and building a shrine, of course, was a common form of dealing with death in past centuries. The grief becomes abnormal, however, when the person's life is affected to such an extent that they cannot continue with normal activities or rebuild a new life.*

Worden (1983) identified four similar situations where abnormal grief may be indicated:

- *chronic grief;*
- *delayed grief;*
- *exaggerated grief;*
- *masked grief.*

These are self explanatory, but the masked grief is particularly important because often a bereaved person is unable to express their feelings overtly and the grief is manifested in some other way. This can often be a physical illness and it is important to recognize this at an early stage. In one hospice, it was recognized that a letter needed to be sent to the GP dealing with the next-of-kin, when a patient died, because the GP might not be aware of the bereavement and it would clarify some problems that might arise.

Finally, it should be reiterated that grief reactions vary greatly with each individual and as Parkes (1972) said, 'Some suffer lasting damage to their physical, mental, social and spiritual status. Some take bereavement in their stride, and others become more mature, effective and well-balanced than they were before they were bereaved'.

HELPING OLDER PEOPLE COPE WITH LOSS

Having identified those people who might be at risk following a bereavement or other major loss, how can they be helped and supported at this time? Do older people have different needs than younger people and how are these to be managed? The main area of work has focused on bereavement counselling and this is considered in detail, but initially the historical context of counselling needs to be considered and reassessed in the light of the specific needs of older people.

Counselling

The great psychologists of the late nineteenth and early twentieth centuries drew attention to the significance of early childhood experience and virtually ignored the development potential of the adult years. Freud (1905) stated that 'psychotherapy is not possible near or above the age of 50, the elasticity of the mental processes on which the treatment depends is as a rule lacking – old people are not educable'. Regrettably, this thinking had a great influence on psychotherapy and the British Psychoanalytic Society had, until the mid 1980s, refused to accept patients over the age of 40. Until recently, the Tavistock Clinic in London also rejected patients over the age of 40 as being unsuitable for dynamic psychotherapy. This influence can also be seen in the literature, where little has been written about psychotherapy or counselling with older people, before the 1970s.

During the mid-twentieth century, other theories began to emerge. Erikson's (1965) lifespan model shows a changing individual operating in a changing society. His stages of development go through to maturity and old age, thus allowing for change and development in later life. He also includes the social, cultural and historical determinants of personality development. This was further developed by Havighurst (1972), who moved from psychosocial tasks to developmental tasks, which arise throughout life. Havighurst brought to light some significant problems of later life, including ageing and attitudes towards death.

This work was taken further by King in 1974, when she published her notes on the psychoanalysis of older patients. King identified five areas of pressure or anxiety which arose during the second half of life and which led some individuals to seek help in later years:

- *Loss of sexual potency and the impact of this on relationships.*
- *Loss of work roles and inability to cope with retirement, including loss of identity and worth.*

- *Loss of children, as they moved away from home and the resulting change in marital relationships.*
- *Awareness of ageing. Loss of health and independence.*
- *Loss of life. Feelings of depression and deprivation at not achieving personal goals.*

Thus, the issues of loss were recognized in later life and the need for help in resolving these issues. Before looking at loss/bereavement counselling, it is important to consider the specific needs of older people and the nature of changes which occur with age and might affect any intervention:

- *Memory performance is often poorer in older people.*
- *Physical problems need to be considered as well as psychological problems.*
- *Individual differences are much wider in older age than in younger people. There is also a wide difference between young–old and old–old, as well as many cultural, social and economic differences.*
- *Older people are often more introspective and philosophical.*
- *Older people have usually established their own successful/unsuccessful ways of coping over many years.*
- *Older people are more likely to be living alone, socially isolated and perhaps have a physical disability.*

Taking these changes into consideration, then some adaptation will have to be made in any counselling or helping process for older people. Thus, in general, counselling for older people will need to take into account the following factors:

- *time limited contract;*
- *explicit, concrete, realistic goals;*
- *need for small, understandable steps;*
- *flexibility in location of sessions;*
- *flexibility in length of sessions;*
- *clear assessment of total situation;*
- *awareness of physical problems;*
- *awareness of social problems;*
- *awareness of effects of drugs being taken;*
- *active rather than passive therapy;*
- *awareness of ageism;*
- *awareness of age differences between therapist and client;*
- *need for formal support and resources to offer;*

- *need to maintain clients' independence;*
- *need to work with carers, as well as client;*
- *review progress regularly.*

Poor physical health frequently goes hand in hand with cognitive deterioration, resulting in reduced social intercourse, loneliness, the incapacity to make decisions, fear of death and yet the lack of incentive to live. Grief, following loss, is a process of relearning the world and for many older people this is made more difficult by such factors as disability, social isolation and loneliness, and the inability to take on new roles and tasks. Anxiety may be increased as they feel unable to go out alone into the world or complete tasks which were previously undertaken by their spouse. There may be a general sense of insecurity. For some, there are intense and persistent panic attacks, which may come from fear of not being able to survive without their loved one or from a heightened sense of personal death awareness. Many people, though, do benefit from bereavement counselling and group work support, when the above factors are taken into consideration.

A comment should also be made on the counsellor–patient relationship when working with older people and particularly the effect of countertransference. In contrast to typical models of transference, in which the client is the subject of most concern, in working with older people, the counsellor may be most 'at risk'. Older clients can stimulate the counsellor's recollections of parents, grandparents and other important older people in their life. Lack of awareness can interfere with effective interventions. Countertransference is often ignored, overlooked or concealed, but in working with older people, it is essential for the worker to be able to confront ageing, disability, loss and grief in their own lives.

The term 'gerophobia' has been coined to show that counsellors often avoid older patients:

> *perhaps because they feel improvement will be limited or that it is more economical to work with younger people, with longer to live, or because of the low status of the elderly, or at a deeper level perhaps because of the therapist's own unresolved fear of ageing and death (Woods and Britton, 1985).*

In working with older people, it is essential to modify the intervention and acknowledge that the process may take much longer. Some counsellors may become impatient with the lack of progress and base expectations on younger clients with other types of problems. Older people, however, especially those working through bereavement, may need continued support in various practical ways for months and even years.

Bereavement Counselling

David Brandon from MIND once dispelled many of the myths and formalities surrounding counselling by saying 'I distrust most terms which describe the process of helping others –

they are high-flown and distant. The ability to *listen*, to *share*, and to *communicate* is more important'. Counselling training is necessary to enhance staff ability, but never let it detract from the basic communication skills that everyone should possess when working with patients. A patient will usually choose to talk to the person whom they trust and not always the designated 'counsellor', so all staff need to be ready to listen.

For many older people, the fact that someone has taken time to listen and just to 'care' for them can be helpful and supportive. With older people, the time taken to readjust may be much longer than younger age groups. In the TV documentary, 'The Life That's Left', there is an example of an older man, who is depressed, negative, refusing help and talking about euthanasia. Eight years later, he was found to be happily engaged in a wide range of hobbies and activities. He estimated that it had taken him 5 years to make his recovery.

Worden's (1983) work has been mentioned in identifying the four tasks or goals of bereavement counselling, but he also provides certain principles and procedures which make the counselling more effective:

- *help the survivor actualize the loss;*
- *help the survivor to identify and express feelings;*
- *assist living without the deceased;*
- *facilitate emotional withdrawal from the deceased;*
- *provide time to grieve;*
- *interpret 'normal' behaviour;*
- *allow for individual differences;*
- *provide continuing support;*
- *examine defences and coping styles;*
- *identify pathology and refer;*

A simpler set of goals may be:

- *Give permission to grieve – tell people it is all right to cry and that you can accept it.*
- *Allow them to express feelings, such as anger. Perhaps ask them to write down their feelings or draw a picture, or make up a poem.*
- *Help them to accept all aspects of the loss – tell you about the silly little things that they miss.*
- *Listen actively. Encourage them to talk about the person – society expects us to be polite and share in relationships. Allow them to be selfish. People often refrain from talking to friends because they fear loss of the relationship if they keep going over the same events and feelings.*
- *Share information about the grief process – it is normal to have these intense feelings, but often people feel they are alone in this experience.*

- *Assist in practical ways. Many of the things you say will be forgotten – write down information, addresses, etc. Leaflets and books may be helpful to give someone. Refer to Cruse or other agencies.*
- *Watch for signs of illness. Get them to contact their GP.*
- *Give permission to stop grieving and help adapt to new roles. Encourage them to become involved in new interests.*

Both of these provide a good framework for bereavement counselling, but the point comes, especially with older people who have a physical disability or who are socially isolated, when the pain of grief has subsided but what does the future hold? How do you go out into the world and rebuild your life? Change for most people is difficult but it becomes even more so in later life. Therefore, small, gradual steps need to be taken towards building a new identity.

Saying Goodbye

One of the hardest things in life is to say goodbye. It is especially hard when someone is dying and when someone has died. Many people need help to say goodbye before they can move on to any kind of recovery. The concept of 'finishing' comes from Gestalt therapy, which holds that any experience in life must be finished or completed. When the past is truly relinquished, then movement can take place. To recover fully from a loss means to finish or completely let go. This does not mean to forget the loved person, but to accept the death and be free to reinvest in life. On several occasions, I have used writing letters, poems or stories by the bereaved person, if they have become stuck at this stage.

Practical Suggestions

Years ago, it was normal for the bereaved person to withdraw from society for a period of time. It was felt that those who had suffered loss needed time to heal. Today, expectations have changed and help might be needed in coping with routines and other people's expectations. As we have seen above, many older people may need very specific goals or plans to assist in their recovery. It may be useful to plan a week's activities, so that routines can be established. Time needs to be available to sit and think, but too much spare time can create problems, as can too much activity. If a person is on their own for the first time, Tatelbaum (1980) has suggested making a list of 'things I can do when I am alone'. Think up a list for yourself.

Another useful practical step in thinking positively is to get the bereaved person to consider any activities that might interest them. Maybe they have wanted to attend a class at a college, or learn to sew, decorate, cook, etc. One man in his 70s, did a parachute jump for charity! You could ask people if there is anything they have wanted to do/see in life that they have not been able to do. A further practical suggestion if a person is not eating well or caring for themselves, is to suggest thinking about a treat – being good to themselves. A little pampering is in order, so help them to think of good things to do. Other professional help, such as physiotherapy or occupational therapy, may be needed if disability prevents an older person from becoming involved in new pursuits or continuing with others.

Many people have used a journal or diary to put down their thoughts. Putting thoughts and emotions on paper is a good way of getting rid of them. Some useful books are available to read, which may reinforce the normality of feelings and emotions. These are included in the recommended list at the end of this chapter.

An often forgotten area with older people is that of physical need. Masters and Johnson (1966) found that there was no age limit for sexual responsiveness and that 7 out of 10 married couples over 60 years of age, whom they studied, were sexually active. Older people are often inhibited or unwilling to discuss their needs, especially in this area, and this is reinforced by family and friends who forget that what has been lost is a sexual partner. It may not be important to marry again or have a sexual partner, but most people do miss the physical contact and closeness of a relationship. With older people, their right to privacy and new relationships with the opposite sex is often ignored or openly frowned upon. People pop in and out to check on them, often using a key to let themselves in and expecting to find them alone. Most women as they get much older will have to face life alone because of the disparity between the number of men and women in this age group, but there still remains throughout life a need to be loved, wanted and to give love in return within an intimate relationship.

Support Systems

Grief is a lonely time, when a person must tread their own path through the pain and in their own time, but it helps if someone is walking beside them. Creating opportunities for using time in a valuable way can greatly enhance survival. Looking at people's support systems and helping them use these effectively is a positive step on the road to recovery. Lund (1989) has drawn together some of the research which indicates the resources which can strengthen a person's position in relation to a bereavement and which can help towards a positive outcome:

- *helpful social supports;*
- *practising rituals and beliefs that facilitate the grieving process;*
- *possessing religious beliefs that foster an acceptance or understanding of death;*
- *knowledge of the grieving process through previous experiences with loss and receiving information on grieving or widowhood from others;*
- *opportunities for anticipatory grieving;*
- *a prior history of good mental–emotional health;*
- *absence of additional losses concurrent with bereavement;*
- *a quality relationship with the spouse (or other) characterized by a healthy degree of closeness, minimal dependency, and lack of prolonged conflict or ambivalent feeling;*
- *perception of the death as unpreventable;*
- *the ability to express grief openly;*

- *belief in control over stressful events;*
- *self esteem;*
- *adequate financial status.*

It may be necessary to put people in touch with organizations or suggest groups that may be available. Older people may often be isolated because of loss of social contacts as they become older or because they have not positively cultivated friendships in middle age. Bereaved men, who have also recently retired, may find that they have lost all their social networks which were involved with their work. They have not been used to long hours of doing nothing or being alone in a house.

Medical help may be requested early in the bereavement to relieve anxiety, depression or insomnia. Short-term use of sleeping tablets, tranquillizers or antidepressants may be necessary and helpful, but should only be used as a temporary measure.

Group Support

Most bereaved people do benefit from individual counselling during the early stages. They need to go over the details of the death again and again, clarifying the situation in their own mind. Then, when they have moved on, a group may help to reassure them that other people have similar feelings.

As with counselling, older people may have difficulty in certain types of therapeutic groups. A less formal setting is desirable. A social group or support group will provide a place for people to come together, talk about common problems, feelings and concerns, and to receive support from one another. Older people enjoy organized outings or practical sessions, where they can discuss problems such as health, gardening, cookery or changing a plug. Transport may be necessary for the less mobile and often most needy members.

Cruse, Age Concern, or the National Association of Widows may be able to provide group support in your area. Days out or holidays can be a particular difficulty, but these may be available through local organizations (like Age Concern) or Saga holidays, which caters for older people.

Support for Carers

In many bereavement situations, where older people have lost a spouse, there may be a carer involved or someone who has to take on that role. Stress and grief are also experienced by carers, especially if they are close family or friends and they may need as much support as the elderly person. Carers can be seen as resources, co-workers or co-clients, but in any role they will need help and encouragement. Some authorities provide support groups for carers and also training programmes. The latter can be useful when practical sessions are included by physiotherapists and nursing staff. Many carers need information on medical or psychiatric conditions, lifting and handling techniques as well as information on services and benefits available and emotional support gained from meeting other carers.

Caring at home puts a great strain on family relationships, especially where there is tension or jealousy among other members of the family. Good communication is essential between all concerned and the carer, as well as the patient or bereaved person, needs to know what is happening. An understanding of the grief process and the differences in grief reactions may help the carer appreciate some of the difficulties arising. In what other ways can you give support to carers? Do you have any leaflets or written material which may be useful or you could collate?

Those Who Refuse Any Help

Many older people do not want help and will resist all efforts to interfere in their welfare. Friends or relatives may recognize the need and request help for them, but independence and individual liberty are perhaps all that are left for many, and these rights cannot be denied.

Case Study: Respecting individual choice

The family doctor referred Mr and Mrs G following the death of their only daughter. As they were not on the telephone, the counsellor called on several occasions, but they were out. Eventually a message was left through the door, stating a specific date and time when she would call. On that day, when she arrived, the following note was pinned to the door, 'Thanks for calling so often, but we go out quite a lot now. Anyway, please do not bother to waste any more of your time as we have decided to try and get over this unhappy episode on our own'.

The pain and suffering is evident, but the message is clear and the decision must be respected. Help has been offered, but rejected. Unless there is serious risk involved, the choice has been made and each person must be allowed to find their own path through grief. Professional staff should make it clear that they are available to offer help and the family doctor or other known support system, such as church or family, should be alerted to the problem.

Support for Staff

Who cares for the carers? What are the effects of working in situations that involve grief and loss on a regular basis? How do professional staff maintain both the quality of patient care and their own emotional wellbeing? This is an important, but often neglected, area.

Grief is a common reaction for professionals involved with suffering, loss and death of patients. The reaction is usually of less intensity and shorter duration than the bereaved relative, but it is constantly reinforced on many occasions. Grief reactions are especially pronounced in working with children, but it is still an important consideration for those working with older age groups. Lerea and LiMauro (1982) surveyed nurses in a 500 bed general hospital and three geriatric centres in America. Mourning was reported by 98% of the nursing staff at the general hospital. The most common psychological reactions included thinking and talking about the patient (92%) and feelings of helplessness (84%). The most frequently reported physical response was fatigue (55%). In the total sample, though, the full range of grief reactions, similar to those experienced by bereaved people, was observed.

Grief reactions of professional staff are complex and reflect multiple losses on many different levels. Working with dying or bereaved patients may evoke intense personal feelings and arouse fears within the individual. Thus, staff working in this area are continually confronted with their own mortality and that of their family and friends. Previous losses may be reawakened and future losses may be anticipated.

Stress in this type of specialized work and also job-related stress in general can lead to 'burn out', when a deterioration in the quality of service, absenteeism, job turnover and personal problems can arise. Nurses, therefore, need emotional support for themselves, for example:

- *A counsellor for the staff would be a valuable support. The Briggs Report (1972) stated that counselling services for nurses were 'an urgent top priority', but these are still not widely available.*
- *Support groups, where work-related issues can be discussed openly.*
- *Occupational health departments.*
- *Preparation and induction courses.*
- *Education and training on loss and bereavement.*
- *On-going regular supervision.*
- *Teamwork. Support should be provided within the team through regular meetings and effective methods of communication.*
- *Developing realistic expectations. Accepting limitations, without feeling guilty, but not avoiding situations because of fear or anxiety.*

Support for staff is essential if quality of service is to be maintained and staff are to continue providing a service that is so necessary for the dying patient and their family. Helping bereaved older people can be a long and difficult task, with few immediate rewards, but gradually the depth of sorrow diminishes and changes occur as the person grapples with recovery. Grief shared is grief diminished and nursing staff have a major and rewarding role to play in this healing process.

Closing Process

There is not always an obvious time to withdraw from supporting a bereaved person. Staff, as well as patients, have difficulty in saying goodbye. In many bereavement situations, it is helpful to support the person through the first anniversary, when they will have worked through the difficult period of their first birthdays, Christmas and wedding anniversary on their own. However, some people may feel they have other supportive networks, such as family and friends, with whom they have close and open relationships. Thus, they may need only minimal outside assistance for a shorter period. For others, it may be a long, slow process and they may need referral to a more appropriate agency for perhaps more social outlets or if there are signs of abnormal grieving, they may need medical or psychiatric help.

It is important to allow the person to grow in independence and move on to other relationships and activities. Nurses or counsellors do not have unlimited time available and preparation for closing contact must be carefully considered and discussed. Gradually lengthening the time between visits and encouraging independence will be the first steps and then a specific time agreed, well in advance, when the person appears to be coping adequately alone. This can be a difficult time for all concerned, but the memory of both the first and last contacts will probably make a lasting impression on the bereaved person and will influence any future request for assistance and ability to share and discuss emotional issues in a positive way. Consider ways of terminating contact and the feelings that you will have and the feelings that the bereaved person will have.

CONCLUSIONS

In conclusion, many older people are able to accept loss and bereavement in their lives, especially where they have a philosophical or positive attitude towards ageing and death.

However, for those who find this a particularly difficult and traumatic time, then they will need the support of the caring professions to identify the need and provide the time and resources to meet this.

CLINICAL DISCUSSION POINTS

What factors may complicate the grieving process?

Depression is more common in later life. How far can this be attributed to loss and grief?

What are the advantages and the disadvantages of using Kubler-Ross' stages of dying and Parkes' phases of mourning as models for looking at loss?

In what ways does bereavement counselling need to be modified when dealing with older people?

What resources are available for older bereaved people? What is available in your area?

SUGGESTIONS FOR FURTHER READING

These are useful, readable books for health care professionals. *Those marked with an asterisk are useful to give to bereaved people.

Buckman, R. (1988). **I Don't Know What to Say.** Papermac, London.
A practical book for the general public as well as professionals. It deals openly and honestly with many

of the emotional and crucial communication problems that arise when someone is dying. It gives straightforward advice and guidance.

*Collick, E. (1986). **Through Grief – The Bereavement Journey.** Darton, Longman & Todd/CRUSE, London.

A clear, readable account of grief as experienced by the author and those with whom she has come into contact. Suitable for professionals, carers and those who have been bereaved, it deals with reactions to grief and offers practical suggestions for dealing with some of the intense feelings experienced at this time.

Cook, B. and Phillips, S. G. (1988). **Loss and Bereavement.** Austin Cornish, in association with The Lisa Sainsbury Foundation, London.

This book has been written for nurses and health care professionals and aims to help them in their work with relatives experiencing loss and bereavement. It is a useful resource book and provides material which should stimulate discussion.

*Grollman, E. A. (1977). **Living When a Loved One Has Died.** Beacon Press, Boston.

An excellent book for those who have been bereaved. Clear, simple, easy to read and keep reading. The most comforting and helpful book to share with people.

*Lewis, C. S. (1961). **A Grief Observed.** Faber & Faber, London.

Autobiography, showing the reflections of a well-known, Christian scholar on the death of his wife. Recently re-made in the film Shadowlands.

Neuberger, J. (1987). **Caring for Dying People of Different Faiths.** Austin Cornish, in association with The Lisa Sainsbury Foundation, London.

This book provides insight into the needs of dying people and their families that may arise from a variety of different religious beliefs and customs.

Penson, J. (1990). **Bereavement. A Guide for Nurses.** Harper & Row, London.

A clear guide to bereavement for nurses. It covers the needs of families before death, at the time of death and particular groups at risk, as well as services available and some good material on communication.

*Tatelbaum, J. (1980). **The Courage to Grieve.** Cedar, London.

A useful book for professional and bereaved people who want a more substantial, but readable book on surviving grief. It is an unusual, self-help book containing positive and creative material to encourage recovery.

*Whitaker, A. (1984). **All in the End is Harvest.** Darton, Longman & Todd/CRUSE, London.

Useful for carers and bereaved people, who may find comfort in the short passages from literature and poetry. Some passages could also be used to stimulate discussion in training sessions.

Worden, W. (1983). **Grief Counselling and Grief Therapy.** Tavistock, London.
A 'must' for all bereavement counsellors and those seeking a good basic text. It covers the theoretical concepts underpinning grief work and provides a practical framework of 'Tasks of mourning' to help bereaved people move through the process of grieving.

Sanders, C. M. (1992). **Surviving Grief and Learning to Live Again.** John Wiley and Sons, New York.
An inspiring and readable book which deals with the grieving process, but also offers support and understanding in helping to cope with the pain and isolation through to the regeneration and continuation of life.

Lendrum, S. and Syme, G. (1992). **Gift of Tears: A Practical Approach to Loss and Bereavement Counselling.** Routledge, London.
A useful book designed to help all those dealing with loss and bereavement. It gives expert, practical guidance on many aspects, including assessment, counselling skills and dealing with abnormal grief.

REFERENCES

Ainsworth-Smith, I. and Speck, P. (1982). **Letting Go: Caring for the Dying and Bereaved.** SPCK, London.

Aries, P. (1993). **The Hour of Our Death.** Penguin, Harmondsworth.

Bowlby, J. (1980). **Attachment and Loss. Vol. 3. Loss: Sadness and Depression.** Hogarth, London.

Briggs Committee on Nursing (1972). Report. HMSO, London.

Buckman, R. (1988). **I Don't Know What to Say.** Papermac, London.

Cameron, P., Stewart, L. and Biber, H. (1973). Consciousness of death across the life-span. **Journal of Gerontology 28**, 92–95.

Cumming, E. and Henry, W. (1961). **Growing Old: the Process of Disengagement.** Basic Books, New York.

Erikson, E. H. (1965). **Childhood and Society.** Penguin, Harmondsworth.

Freud, S. (1905). **On Psychotherapy.** Standard Edition 7. Hogarth, London.

Freud, S. (1953). **Collected Papers, Vol. IV: Mourning and Melancholia.** Hogarth, London.

Havighurst, R. L. (1972). **Developmental Tasks and Education.** David McKay, New York.

Hinton, J. (1979). Comparison of places and policies for terminal care. **Lancet 1**, 29–32.

Hockley, J. (1983). An investigation to identify symptons of distress in the terminally-ill patient and his/her family in the general medical ward. **Nursing Research Paper 2.** City of Hackney Health District, London.

Kalish, R. A. and Reynolds, D. K. (1976). **Death and Ethnicity: A Psychocultural Study.** University of Southern California Press, Los Angeles.

King, P. H. M. (1974). Notes on the psychoanalysis of older patients. **Journal of Analytical Psychology 19,** 22–37.

Kubler-Ross, E. (1970). **On Death and Dying.** Tavistock, London.

Lerea, E. L. and LiMauro, B. F. (1982). Grief among healthcare workers: a comparative study. **Journal of Gerontology 37**(5), 604–608.

Lindemann, E. (1994). Symptomatology and management of acute grief. **American Journal of Psychiatry 101,** 141–148.

Lowenthal, M. and Haven, C. (1968). Interaction and adaptation: intimacy as a critical variable. **American Sociological Review 33,** 20–30.

Luborsky, M. R. and Rubinstein, R. L. (1990). Ethnic identity in later life: the case of older widowers. In: J. Sokolovsky (Ed.) **The Cultural Context of Aging,** pp. 229–241. Bergin & Garvey, New York.

Lund, D. A. (Ed.) (1989). **Older Bereaved Spouses.** Hemisphere, New York.

Masters, W. H. and Johnson, W. E. (1966). **Human Sexual Response.** Little Brown, Boston.

Parkes, C. M. (1972). **Bereavement: Studies of Grief in Adult Life.** Tavistock, London.

Parkes, C. M. (1978). Terminal care as seen by surviving spouses. **Journal of the Royal College of General Practitioners, 28**(186), 19–30.

Parkes, C. M. (1990). Risk factors in bereavement: implications for the prevention and treatment of pathological grief. **Psychiatric Annals 20**(6), 308–313.

Parkes, C. M. and Parkes, J. (1984). Hospice versus hospital care – re-evaluation after ten years as seen by surving spouses. **Postgraduate Medical Journal 60,** 120–124.

Simos, B. G. (1979). **A Time to Grieve.** Family Service Association, New York.

Tatelbaum, J. (1980). **The Courage to Grieve.** Cedar, London.

Weiss, R. S. (1974). The provisions of social relationships. In: **Doing Unto Others.** Prentice-Hall, Englewood Cliffs, NJ.

Woods, R. T. and Britton, P. G. (1985). **Clinical Psychology with the Elderly.** Croom Helm, London.

Worden, J. W. (1983). **Grief Counselling and Grief Therapy.** Tavistock, London.π

Chapter Seven

Individual Responses

John Dean, Glenys Dean and Mary Savage

Core Themes in Gerontological Nursing

Ageing Matters	*New Social World*	*Lifespan Perspective*	*Health and Old People*
Illness and Dependency	*Quality Nursing Care*	*Therapeutic Intervention*	*Politicizing Gerontological Nursing*

Key Words

Mixed Economy of Care • Caring Relationships •
Residential Care • Choices • Risks

INTRODUCTION

Over recent years the emergence, or increasing recognition of, a mixed economy or pluralistic approach to care provision has taken place. While some would argue that care provision has always been made through a variety of different arrangements and agencies, there is no doubt that there is currently a massive drive behind moves to spread responsibility for care over a wider range of providers. There may have been implicit recognition in the recent past that much, if not most, care was provided by family members (mostly women); that recognition is now becoming explicit and exploited. Purchasing authorities are now required to make the maximum possible use of private, voluntary and informal providers of care (National Health Service and Community Care Act 1990).

Much has been written about the fiscal and ideological origins of the (re) emergence of welfare pluralism. The interested reader will find some suggestions for further reading at the end of this chapter. The purpose of this chapter is to examine other issues surrounding the provision of care by people and agencies other than the state sector. There are clear implications for the quality of life of both carers and cared for when primary responsibility for care provision is devolved from the level of the state. Some of these implications are not new. Arguably a plurality of care provision has been in existence for many years, predating the modern National Health Service. Indeed, the National Health Service was founded, in part, on the assumption that welfare pluralism was an essential prerequisite of a Welfare State.

> *... the welfare state was portrayed as an 'extension ladder' built upon a universal infrastructure or 'national minimum', which sought to extend a superstructure of private, voluntary and statutory services that enhanced individual needs selectively by means of more diversified provisions.*
> **(Hewitt, 1992; p.27)**

This chapter examines extent to which this diversified provision has enhanced individual needs. Other sections of this book deal with one area of that care provision, namely the state sector and the professions which operate within it. The purpose of this chapter is to examine the concept of caring as provided by those who are relatives or those working in the private residential care sector. In order to explore some of the issues that arise more fully, personal experiences are described by two people with extensive experience of caring in different contexts. Both accounts have been reproduced faithfully, as written by Glenys Dean and Mary Savage. The value of the two accounts is that they offer the reader an opportunity to examine the complexities of caring under different circumstances. Neither account is intended to be typical of everybody else's experience; indeed, it is the uniqueness of each account that emphasizes the importance of culture, biography, special relationships, economic and other circumstances in establishing a caring relationship which endeavours to account for the needs of the cared for and the caring.

This chapter engages the reader in discussion and critical thinking. While both are important it is not our intention to 'over-intellectualize' the concept of caring. Suggestions are made at the end of the chapter for further reading on the more academic and philosophical issues surrounding the subject. A number of activities are included within the chapter which are intended to help you to engage in the discussion and reflect upon the experiences described.

This Chapter aims to explore the following issues:

The impact of the diversification of care provision on carers

---

The concept of informal caring.

CARING

Contemporary society offers a wide range of caring services. These include the care offered by professional or paid carers who offer a service in return for financial and/or other forms of return family carers who provide care for relatives in need and volunteer carers working for charitable foundations or community groups. In the case of paid carers these may be working within the formal state sector of health care, the National Health Service (NHS) or the private sector of health care funded independently by the person in need of care. These apparently straightforward distinctions have become less clear over recent years for a number of reasons:

- *The relationship between the state sector and the independent sector has become closer when both are viewed as collaborators in health care provision.*
- *Some private providers of health care have assumed some of the characteristics of the state sector including size, relationships with purchasing authorities and range of care provided.*
- *The state sector has assumed some of the characteristics of the private sector including the introduction of consumerist policies, flexibility of provision and management of human and financial resources.*

The characteristics of professional caring in either statutory or private settings might be seen to be very similar. These characteristics include:

- *skill based on theoretical knowledge;*
- *the provision of training and occupation;*
- *tests of the competence to practise;*
- *organization;*

- *adherence to a professional code of conduct;*
- *altruistic service.*

(Williams, 1993)

These characteristics suggest not just the status held by the professional person but also the relationship that the professional carer has with the client. So, for example, the characteristic of skill based on theoretical knowledge suggests that the carer is able to offer 'expert' advice or skills to clients in need in a way that a relative is not. Adherence to a professional code of conduct implies the need for external (from the individual carer) standard setting and monitoring of behaviour.

The formalized nature of professional care is further reinforced by the need to ensure 'value for money' and the requirement to reach the standards of, for example, practice, ethical behaviour, record keeping and specialization required by registration authorities. For these and many other reasons there is a clear distinction between the role of paid, professional carers and others who contribute to the mixed economy of care.

There are other descriptions of caring which place less emphasis on the professional or other status of the carer. Brykczynska (Jolley and Brykczynska, 1992) refers to a number of constructs of caring which are of importance whoever provides care. These constructs are:

- *compassion*
- *competence*
- *confidence*
- *conscience*
- *commitment.*

Compassion is often associated with nursing but not necessarily with nurses. Its presence is a tangible reality and its absence is readily perceived by the client. Competence is not just about proficiency in particular clinical procedures but also about critical thinking and modifying behaviour. Confidence is about trust and is the very foundation upon which meaningful caring relationships are built. Conscience refers to the extent to which the carer distinguishes between that which is right and that which is wrong in an informed way rather than through blind adherence to policies and codes of conduct. Commitment here refers to the commitment between two people, the carer and the cared for. It requires us to give; not just time and effort but honesty, skill, judgement but not judgementalism, and courage.

We have already stated that this chapter is not intended to provide a 'typical' picture of carers but it is possible to examine some of these principles in the personal accounts provided. It is also possible to seek out some principles of good practice that could and, perhaps, should be extended into the arena of professional care. At the same time it should also be possible to see where, regardless of the nature of profession education, there are areas where there is no perfect substitute for the qualities of loving family carers.

The first account of caring for a relative is provided by Glenys Dean. She describes some of the issues arising out of the care she gave to her stepmother, Mrs Morgan, until her death. Read her account and consider the questions at the end. Allow yourself plenty of time to read it through without interruption.

Case Study: Glenys and Eunice Morgan

My father died in 1985 and from then on I assumed responsibility for the care and support of my stepmother then aged 86. This continued until her death some 5 years later.

The change was not as abrupt as these words may suggest: my father had been in failing health for many years and although my stepmother cared for him exclusively I was required to be in attendance each weekend, chiefly to receive confidences from each of them and (as I reflected in occasional bitter moments) to assume the role of Aunt Sally. For upwards of 10 years. I drove to South Wales from London each weekend, to visit two cross, critical old people to whom I was simply a pair of hands and a pair of ears. My stepmother was always my liveliest critic, ready always to support my father's negative view of myself and my beloved and modestly successful family.

When my father died, and I became responsible for the care and support of my stepmother, I viewed the prospect with some dismay. My husband retired soon after and it became clear that we should move away from London to settle nearer to Mam. We bought a house about 5 miles away from hers and assumed that eventually we would have to share it with her. As things stood, however, she was emphatic that she wished to stay where she was, that she required no help; that she could manage perfectly well as she was.

This was manifestly not so, but we decided to accede to her wishes while at the same time quietly supporting her. In hindsight, it worked very well. As we considered the situation, some guidelines (it appeared to us) were already in place. Some areas would remain, unquestionably, Mam's domain. She was an expert housekeeper, a frugal shopper and took great interest in her garden. In these areas her word was law.

In financial matters my father had usually taken responsibility. Mam was more than ready to allow my husband to take over this role. Even when he wished her to make certain changes (though careful not to voice any criticism of my father) she was most co-operative. We had found that most of their capital had been invested in a manner that paid interest only at the end of a long period of time and that direct access to the capital was difficult. Derrick (my husband) reinvested the capital so that interest was paid half-yearly to provide some money for ready use, while the capital was accessible should it be required, for example to pay for medical treatment or necessary repairs to the house.

We decided that her savings were to be used for her comfort and to provide small luxuries, which could not be bought from her pension. This proved impossible to implement. We had reckoned without her frugality, which never deserted her. She made every penny do its work and existed within the confines of her meagre pension with always something left over at the end of the week. She refused to buy any labour-saving gadgets. Her vacuum cleaner had been bought many years before, lovingly cared for by my father and it did a terrific job (I use it still). She had the greatest level of sales resistance that I ever met. Underclothes and stockings were darned neatly; sheets turned sides-to-middle, then into pillow cases and tea towels and finally into dusters and so on. Holidays were taboo; she would never agree to being away from home for even one night. Outings were acceptable provided there was a good reason for them – pleasure on its own was not sufficient. We became expert at coaxing her out for a drive to Radnorshire, with an appetizing picnic in the boot, to look at an organic poultry farm. Were the chickens, in her opinion, worth buying?

We frequented carboot sales in the cause of charity, or garden fetes in the grounds of the local hospital. An hour or two was sufficient and she was then ready to return home. She was not a gregarious lady, so pensioners' socials and outings held no attraction for her. It seemed to me that the small 'outings' that I have described were of importance to her wellbeing. When a friend visited, she was able to hold her own in conversation and add her own points of interest to the discussion. She also enjoyed watching television programmes, especially the political ones on which she commented with a trenchant wit. A keen and intelligent mind uncovered itself and I reflected sadly on a long life when such things had to be hidden away because of the customs of the day.

The highlight of the week was unquestionably the Friday morning visit to the local supermarket. Preparation began on the Thursday evening when a list would be written out on a strip of cardboard cut from an empty cereal-box. On Friday, we would first drive to the Post Office to collect her pension, then to the surgery to renew the prescription and on to the chemist who greeted her effusively and plied her with outrageous flattery, which she greatly enjoyed. I kept well into the background while she held these little courts: they were important to her and she re-examined every comment when she returned home.

We next hit the supermarket and moved, always in the same sequence, from one area to the next. She shopped confidently and well, utterly impervious to the wiles of the advertiser, although she was always interested in new products, especially in house-cleaning preparations. Having selected her purchases, she would retire to sit on a bench at the front of the store while I dealt with the check-out and loaded the goods into the car. Later at home, the list would be rechecked and the goods put away, always in the same order.

Simple as the routine sounds it was of great importance to her contentment. It was her 'finger on the pulse' and worth any amount of patience on our part. It was also a fragile situation as we found one week when the bench had been removed to make room for yet another advertising display. I asked for a seat for this frail old lady, but it was not forthcoming. Seeing her distress I became disproportionately angry. I could see that this small but vital component to her welfare was being denied by greedy people. I wrote to the head office of the company and sent a copy to the local branch and long before the apology had been received from the firm the bench had been restored to its accustomed place.

Her circle of friends was small, most of them of life-long standing. A member of the chapel sisterhood visited each Wednesday evening and another rather eccentric lady came on another day, usually with a load of troubles which she would pour out, quite forgetting Mam's deafness. Afterwards, she would go away, feeling cheered while Mam would mischievously confess to having nodded off once or twice during the recital. She became very friendly with a widowed lady who lived across the road and they saw each other at least every day.

Chapel had always been an important aspect of her life and we encouraged her to continue to subscribe to the congregation of which she was a member. We were grateful to the chapel membership for keeping its end of the bargain and visiting her and taking an interest in her welfare. She found the services difficult because of her deafness; we never could find a suitable hearing aid. I acted as her deputy as often as not and reported back to her.

Each Sunday she came to us for lunch, the traditional roast meal that she greatly enjoyed. She always took pains with her appearance and my husband always commented on how well she looked, which gave her great pleasure. She took a small glass of sherry (a huge indulgence for her) and chatted with my husband while I put the meal on the table. I always laid the table with care and she was aware of being a welcome guest. I felt that she was entitled to a little spoiling after years of looking after my very difficult father.

She was less easy when we had visitors, especially our children and grandchildren. She said that she was unable to follow the conversation because of her deafness, but this deafness was rather selective and I knew, from my own childhood, that she did not really like children. We decided, however, that we would not alter anything, allowing Mam to decide whether to visit us or not, thought she was plainly angry with us if we told her that visitors would be present. I did not feel that we had ever resolved that particular clash.

Her health was of prime importance to us all. We knew that if she became less mobile she would quickly lose heart. On one occasion, after my father's death, she had an attack of gastroenteritis and I bought her to our home to nurse. It was winter time and she had been thoroughly chilled in her house which had no central heating. Although she was so ill, she fretted greatly about being away from home and I meanly used this as an inducement to her to eat just a little as she improved. Her delight when she at last improved sufficiently to visit the house was touching and she soon was able to return there.

Each fortnight we visited her older sister who lived in a nursing home some distance away. We spent about an hour there admiring the garden and the comfort in which she lived. On the journey home she always spoke of her satisfaction in living in her own home and 'being beholden to nobody' as she put it. My husband and I always grinned at each other at this point, but we were reassured that our 'care plan', though not as posh as the nursing home, was at least on the right lines.

When she needed medical care, we both insisted that her savings should be spent on private treatment. It proved a worthwhile investment, chiefly as regards the saving of time and in the assurance of privacy. An attack of polymyalgica rheumatica was dealt with immediately and the course of steroids begun without loss of time. A tiny cyst on her face just where her spectacles rested was removed gently without fuss. On the other hand we received kind and sensitive care from the young audiometrician who showed her how to use her new hearing aid at the local hospital.

The only other health back-up she received was from the chiropody service, about once a month. Perhaps they had reports on her through her GP, but certainly nobody contacted me even to check that I was carrying out the job of 'carer' properly.

If I were to sum up how we cared for Mam, I would say that we respected her wishes and tried to help her maintain the kind of life she wanted with as little intrusion as possible. We did not wish to take over or to make sweeping changes that could only cause distress. She, in turn, did her best to keep active and did not take undue advantage of any offers of help.

During one of my father's many illnesses, we had a telephone fitted in the bedroom. Perverse man that he was, it had been removed almost at once. Mam would not allow one to be installed for her benefit because father had not thought it necessary. Thus it was when she woke in the small hours with an acute chest pain, she had to struggle downstairs to telephone us. We found her slumped over the kitchen table having had a heart attack.

We decided that she should remain at home, supported by her family doctor and nursed by me. She was made warm and comfortable in the large recliner chair and we sat with her through the day. The doctor visited twice and one or two friends came in for a word. She was pain free and remained clear in her mind. Though I never recall a loving embrace from her during my whole life, she roused a little as I tucked her up, smiled at me and raised her hand to my cheek. Derrick sat holding her hand as she slept and in a few more hours she died peacefully.

After she had died we followed her wishes meticulously as a mark of respect to her – or indeed of caring.

You should now reread the section, giving particular attention to the following questions. Where possible find the evidence for your answer in the text and develop it using your own experience:

■ *To what extent did the previous family relationship between Glenys and her stepmother (Mrs Morgan) influence the caring relationship?*

■ *What was Glenys able or indeed unable to do as a result of this relationship that it would have been difficult for another person to do?*

■ *How did Mrs Morgan benefit from Glenys's care? Were there any instances where other types of care provision might have benefited Mrs Morgan more? What were her needs and how were they met?*

■ *How did Glenys benefit from the experience and what were the penalties she paid?*

Inevitably, you will have constructed your own answers to the questions. The following points are intended to pick out some key points. In answer to the first question you may have begun with the description of Glenys's visits to her father and stepmother and the role that this imposed on Glenys as confidant, support and 'Aunt Sally'. You have knowledge about how Mrs Morgan performed in the house; her strengths and limitations, those things she did well and those things that had always been done by her husband. You have enough knowledge to be able to suggest some activities and not others, for example understanding Mrs Morgan's relationship with her sister; knowing how Mrs Morgan had lived her life and wanted to continue living her life.

There were certain areas where Glenys was in a 'privileged' position. This enabled her husband Derrick to make adjustments to her financial circumstances in a way that would have been very difficult for somebody in an official capacity. Whilst worrying about Mrs Morgan's safety, Glenys was able to let Mrs Morgan take risks in a calculated way that allowed her freedom. This too would have been difficult for somebody in an official capacity to do. Ultimately the decision to let Mrs Morgan die at home was only really possible because Glenys and Derrick were with her.

Mrs Morgan benefited from the situation primarily because the care was centred around her and nobody else. She was able to organize her carer in a way that would have been impossible if her carer had other patients to care for.

Glenys benefited from the experience by getting to know her stepmother better than she had done before; the closing paragraphs of her account suggest that. What was the cost to Glenys? The cost included the move to Wales from London, the weekly shopping trips, the night calls or lack of them, the reluctance of Mrs Morgan to share Glenys's family and many other things, perhaps not mentioned here.

Mary's account is by way of a series of case studies of some of her residents together with some concluding notes. She introduces herself in the next case study. Read Mary's account of caring in a residential home. As before, allow yourself plenty of time to be able to read it through without interruption.

Case Study: Mary Savage

I am fast approaching the age group known as 'elderly'. As the owner and manager of a residential care home for older people I probably have more in common with my residents than the younger care assistants. However, it is not easy to imagine the emotions and feelings when a home is given up.

The following case studies are of a group of people who have lived or are living with me in my care home. Their life styles were different and I think that this shows in their responses to growing old and to residential care.

Circumstances forced the decision in some cases with relatives often making the final decision when the person was no longer able to understand the situation due to senility. Choice does not always exist for the older person as pressures from family and other agents make the choice for them.

EMMA
As a small child aged 3 years, Emma was taken to Canada by her father. She was put into an orphanage and abandoned. At the age of 12 years, Emma stayed on at the orphanage working as a domestic help. Aged 20 years, Emma was taken into the home of the retired cook from the orphanage and they returned to England. For the remainder of her working life she was in service in several large houses. Her life was hard and she lacked affection.

She had to get up early to clean out and make up the fires and spent most of her day cleaning and performing menial tasks.

At the age of 70, Emma retired and was given a single bedroom flat by the council. Some years later Emma met and befriended a young mother with two children and a dog. The dog was the catalyst in the friendship. When Emma needed residential care this young friend encouraged her to come into my home.

With this background of hard work and very little affection, Emma accepted residential care as just another episode in her life.

Emma is a small thin person with no dentition. She is very active and self-caring and requires minimal help. On admission she appeared to be very institutionalized, and obviously used to authority. It is very informal in the home and we are all on first name terms. Emma calls me matron or the boss, and runs in to tell the other residents when I come in. She likes to talk about her life and has a good long-term memory. Sometimes she complains that other residents are hitting her and she often has arguments with other residents. She has not made friends with anybody in the home.

Emma accepts care without giving any idea about what she feels. She likes her food and her bed, preferring to share a room. She loves to go out for walks and shopping. When a group of residents go out for the day she shows that it is appreciated with many thank yous.

On Emma's 90th birthday we bought her a wrist watch because she said that she had never owned one. Her delight was lovely to see. She loved to be asked the time. Emma is a woman very simple tastes and is very easily pleased.

She was consulted about coming into care and appeared to be in full agreement with it. It is a role-reversal for this lady as she is now being cared for. Her friend still visits her regularly and sometimes takes her home for a meal.

Emma still enjoys helping and assists staff in giving out teas and collecting empty cups. She also likes to help hanging out washing to dry even if it only means holding the pegs.

JOHN

When John came to live in the home it was arranged by mutual consent between John and his two daughters. He had lived with one daughter for several years but had recently become very confused. He suffered from hallucinations during which he would barricade his bedroom door against imagined intruders.

John's family background was very sketchy; his two daughters knew very little of it. He had been in the forces during the war. After the war he worked for a firm which took him abroad for the greater part of his working life. Most of his work was 'pipe-lining' in oil producing countries. John adapted well to communal life whilst still remaining a private person. He liked to go out for walks and often called at both daughters for coffee or a meal at weekends. Sometimes he was missing from the home for 3 or 4 hours but always found his way back. He carried a card with his name and address in his pocket. This caused us all some concern; however, in consultation with John and his family it was considered a calculated risk.

John was killed when out on one of his walk. He was not crossing the road but was struck by a car which mounted the pavement. After his death his family found out a great deal about their father's life. During the war John had been in the Parachute Regiment. He was considered a hero and was decorated. He was dropped behind enemy lines to bring out prisoners of war. One such man attended John's funeral along with other colleagues from the Red Berets.

John often visited the British Legion where, for several years, he was President. Learning of his past helped us to understand his behaviour. Perhaps his disturbed nights and violent dreams were a legacy of his past.

EVA

A woman with quiet, genteel manners, Eva was brought up in a well-to-do family. She was the second born of six children, four girls and two boys. When Eva came into residential care, she and a younger sister were the only survivors of the six children. They were a close-knit, loving family. Her father was a well-known jeweller and pawnbroker in the locality. The family lived in a large house with another house on the coast for holidays. They employed a daily help, a maid and a gardener. Only three of the children married, the youngest boy and the youngest girl. They both had children. The remaining members of the family stayed together until the oldest daughter was married in her fifties to a widower.

Eva had taken up a career in the Post Office and was the manager of the General Post Office in her home town when she retired. She went to church regularly and sang in the choir. She also sang solo, giving local concerts.

Eva accepted life in a care home. It seemed an extension of her life where there had been servants to care for her. She praised or criticized gently the care that was given to her. As a member of a group within the home she did not make specific friends but seemed to accept other residents as family.

Eva liked to go out for walks and often dropped into the local golf club for morning coffee. On one such excursion she was knocked down whilst crossing the road, suffering a fractured pelvis. On recovery from this injury she was unable to go out unescorted and indeed seemed to lose the desire to go out. Eva surprised us all by her lack of inhibition when either dressing or undressing, or going to the toilet or bathing.

Eva had few visitors, her closest relative being her elderly sister who was in another residential care home. She had two nieces, one of whom visited her infrequently.

Eva was 92-years-old when she died. She never lost her air of gentility.

ANNIE

Annie was a well-known person in her town. With her husband she ran a public house for many years. When they retired her only son took over the business.

When Annie came into care she was in her late eighties. She had senile dementia and was causing anxiety to her family. Annie would wander out during the night and the police were often involved in bringing her home. Her son and daughter, on the advice of Annie's

GP, decided to put their mother into care. On admission to the home Annie was a fit, active, older woman. She objected strongly to her new environment and did not appear happy about the arrangements. As a publican, Annie would be used to calling time in the public house. During the first weeks in care she would march around the sitting room berating the other residents. She would threaten to call the police if they didn't drink up and go home.

Annie objected to any help given and became aggressive to the care assistants, showing a fiercely independent spirit. Her daughter visited daily showing distress at her mother's behaviour.

Annie had no choice in what happened to her, no alternatives were considered. Because of her mental state family and doctor decided what would be best for her.

Annie did not respond to other residents and did not make any friends. When her granddaughter visited, bringing her young family to see Annie we saw a different side to her. She was gentle and loving to the children and always welcomed them, sharing with them the chocolate she so loved.

JENNIE

Jennie came into care from hospital aged 79 years. She was a stroke recovery patient. A widow of many years she had twin sons, both of whom were married with children. Jennie appeared alert and walked well with little support Family relations seemed normal and Jennie appeared to have little regret about coming into care. She was the oldest of four children with only two survivors at this time; Jennie and a younger sister.

The family was poor with both parents having to work hard to provide. Early in life Jennie took on responsibilities of caring within the family. This caring role as she grew older spread into the extended family and friends. Sometimes her efforts to help were seen as interference by her neighbours. However, it was evident that she gave her time and support to all who she thought needed it.

When she became ill and was unable to care for herself she came into care after consultation with her family. We soon realized that Jennie was planning only to stay until she had further recovered from her stroke. When it became evident that she was not fit to live by herself she became bitter. There was not a satisfactory package of care that could be offered to keep Jennie in her own home. Her council house was given up and her furniture disposed of. Her two sons arranged all this without full discussion with their mother. Jenny's response to this was to become aggressive with her family. She complained bitterly that her sons should have taken her into their homes and looked after her as she had helped other people in the past. Each visit became an emotional battle and gradually the two sons visited less and less until one son stayed away for several months. Her sister, however, came to see Jennie at least twice a week, usually sitting quietly while Jennie complained incessantly to her.

She made no friends with any of the other residents and unsettled one or two of them by always complaining to them. Not one gesture of care that we gave to her appeared to be appreciated by her. Jennie was caught up in a situation beyond her control. She resented *deeply that she had to give up her home and would not accept that she could not run and maintain her own home again. Jennie never stopped talking about putting her name on the council list for a bungalow.*

JAMES

I first met James when I had a call from the geriatric unit of the local hospital. James was a patient who had decided that he needed residential care. I visited him on the ward and James joined us in the home a few days later.

James was 93-years-old. He lived alone following the death of his second wife 6 years previously. He had no immediate family but had two friends who cared for him. One friend was elderly and somewhat reluctant to still be responsible for his affairs. The other friend was younger and had given James several years of friendship.

James had been a company director. He had been married twice with both wives having died as a result of breast cancer. He had nursed both wives at home with help. There were no children from either marriage. James had travelled widely and had lived in New Zealand for a time.

When James came into residential care he made the decision and accepted it fully. He was mentally alert and soon settled in. James always said he was very happy in the home. He wrote many letters to friends both in this country and abroad telling them how happy he was to be cared for. He was accepted by the women and well looked after by Mary who sat next to him. As he settled in he became more assertive in his behaviour and whilst accepting the fussing from some of the women, he took on a role of male caring within the group. James appeared very settled and content within the home. He joined in all the activities within the home, enjoying it all.

His friends visited frequently giving him great pleasure. After some months James decided to sell his home and make arrangements to stay with us on a permanent basis. Whilst such arrangements were being made James died very suddenly from a heart attack.

Looking at these case studies the question that begs to be answered is – does old age cut across gender and social uniqueness in a care home? All the evidence points to no. Although the lifestyle of a group of people in a residential setting becomes similar, in that the residents are sharing facilities, these elderly people keep their uniqueness and their values gained through life experience even though it may appear to the outsider that they have lost this uniqueness.

It becomes evident that not all older people retain their rights of choice. Decisions are often made on their behalf without consultation. This consultation may be lacking for several reasons:

- *they are at risk living alone;*
- *a package of relevant care is not available;*
- *families cannot provide the relevant care;*

■ *they are unable to participate effectively in any care plan due to mental health breakdown.*

However, several residents made their own decision to come into care and indeed chose the home. With the help of supportive friends and relatives they made all the necessary arrangements. When this has happened the resident is more likely to settle into the home than when the older person is not involved in the decision.

Creating an ambience for older people within residential care is not always easy. We are urged to create stimulation and a variety of activities for our older clients. Remembering, however, their uniqueness we have to find activities to suit all levels of difference. Several areas of similar tastes may be found. The majority of people like music of some kind. The older person of today lived through some traumatic times including at least one world war. Music of this era is recognized and impromptu sing-a-longs are enjoyed.

Older people generally have children and staff and relatives are encouraged to bring in smaller members of their family. The Brownies from the local Church come into the home at Christmas and Easter and sing appropriate hymns and songs. Animals are generally liked by most people and most residents have had a pet at some time in their life.

Handicrafts are more difficult to organize as some older people can no longer handle knitting or sewing because of loss of eyesight or loss of the use of hands. However, we have a small group of residents who are involved in producing a variety of fancy goods which are sold at our garden fetes.

Outings are sometimes arranged. Full days out to the seaside or shorter trips to places like Blackpool illuminations are appreciated by those who are well enough to go. Others prefer not to.

We have found that the majority of older residents prefer not to be involved in domestic activities. They seem content to let someone else have the hassle of shopping, cooking and cleaning. Even when offered the opportunity they decline.

Some friendships develop within the home, usually between two or three people involved rather than one-to-one. However, men present a different social place within the home. There are fewer older men in care than women. They alter the social structure in that the women take on a caring role towards the men and are often more chatty and sociable.

Tensions are normal within groups of people and there are often factions and disagreements between older people living together. One of the problems that we have met is that there is a risk of learned helplessness by the resident in care. People should be encouraged to live life to their full potential. This sometimes involves taking calculated risks.

These opinions and reflections are our own, based on the observations made whilst living with a group of older people over several years. One factor that we have observed is that there are no halcyon, golden, olden days – our residents dispel this. Old age is not always nice.

Now re-read the section, giving particular attention to the following questions. Where possible find the evidence for your answer in the text and develop it using your own experience:

- *How does Mary benefit from the relationship that she has with her residents?*
- *Look at least two of the care studies and identify what you think the needs of the residents were. How were these needs met?*
- *How do the residents in Mary's home benefit from the relationship?*
- *Were there any instances where other types of care provision might have benefited the residents more?*

CONCLUSIONS

In some respects the two accounts are very different from each other. Glenys's account is essentially about the relationship between two people which has its origins many years ago. Mary's account is about a range of different people whose backgrounds and experiences are as diverse as their reactions to residential care but whose introductions to her have been comparatively recent.

In other respects the accounts throw up certain essential characteristics of a caring relationship: the importance of biography in understanding people's needs; the need to offer choice where possible; the importance of risk in caring even, as was the case for two of Mary's residents, when it has serious consequences; and the consideration of the whole person in providing care rather than the consideration of one aspect of a person. The emphasis, in both accounts, seems to be primarily about helping people to live and live well rather than about 'managing' an illness or disability. In fact, there is very little specific reference to managing ill health in either account but a great deal of emphasis on enabling life to be lived as the person wishes to live it.

The constructs of caring as described by Brykczynska appear to be highlighted here as those elements of care which rise above the distinction of professional and unpaid care. They provide the basis for a set of values and beliefs which will serve the client well when served by carers of all distinctions. To assert that family carers are better placed to care because they love their relative is to deny the complexity of family relationships over a long period of time. To assert that professional carers are devoid of equally strong feelings toward their patients is equally inaccurate. Brykczynska (Jolley and Brykczynska, 1992) states 'Feeling compassion towards a stranger followed up by an empathetic approach is a necessary prerequisite for true caring to take place.'

Whilst compassion is not a replacement for love, it is certainly the case that it requires the establishment of a close personal relationship with the client and cannot be achieved by a cool professional aloofness. The continued development of a mixed economy of care is assured.

The oil shocks of the 1970s and the consequent recession that followed produced an economic climate that predisposed political systems to consider fundamental reforms. The demographic arithmetic in many countries did the same. Governments faced both declining births among the younger age

groups and a growing older age group that will become even more significant in the next century.
(Drummond and Maynard, 1993)

Whether the motivation to explicitly recognize and exploit the informal carers and the private sector is primarily economic or not, there is no doubt that care in this area will increase considerably as the direct involvement of the state as a care provider diminishes. The pressures that this will place on family members, especially women, and the extent to which relationships will be able to stand these pressures, has yet to be seen. What is certain is that failure on the part of the family or the private health care sector to provide during the following years of demographic change will have the most profound implications for the health care of the population in the UK. As the state withdraws from its direct involvement in care provision it may well need to increase its indirect involvement in the care and support of families and other care providers.

SUGGESTIONS FOR FURTHER READING

Hewitt, M. (1992). **Welfare Ideology and Need; Developing Perspectives on the Welfare State.** Harvester-Wheatsheaf, Hemel Hempstead.
This text offers a useful overview of the development of welfare pluralism including the origins, the political and economic imperatives that have surrounded it.

Ford, J. and Sinclair, R. (1987). **Sixty Years On.** Womens Press, London.
Very personal accounts of women experiencing old age, developing their own identity.

Jolley, M. and Brykczynska, G. (1992). **Nursing Care: The Challange to Change.** Edward Arnold, London.
Gosia Brykczynska's chapter on caring is an excellent and impassioned debate on the important elements of caring.

The Hen Co-op (1983). **Growing Old Disgracefully.** Piatkus, London.
A creative group of people who challenge the accepted views of growing old.

REFERENCES

Drummond, M. F. and Maynard, A. (1993). **Purchasing and Providing Cost-Effective Health Care.** Churchill Livingstone, Edinburgh.

Hewitt, M. (1992). **Welfare Ideology and Need; Developing Perspectives on the Welfare State.** Harvester-Wheatsheaf, Hemel Hempstead.

Jolley, M. and Brykczynska, G. (1992). **Nursing Care: The Challenge to Change.** Edward Arnold, London.

National Health Service and Community Care Act 1990. HMSO, London.

Williams, J. (1993) **What is a Profession? Experience Versus Expertise in Health, Welfare and Practice.** Open University Press, Milton Keynes.

Section 3

Nursing Perspectives

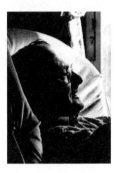

Developments in Nursing Older People: Past, Present and Future
Lesley Wade

Developing a Knowledge Base in Gerontological Nursing: A Critical Appraisal
Mike Nolan

Rehabilitation
Karen Waters

Advanced Practice: The Case of Leg Ulcers
Yvonne Awenat

The Challenge of Advocacy: A Moral Response
Kevin Kendrick

"Life is a country that the old have seen and lived in.
Those who have to travel through it can only learn from them."

Joseph Joubert, (1842) *Pensées*, 6.32 tr Katherine Lyttleton

This section reflects the state of the art and science of gerontological nursing, paying particular attention to the past, present and future.

Our present is always influenced by our past, so we start the past in Chapter 8. Lesley Wade traces the development of elderly care nursing, drawing on historical insights to illuminate the current context of gerontological nursing and tracing the probable path of future gerontological nursing.

In Chapter 9, Mike Nolan challenges the reader to consider how and why a knowledge base for gerontological nursing should be developed and suggests how this might be done.

Chapter 10 focuses on a field of nursing which is gaining increasing attention and becoming more important as the demand for effective health care increases – rehabilitation nursing. Karen Waters concentrates on the nursing contribution to rehabilitation nursing with older people. The importance of clarifying and developing the nursing role is emphasized.

Chapter 11 is a case study of one specialized area of gerontological nursing – the management of clients with leg ulcers. By tracing the development of this field, we illustrate how nursing has advanced to the benefit of older people. This chapter includes specific clinical information, giving us a window on the depth as well as the breadth of gerontological nursing.

Chapter Eight

Developments in Nursing Older People: Past, Present and Future

Lesley Wade

INTRODUCTION

Present day practice has evolved from a rich variety of community and hospital based care, its development and future shaped by ordinary people who, according to their era, nursed older people within a variety of models and packages of care. Emphasis is placed on the impact that politics and the economy had and continues to have in this nursing speciality. Previous images about nursing older people often lack this essential dimension. A further challenge to nursing within this chapter is to reflect whether gerontological nursing was and continues to be the pivotal force that develops nursing. In revising our approaches towards the development of nursing older people accurate historic sources will be used, to challenge some cherished beliefs. Contemporary developments within nursing such as nursing development units, and clinical leadership will be analysed. Today, gerontological nursing tends to emphasize the needs of groups of older people and their personal views. This chapter celebrates the growth and development of nursing within this field and the increased skills and diverse opportunities ahead for gerontological nursing.

This Chapter aims to:

Develop an analysis of nursing older people through a sociopolitical perspective, encouraging greater use of research within this area

---

Recognize and utilize previous nursing activities that could inform present practices in the care of older people

---

Examine some contemporary and future developments within this area.

To meet these aims, this chapter has been divided into three parts:

- *previous views of old age;*
- *past frameworks of care;*
- *contemporary developments in the care of older people.*

PREVIOUS VIEWS OF OLD AGE

Looking at pre- and postindustrial attitudes towards old age we can see that societies have always faced the issue of how to treat older people. Historically, older people have had mixed fortunes. In the Old Testament older people's hands had to be kissed by anyone who entered the house. With the Athenian empire and the worship of beauty, the old were ridiculed. The

Renaissance revived all the Athenian love of beauty and distaste for age. Leonardo's grotesque drawings show a fear of growing old (McKee and Kauppinen, 1987) whilst in England, Shakespeare represented the old in unforgettable metaphors. One of the first primary sources that allows us to analyse the position of older people and the control of poverty under the auspices of social policy is the Elizabethan Poor Law Act of 1601. In a clause from this act it appears an unequivocal statement that individuals were to look to their immediate relatives for help and these relatives were expected to provide it:

> *The father and grandfathers, mother and grandmother and children of every poor, old, blind, lame and impotent person, or other poor person not able to work being of sufficient ability, shall at their own charge relieve and maintain every such poor person, in the manner, and in according to that rate, as by the justices ... in their session shall be assessed*
> **(Leonard, 1900; pp. 133–134).**

This act remained the mainstay of public welfare provision until its repeal in 1948, when no wide ranging statutory restatement of the duties of relatives was made. Although it appears clear cut that a transition was made from *family* responsibility to *state* responsibility, the above clause is a small part of the larger document, whose prime purpose was exactly the *opposite*. In reality, this act was designed to formalize a system of public responsibility for the needy; only in *certain* limited and specific circumstances would relatives of poor people have to share the responsibility of care (Pelling, 1991). Familial obligations focused on children who bore a legal duty to offer assistance. Brothers, sisters, nephews, nieces and grandchildren were all exempt. Children were only expected to assist if their parent was 'destitute' not just simply poor or needy and the child had to be of 'sufficient' means.

Obligations to parents ceased upon a female child's marriage. Even if she was to marry a wealthy man, obligations did not extend to grandparents even if they had raised a child from birth. Sons and unmarried daughters could not be compelled to offer services of any kind to their parents. They could not, for example, be compelled to take an older person into their own home. Basically, if an older person was destitute the Poor Law authorities would support them, but could take legal action against the son or unmarried daughter to recoup some of the cost. Quite simply it was 'un-English' behaviour to expect children to support parents (Pelling, 1991).

The accepted view of the Poor Law is that at all time and in all places it was harsh and miserly. However, this view may not be valid and it is important to see what the Poor Law actually did rather than what was said of it. In the mid nineteenth century, in the years following the Poor Law reforms of the 1830s when Victorian values of familial duty were supposedly held with fervour, the majority of all older persons in England were maintained by the Poor Law. They received weekly pensions that had a relative value in excess of pensions paid by the late twentieth century welfare state (Pelling, 1991). Victorian Poor Law handouts are often discussed as derisory pittances. Compared to the total income of the working population, a Victorian pension gave the older person the spending power of 70–80% of the younger average adult of the 'working class'. When matching twentieth century pensions to earnings, the state retirement pension has retained a worth of only 40–45% (Thomson, 1983). While the new Poor Law was passed in 1834, it was not implemented to take effect as far as older people were concerned until the period after 1860. Evidence has previously indicated that up to the middle of the nineteenth century older people fared better relatively to younger people. But after 1863 Poor Law pensions were slashed and the plight of the older working class became the focus of political concern. A case is therefore made that our historical perceptions regarding care of the older people too often dismiss our heritage as a nation in providing community care. An example of how communities supported older people with a less formalized approach towards organized community care can be seen by studying official statistics and matching census records and Poor Law records.

An Early Model of Community Care

Midway through the Victorian era a place called Ampthill had a thousand older people. This area had one of the lowest per capita levels of Poor Law spending for the country. Two in three women aged 70 or more, and one in two men, were Poor Law pensioners. They received an allowance generated by a local property tax. Once granted a pension it was seldom lost before death and the proportion of the population who received such support through old age was high. Payments were made to all forms of households, to older people living alone, with a spouse, with other pensioners, as lodgers with children, married or unmarried. Extra payments were made for special diets, medication or provision of a nurse (Wright, 1992).

Reflecting on your practice, how sympathetic has present-day social policy been to older people? In helping you to reflect, consider these three views of the care of older people, two from the consumer's perspective and one from a student nurse.

Case Study: Harold's plight

Harold Abraham still recognizes his wife when she visits him in hospital, despite his absence of speech following a stroke 4 months ago. Harold was born in 1918 and was thus an infant when nursing won the battle for registration but old enough to remember the depression of the late 1920s, fight in the Second World War and be in receipt from the welfare state. Under the rationalizing programmes of the new Trust board, Harold's wife has been told he is to be moved, either into the community or a private nursing home. Harold has grown old in the security of a welfare state which promised care from the cradle to the grave. If Harold could speak he could tell us about the tremendous changes in health, medical and nursing standards that promised a continuity of care.

It is important that nursing elicits the views of older people if we are to evaluate our development. History can too often be the story of powerful people producing a one-sided biased account. One project that I undertook as a joint appointee within a nursing development unit in the mid 1980s was to get my students to take oral histories from clients in their care. Below are two extracts. One is from Sister Brownlow a 78-year-old ex-nurse, who recounted what care of older people was like in her training in the 1930s in Bolton, Lancashire. The other is from Mary an ex-pawnbroker who used to regularly come in to hospital for respite care.

Case Study: The nurse's story

Mrs Brownlow: It was 1931 and the day after New Year, we all had to attend Matron's Office. We stood, hands behind our backs, being told where we were to go. You girls will go on to the old people's wards and if with luck you survive this, you will proceed with your training.

Interviewer: What was it like?
Mrs Brownlow: Long rows with what appeared to be skeletons in beds. This was the female ward, but many of them still smoked clay pipes and it was my duty to light them. They were dressed in light cotton gowns that did not fit correctly and the women desperately tried to cover themselves up.

Interviewer: What was your job, what nursing did you do?
Mrs Brownlow: Well the nurses were quite kind because some of those people came into hospital in terrible conditions, with vermin and dreadful pressure sores. I was told to treat them kindly, we all had a mum.

Interviewer: What sort of instruction did you have?
Mrs Brownlow: None, None at all, till we did medicine.

Case Study: Mary's story

An oral history taken from Mary, a respite patient cared for within a nursing development unit, is testimony to the developments and comfort nursing in hospital can bring.

Interviewer: Is there a difference in nursing now than when your parents were alive?
Mary: I'll say there is, they lived in fear of the work house, it was a sign of disgrace if you were in there.

Interviewer: Has the hospital or nursing changed that much?
Mary: Without a doubt, it was do this and do that, people in long rows and no one talking to the patients.

Interviewer: What's changed?
Mary: The nurses – they are much more friendly, they get to know you and you get to know them. They seem genuinely interested in you . . . You miss it when you get home.

Thompson (1990) argues that the history of ageing in this country has still to be written, silence is itself significant as it reflects powerlessness and ambivalence. A case is made here that if nursing does not record and evaluate the feelings that older people themselves have of nursing developments, this loss will be detrimental to each.

Past Frameworks of Nursing Care

Whilst much of the history of medicine and nursing focuses on institutions, we cannot omit the care older people were given by domestic nursing during the nineteenth century. One of the features of Poor Law medical relief was that the poor and infirm could be nursed at home. For example, the records of applicants for nursing posts during the Crimean War reveal a Poor Law nurse whom Florence Nightingale wrote was 'active, clean, useful, kind and industrious but wholly unfitted by the impropriety of her manner for a military hospital' (Summers, 1993). Therefore the image of the Poor Law nurse, the majority giving care to the elderly, does not fit into mainstream nursing tradition. If the public esteem was low, so was remuneration. In an attempt to expand and systematize the Poor Law nursing service Edward Sieveking, a German trained doctor, and Louisa Twining produced various schemes to improve care. Twining argued that the punitive aspect of the new workhouse regime was completely inappropriate for the aged. Twining and her workhouse visiting society attacked the inadequate and insanitary conditions of workhouses and infirmary wards condemning the workhouse nurse as incompetent, and uncaring to the point of cruelty. Summers (1993) points out that Twining identified one of the chief tasks of nursing as the maintenance of order through the imposition of authority. Significantly, Summers argues that previously what might have been understood as neighbourhood help with assistance and comfort, freely contracted between the carer and cared for and liable to be reciprocated at a time of future need, is now being portrayed as a relationship of power. When nurses write their own history of this period, this is often described as the dark ages. In articles, reports and commissioners' investigations these pauper nurses are spoken of in disparaging terms, particularly the inferiority of their character (Davis, 1978). In an atmosphere of increasing agitation against the Poor Law nurse, the Poor Law Board recommended that trained and paid nurses should be employed in preference to pauper nurses.

Quite clearly, the last part of the nineteenth century saw a drive towards institutional care. The conclusion one could make, is that the nineteenth century home nurse and the workhouse nurse were marginalized by notions of progress, which were and still are hardly questioned by their contemporaries and by patterns of public expenditure. A problem for anyone studying the development of nursing, especially gerontological nursing, is to accept that the new model of nursing created successfully by Nightingale coexisted with effective patterns of lay care. Much of the history of nursing rests upon a knowledge of the administrative framework in which nurses were required to work, but is incomplete without an account of the care given.

Victorian Nursing Practice

A nursing report from a workhouse in Northamptonshire during the late nineteenth century, provides evidence of clinical skills employed within an early form of gerontological nursing (Adams, 1991). The majority of the nursing reports concern bowel care, treatment to prevent pressure sores and wound care. The most frequently given aperients seem to have been magnesium sulphate and enemas. The nurses at Thrapstone noted when pressure sores became red and recognized that the best way to avoid continued pressure was to change the patient's position frequently. Older patients required careful attention to their nutritional needs and culinary skills were an additional requirement of gerontological nursing. Warm milk and Bovril were given to ill-nourished patients, whilst patients with diarrhoea were given arrow root and sugar mixed with milk (Adams, 1991).

Examinations of workhouse records show the mixed nature of Poor Law nursing. Nurses had to deal with patients who were 'fitting together with those suffering from mental illness whilst others sobbed the greatest part of the night'. Providing comfort and easing pain were given a low priority. Patients who complained of pain had it soothed by the application of hot flannels, whilst those with circulatory disorders had their suffering eased by using hot water bottles.

Some joint husband and wife appointments to the post of administrator and matron also enlighten our view on gerontological nursing. Clearly, the hierarchical culture meant that master and matron set the climate, but as oral histories are beginning to reveal, the staff were happy family, no matter what people said about the old Poor Law. 'If there was a good master and good matron you had happy inmates, it emanated from the top' (Adams, 1992). One interview from a Mr Lewis, a former master gave us this information: 'My wife in particular used to know everyone in the place by name, even though there were sometimes nearly three hundred people there. It was very personal and I think this permeated right down to the residents' (Adams, 1992).

Assessment of the value of nursing in these institutes has been called for by White (1978) who argues that these nurses were able to defend the interest of the long-term sick, the old and demented. The premise on which this defence is built is that these nurses treated older people and the long-term sick as people and individuals rather than cases or write offs.

From the twentieth century it is difficult to assess objectively the quality of care in these institutions, clearly it depends on the climate created by the master and matron who could be either paternalistic or draconian. Suitable personnel were furtively sought and the character of the individual meticulously assessed against nineteenth century morals. Dingwall *et al.* (1988) stated that both physician and philanthropist wanted the respectable strata of working class women from whom the better sort of domestic servants was recruited. The ideology of domesticity and motherhood were intended to act through women to influence the public domain of men, the rough edges of working class life smoothed to a pattern of compliance with an upper or middle class vision of harmonious social relationships (Dingwall *et al.*, 1988).

It could be argued that the Nightingale model of nursing did very little to advance the care of older people. Acknowledged as a dynamic leader and one of the first nurses to intellectualize and write up theories on nursing, Nightingale's process of nursing became the universal model for much of the Western world. A gifted scholar, creative thinker and persuasive leader, nursing became a victim of her success. To the working class she was the ideal of Victorian respectability. However, it is important to assess how far the Nightingale school of nursing improved the wellbeing of older people. Even today, the remnants of the Nightingale style continue to dominate practice. With the introduction of the National Health Service one can surmise that much of the Nightingale style was introduced into gerontological nursing. Uniform dress codes served to identify not so much the individual but the profession of nursing; length of uniforms, cuffs and collars were hardly appropriate for work activities. Deferring to others at all times and long hours on duty were contextualized around the idea of altruism; there was little room for autonomy or independent thinking.

Collective Responsibility

A further issue to address is the place of residence of older people in the past, where they were nursed and who nursed them. The mechanisms that supported those that needed care, especially older people and the infirm, were derived from institutions. The church could be seen as the equivalent of 'public sector' care and also kin. How this kinship network gave care is still under researched; our lack of knowledge about the fluctuating demographics of the past makes it difficult to assess to whom the caring fell. According to recent evidence, those who were in need of social and financial support, older people and widows, did find the care they needed in preindustrial society, and they were cared for through collective responsibility (Dalley, 1988). Thompson and Golding (1975) state that towards the end of the middle ages it was not uncommon for persons of moderate means to arrange a kind of old age insurance for themselves by signing over their property to a charitable foundation in return for board, lodging and medical care for the remainder of there lives. They refer to this group as superannuated pensioners. In 1782, parishes were permitted to provide workhouses for the exclusive use of children, the aged and the sick, with little differential made between the sick and able-bodied in eligibility and receipt of relief. However, the image we have of older people in workhouses is a mid twentieth century reality and not true of the nineteenth century. Thomson (1983) reached the conclusion that few older people, perhaps one in ten, would ever have seen the inside of a workhouse, and those that did so would stay in for a matter of a few weeks or months. Interestingly, females were less likely to enter a workhouse than men, the reverse of the present situation in institutional care. Basically, institutions such as workhouses played a minor part in the actual day to day provision for older people.

Studies on widowhood during the eighteenth century indicate that a high proportion of this group maintained their own households. Many older people had their own resources or were given support from kin and informal and formal charities. That there were well-established mechanisms within the community is also supported by recent historical evidence. Wear (1986) points out that in most parishes there seemed to be a system of welfare by contract developments, the parish authorities not forcing families to pay but often paying individuals to nurse the sick and the old. Accepted wisdom until recently suggested that in preindustrial societies, those in need fell back on the support of their families. Current studies in the history of old age and care provision suggest the opposite. Smith (1986) suggests that in times of demographic pressure the individualistic or family-orientated solution proposed for the treatment of older people triumphed; however, from a very early period in English history and in other parts of northern Europe care has centred on the community rather than the family. Although institutional arrangements have varied over time with the source of relief shifting from manors, churches, gilds, parishes and Poor Law unions and eventually the state, emphasis has always been on extra familiar locus of welfare institutions.

European visitors were impressed by this collective support. Himmelfarb quotes Franklin in 1766 stating: 'There is so many almshouses for the aged of both sexes, together with a solemn law made by the rich to subject their estates to a heavy tax for the support of the poor' (Himmelfarb, 1985; p.5).

Also, in quoting from the eighteenth century, de Tocqueville, a French observer on English life, echoed the same views. Significantly, both commentators felt this altruism detrimental to the general economy of the country. Even after the National Insurance Pension Scheme of 1911, and inception of the welfare state after 1945, the value of pensions relative to the average working class income never reached earlier levels. Interestingly, Thomson directly relates the fall in pensions at particular periods to the number of older people entering residential care and the shift in balance from a predominantly male residential population to a female one.

The Medicalization of Nursing Old Age

From the nineteenth century onwards, the profession of medicine and nursing has re-examined the role it plays in the care of older people. To some extent all professionals who choose a career in the care of older people are seen as risk takers as previously geriatrics suffered from a lack of research and kudos. As a consequence, disease in old age did not warrant special attention and gerontological wards were seen to be the Cinderella of nursing. For over 100 years we have been under the spell of a movement towards increased technical specialization in medicine. By the eighteenth century, with the rise of scientific medicine, there was already a distinct disparity in the treatment of younger age groups as compared to those in middle and old age. In an attempt to apply a scientific model of medical progress, the life course of a human being was now seen as peaks and troughs. Naturally, the peaks were from childhood and the trough was old age. This degenerative approach dominated much of nineteenth century medicine's attitude to old age. The most comprehensive and influential concept for the medicalization of old age is that of 'Marasmus Senilis' or wasting fever. This wasting disease was seen as part of the normal order or naturalness of the life cycle. Suggestions for rehabilitation within old age therefore remained inconceivable for many years.

The emphasis on the scientific approach to old age is confirmed by Sir Francis Galton's statistical research which demonstrated that certain abilities vary with age (Harris 1990). However, it was a Russian, Metchnikoff, who in 1903 proposed that there should be a new field of study into ageing which he called *gerontology*, predating the term *geriatric* medicine by 6 years. The dominance of geriatric medicine during the early part of the century demonstrated the dominance of the youth model or the infantalization of care that remains with us today (Hockey and James, 1991). As old age could not be reversed, medicine either tried to stop you getting old or prescribed care that was more appropriate to younger age groups. As the body was seen to have limited ability the medical view supported the idea that investigation into old age was futile and risky. Evers (1990) charts the development of geriatric medicine as a speciality, and identifies Marjorie Warren as one of the major leaders in changing medical care. Her contributions were summarized as:

- *classifying patients;*
- *improving the environment;*
- *establishing a multidisciplinary team.*

In the early twentieth century, groups of writers and publicists began to talk and write about social hygiene. By this they meant the improvement of the quality of the population by a conscious intervention in the biological laws that governed its growth, development and reproduction. This discussion led to the foundation of several social hygiene organizations. They based their policies on two foundations: the elimination of the unfit and the improvement of the general level of industrial and personal efficiency among the working class. How far some of these beliefs affected older people, with respect to resources, provision of care and negative attitudes, has yet to be explored.

It took two world wars to create an impetus for changing attitudes towards older people. After the Second World War there was a growing realization of the social and medical implications of an ageing population. This, alongside an awareness of the low level of care to older people and the creation of the National Health Service, forged a new deal for older people. The Beveridge report of 1942 was the first modern social planning document to recognize the importance of the 'problems' of older people. They were seen as the most rapidly surviving 'unfit' group in the population and British civilization seemed to be threatened with extinction through childlessness and dependency.

The Effect of Institutional Nursing Care on Older People

The state of institutional care for older people was fully exposed during the Wartime Hospital Survey. Numerous reports showed that accommodation was of the 'most primitive type' of 'unsuitable design' and incapable of satisfactory improvement. Prolonged exposure to institutional environments has long been known to increase mental and physical dependency (Goffman, 1961) In his analysis of institutions, Goffman highlighted four main characteristics: rigidity of routine; block treatment of staff; depersonalization of residents; and social distancing between staff and patients. In examining admission procedures and ward organization, Goffman noted that people within institutions assumed socially inferior roles. This has been substantiated by Miller (1989) who noted that admission to hospital encouraged loss of independence. If older people's health was poor, their expectations were even lower.

Evers (1990) argues that there is no precise chronology associated with geriatric medicine's development. Developments, if any, were patchy, it having more of a custodial image of warehousing. Its unique contribution came from its clinical presentation of illness and its expertise in rehabilitation. Tensions about the development of geriatric medicine revolve around the idea of having either a residual service, an integrated service or an age-related service. The former, in a period of sociopolitical and demographic change, has been forced to change. The second option, an integrated service, addresses the need to give older people access to technology. In a paper put forward in the *Lancet* the concept of an integrated service that guarantees older people access to the same facilities as younger individuals was put forward MacLennon (1993). The argument for an integrated service is that the medical and nursing staff are more likely to be up to date with recent advances, improvements and changes. 'This integrated service provides all members of nursing and medical staff with insight and experience in care of the elderly' (MacLennon, 1993). There are considerable differences of opinion as regards the fusion of these units. The most obvious criticism lies in the fact that the ward environment and staff may not have a gerontological perspective, creating a non-therapeutic environment; dehumanization and institutionalization can take over rapidly. It can be appreciated that the staff working on the wards have to want to care for acutely ill older people.

The third option, the one that this author feels comfortable with, is the development of a specific age-related service, offering comprehensive acute, rehabilitation, and community involvement with continued responsibility for patients. As far as nursing is concerned, this is an exciting opportunity for it to take a lead role in many of these new developments. Increased knowledge and skills in gerontological care nursing can be illustrated by using a historical perspective and considering the care required by an older person hospitalized for a cerebovascular accident. In the 1950s attention to personal hygiene, comfort and safety needs of the patient were emphasized in nursing practice. In the 1990s, nurses require additional knowledge and skills related to family counselling, client education and rehabilitation and ethical and legal issues. More importantly, nurses need to learn in appropriate clinical learning settings.

THE CONTEMPORARY DEVELOPMENTS IN GERONTOLOGICAL NURSING

Nursing has come a long way since the days of battling against communicable diseases, long stays in hospital after surgery, and custodial care. Nurses caring for older people have continually pushed back the frontiers of nursing. It has been suggested throughout this chapter that gerontological nursing has been the vanguard of change within nursing. Every vanguard needs supporting mechanisms to maintain and develop new skills. The boundaries that gerontological nursing has traversed can be demonstrated by the backgrounds of course members on the English National Board's framework and higher award. Macmillian breast care specialists learn core skills alongside nurses working in accident and emergency, gynaecological wards and a variety of other areas. The English National Board's 941 course and the longer clinical course, the 298 in elderly care, offers a pathway within the 10 key characteristics of the ENB framework, to develop clinical practice and academic creditation.

What makes these courses special is the tripartite nature of the relationship between manager, course member and educationalist. Learning contracts are individualized, recognizing the specific area of clinical practice and development of the nurse. Increasingly, older people are part of the curriculum development team itself, sitting alongside managers and educationalists. Therefore this lateral dissemination of gerontological practices crosses and enriches boundaries within various nursing directorates, older people themselves contributing and informing nursing practice. Nurses caring for older people should also take the advantaged of gaining professional academic credit for previously undervalued skills. Acquired prior learning (APL) and acquired prior experiential learning (APEL) recognize personal and professional development and skills. If the nurse wishes to have previous work credited, achievements have to be supported by evidence and the developing of portfolios. With the wealth of experience in developing practice there is every opportunity to maximize and 'cash in' on previous and ongoing innovations, particularly as some educational curricula and guidelines change slower than developments in practice.

Nursing Development Units

Pioneering work within nursing development units (NDUs), nursing-led beds and nurse practitioners, represent a small proportion of innovative practice within the field of gerontological nursing. Developing nursing through the concept of NDUs has been one of the luminous lights within gerontological nursing over the last decade. Wright (1987), one of the first consultant nurses in the care of older people, stated that you cannot develop nursing without first developing the individual nurse. Therefore, an NDU has a strong emphasis on the professional development of staff regardless of grade or qualification. The track records within NDUs evaluated by Shaw and Bosanquet (1993) and Black (1993) demonstrate this strong commitment to education, research, innovation and risk taking. This commitment has been witnessed in NDUs not only in Brighton and Southport but throughout the UK and beyond. NDUs have been both the crucible and the catalyst for change in nursing practice. Malby (1992) identified 11 characteristics of an NDU which covered areas such as increased nurse autonomy, shared knowledge of new ways of practice and challenging, planned change. Nursing-led beds, access to patients' notes and self-medication trials have their roots in these units that specifically care for older people. To some extent NDUs and primary nursing have been the quite revolutions within gerontological nursing. How and why these initiations paved the way for the entrepreneurial nursing roles of the future may lie in dynamic clinical leadership and a growing confidence in nursing skills.

Primary Nursing

Primary nursing is a concept that gives increased accountability and autonomy to the nurse, facilitating the development of both clinical and managerial skills. Below is an extract which looks at the impact of primary nursing on older women (Wade, 1992). Consider how Sheila, the primary nurse, interacts with Ivy, her patient.

Case Study: Sheila's story

Interviewer: What do you see, Sheila, as one of the benefits of using primary nursing?
Sheila: I see it as an opportunity to really get to know my patients, the patient with the nurse and the nurse with the patient. By becoming that bit closer, you get that bit more observant and the more you get close, the more you work in harmony.

Interviewer: How did you form a relationship with Ivy then?
Sheila: By being interested in Ivy. If you are interested in her, then she will be interested in you. She shares her life with me and I share my life with her.

Interviewer: How do you think you help her?
Sheila: Well, Ivy has a lot of pain, but it's no good insisting she has more medications, so we change her position, massage her back and are very careful when helping her out of bed in the morning. You see, Ivy has come to trust me and she says only I know how to move her.

This interaction demonstrates how nursing is identifying the processes by which good care is delivered. Sheila's conversation is sensitive, demonstrating a feeling of togetherness and reciprocity and this intimacy allows alternative ways of giving care. Shelia's gerontological perspective combined with the one to one relationship primary nursing offers, shows advanced knowledge of touch, pain control and communication. Benner (1984) described aspects of advanced skills within clinical practice as 'presencing', being there for the patient, acting as an advocate, maintaining independence for the client, which in turn the client trusts.

FUTURE DEVELOPMENTS

Much of the evidence for self development within specialized settings for older people has been supported by clinical supervision and encouragement from enlightened management. Nurses within these settings may be comfortable with their expanded role, focusing on the nurse–client relationship. However, *The Scope of Professional Practice* (UKCC, 1992) emphasizes both the expanded and the extended role of nursing practice. These include areas such as administering intravenous drugs, access to arterial lines and suturing. In combination with clinical supervision this offers the chance to change the boundaries between nursing and other allied professions. Anxiety that 'hi touch' may be replaced with 'hi tech skills' may be a problem of perception rather than reality. Gerontological nursing traverses the boundaries between high touch and high technical skills; this is part of the unique quality required from nurses caring for an increasing older population. Clinical supervision as an exchange between practising professional to enable the development of professional skills' (Butterworth and Faugier, 1992) is a concept that assists nursing to develop within an environment that constantly asks for skills to be redefined. Highly motivated, educationally supported and competent nurse practitioners can benefit older clients. Take, for example, the increasing numbers of older people using accident and emergency services. Triage systems of nursing are recording increasing numbers of older people with falls, whether at home or during leisure activities (Home and Leisure Accident Report, 1988). In response, trials in nursing-requested X-ray systems have been seen to speed up admissions and reduce the waiting and anxiety of older people. Similarly, clinical nurse specialists are developing skills in thrombolytic and electrocardiac monitoring, cancer care and orthopaedics (orthogerontology). Reduced iatrogenesis, by teaching older people to self medicate, assisting with cardiac pacing or dialysing older renal patients all demonstrate the range and depth of this type of nursing.

Joint teaching and clinical roles have been pioneered within specialist units for older people, building bridges for further development. It may be argued that nursing older people has been at the centre of activating and transforming nursing practice. This is demonstrated clearly in Chapter 1, which examines the use of reflective practice and journal writing within the framework of a joint appointee role.

Nursing-led Initiatives

The development of nursing beds, (Pearson *et al.*, 1992) in conjunction with clinical skills demonstrates the value of gerontological nursing. Nursing beds are essentially those established where nursing is the chief therapy. However, for nurses to operate therapeutically with older people they need high levels of skill in promoting physical and psychological comfort. The development of nursing-led units for older people has proved to be effective in reducing length of stays and increasing patient satisfaction, focusing on specific therapeutic intervention advanced skills in rehabilitation, emotional support and technological competence. Different patterns of care and the increasing consumerism of the older population require even more varied practice.

Skills in nursing older people undergoing day surgery have to address issues like communication, pain control and post-discharge care. 'Blitz' programmes, such as cataract programmes that could cover 40–60 operations per day, could be facilitated through day case surgery (Day Surgery Task Force, 1993). The gerontological-orientated day case nurse, will need to contact local voluntary organizations such as Lions Clubs, WRVS or the Red Cross, to arrange a befriending, escort and transport service for specific older people. The Task Force's assessment on day surgery predicted that within the decade, 50% of elective surgery will be performed on a day service basis. With a growing consumer-orientated older population, gerontological nursing will need increasing skills in this type of surgery. It will need experience in screening and assessing safe client selection, knowledge and skills in anaesthetics, operating techniques and recovery room skills. Liaison and support for clients and carers will be essential as older people will increasingly become the 'day trippers' of hospitals.

The Role of Self Care and Self Help Groups

The movement for self health care has emerged with vigour over the past decade. There are two levels: first, the increasing interest shown by individuals in taking positive action on behalf of their own health. This group is concerned with self care. Second, there has been a proliferation in the setting up of groups of people sharing particular health and social problems – these are known as self help groups.

The forces behind these expansions in self health care in older people's health are varied. Some of the most important reasons are:

- *greater awareness and interest in preventive medicine;*
- *the prevalence of chronic health problems;*
- *disillusionment with professional medical care;*
- *the resurgence of various forms of alternative medicine;*
- *awareness of the value of mutual aid and support.*

To some degree these developments also reflect the opinion that health issues need to be debated within the community as a whole, and that individuals should take a more direct input with environmental and service provisions, which affect their health.

Self care and self help, viewed in terms of individuals defining, planning and being responsible for health behaviour, is certainly not a new idea. Social trends during the 1960s and 1970s, both in America and Europe, provided a fertile base for the growth of these ideas. Some of the most important of these trends were:

- *the growth of the women's movement;*
- *the emergence of a powerful consumer lobby;*
- *the questioning of the medicalization of later life;*
- *a preoccupation with health and physical fitness.*

Kitson (1991) proposed a theoretical framework for gerontological nursing using the self care concept advanced by Orem (1971). In a critical analysis of Norton's geriatric nursing model, she moves away from the emphasis on medical diagnosis towards a more advanced nurse practitioner. In order that older people may be empowered to take up self care and be part of self care groups, individual clients need to:

- *learn more skills in observation;*
- *apply basic medical knowledge about common health problems;*
- *use health care resources effectively.*

All this may require a conceptual shift in both gerontological nursing programmes and within older people themselves. Self care education programmes could be staffed by disciplines other than nursing. Rather than have professional rivalry, it may be more productive to consider new roles in gerontological nursing such as the community health facilitator. This person would need to communicate effectively with a wide range of groups and individuals organizing and co-ordinating resources, acting as a mediating link between lay people, community organizations and health workers. Gormley (1994) sees self care in relation to older people as a return to negative nineteenth century values, seeing the introduction of quasi internal markets detrimental to older people who will be at the beck and call of philanthropy. However, accurate historical research of gerontological provision within that century does not confirm this. It perhaps is more accurate to question the impact of professionalization on the welfare and nursing care of older people within the twentieth century, if we are to begin to consider the impact politics and the economy has on nursing.

Social and Medical Policies

To some extent, new roles in gerontological nursing are emerging as a result of changes in national and local approaches to community care. The roots of these changes can be traced back many years, but the recent history starts with the House of Commons Social Services Selected Committee Report in 1985, followed by the Audit Commission's Report *Making a Reality of Community Care* in 1986. The most influential report, the Griffiths Report *Agenda for Action* appeared in March 1988. It immediately caused debate, with its transatlantic management system and its emphasis on local authorities being given responsibility for community care. During 1988, the Government issued a White Paper *Promoting Better Health* on primary care covering particularly the role of general practitioners. Arising from two further White Papers *Working for Patients* (1989) and *Caring for People*, new forms of care management systems were introduced.

Some have seen the *Caring for People* White Paper as being predominantly of interest to local authorities and *Working for Patients* as primarily of interest to the health service. The thrust of Government policy is to establish competition among the providers of health and social care, giving health authorities and local authorities an enabling role as commissioners of health and social services. One major dichotomy that has arisen is the issue of social care versus health care, which was laid at the feet of local authorities. Local authorities took responsibility for all social care, including purchasing and provision for residential and nursing homes. The gerontological nurse often acts as the 'go between' in these situations. It is desirable to provide community services to help people to continue to live in their own homes, but there has been an underplay on the need for appropriate residential and nursing home care.

In the health service the commission/supplier relationship is seen predominantly in the planning agreement established between district health authorities and their providers' units. Basing services on a range of contracts has both advantages and disadvantages. In principle, the nature of the contract depends on what the authorities, which may be the district health authorities, family health service authority or local authority, believe are needs that must be served. Often those needs are seen in different ways by different organizations.

A good example of how differing groups view need is the issue of older people and high technological therapies. In the past there has been the assumption that high technology was mostly used for younger clients, overlooking the appropriate need that many older clients have had for acute medical care. Any policy that could lead to rationing of high technology could disadvantage the older client, limiting access to necessary treatment. However, when older people are asked about technological interventions, such as cardiopulmonary resuscitation or dialysis, their goals are no different from the rest of the population.

Case Management

Case management in some ways can be seen as a Rorschach test for those who hear it. Each professional group tends to have an understanding of it based on his or her own setting and experience. Many see that it is a way of overcoming the fragmentations of service and duplication of care programmes, thus increasing co-ordination. Øvretveit (1993) sees case management as a natural progression from working within a team concept. In the Griffiths Report (1988) it was implied that case managers would carry out the process of care management; screening for priority clients; organizing a full assessment; planning; and co-ordinating how that plan was carried out. If nursing sees itself as the leading professional group to take this role on, then specific skills are required. At present, many models still require evaluation. Individual case management systems need to be designed to meet local circumstances. The benefit of case management for older people lies, it is thought, in individualizing care, helping clients to gain access to a compendium of services whilst staying at home. Callahan (1989), reviewing the research on case management in America, found it an inappropriate panacea, often motivated by reducing cost. Often in the push to promote case management styles, the consumer – the older person – is forgotten. Integrated care pathways are case management tools that involve the whole multidiscplinary team. Using a single plan of care the client will receive care from the multidisciplinary team in a co-ordinated manner.

Integrated Care Pathways or Care Maps

The idea is that an integrated care pathway, with mapping of care, identifies the nursing, medical and paramedical activities. This in turn informs all colleagues of what each member of the multidisciplinary team is doing. An example of a sample pathway is an integrated care pathway of a client who has had a myocardial infarction. The pathway is an attempt to amalgamate on one document and in practice all the core elements of care and treatments given by all disciplines. The pathway includes elements related to time, for example when to insert and remove a venflon, or when to take cardiac enzymes, but the client's care is not confined to the pathway and the individuality and condition of the client is recognized and cared for. When a client deviates from the pathway or care map, any such variances are documented, coded recorded and evaluated. Resulting information is used to assist in clinical audits, giving instant feedback to staff. The natural step is that the case manager who co-ordinates and manages that care is a nurse with the relevant clinical expertise. Skills are needed througout the care experience from before admission, to implementing care and engaging in discharge planning. If case management is to be employed within a setting that comprises older people new gerontological roles within a variety of settings are needed. These new gerontological nurse practitioners would have to:

- *be an identified case manager (a nurse) who has previously been a primary nurse, heading up case conferences;*
- *have skills in multidisciplinary integrated care mapping, organizing agreed pathways and variances which including a gerontological nursing perspective;*
- *be skilled in providing 'feedback systems' that looked at reasons for older patients deviating from pathways;*
- *be responsive to altered needs, that benefited the older client; these may include greater technological and social skills.*

The new gerontological nurse of the future will be multiskilled, taking a lead role in focusing care specifically to the needs of individual clients.

SUMMARY

Using primary sources, this chapter has replaced some of the myths surrounding previous views of old age. Legislation such as the Poor Law, patterns of care within families, and previous models of nursing care have been examined for their actual impact on older people and nursing. Oral histories and case studies have demonstrated the lack of a golden age of care. Nursing older people has always been complex, comprising diverse skills such as political awareness and manual dexterity. Many of the primary sources have produced positive examples of care, which have been sensitive and highly organized. An emerging theme from assessing the development of nursing older people within the community is the evidence that local communities had a collective responsibility towards older people that complemented and supported nursing initiatives. Gerontological nursing often forgets this heritage and should re-examine the close ties it has with the community. Past frameworks of caring, positive role models can be seen in workhouses and local models of nursing. The development of frameworks of nursing can, throughout the centuries, be seen to be at the behest of political social and economics change. This becomes more evident and creates tensions exacerbated by increased scientific and medical knowledge. Contemporary developments in the care of older people are exemplified by proactive nursing, with dynamic changes in nursing practice. During the last decade, developments such as nursing development units and primary nursing have increased the speciality's self esteem, benefiting patient care. This has been assisted by laterally thinking management and well-educated nurses, who spearhead new roles, thus developing new skills. The gerontological nurse practitioner is know poised to take on case management, cross boundaries and network globally.

CONCLUSIONS

Living and nursing within an environment of discontinuous change requires radical ways of thinking, planning and alterations in skill. Advancements in technology, economics and biotechnology will continue to challenge and develop gerontological nursing. Handy (1990) coined the phase 'upside down thinking' to describe changes in the way people need to think, plan, communicate and learn. Gerontological nurses are no exception, having greater experience in 'upside down thinking'. This chapter has demonstrated a heritage of radical thought through varied community care programmes, nursing development units and clinical research skills. Therefore, the future of gerontological nursing lies not just in crossing boundaries between disciplines but thinking and practising in varied ways. Sound sensitive computers, compact discs and video will radically alter the way gerontological nurses access information and plan care within a technologically sophisticated older population. Using various forms of networks, nurses may internet by superhighways, electronic mailing and video phoning to an array of disciplines and clients. This change in skills and practices will facilitate differing ways of problem solving, client monitoring, teaching and counselling. Where, and to whom, nursing takes place will change, nurses may use their own home, using a computer and facsimile to selected caseloads that could be international. Expertise invested within the gerontological nurse could then be disseminated and used in a far more effective way. This future would result in clients being more informed, with a plethora of expertise co-ordinated through a named nurse that is very easily contacted.

The uses of technology within gerontological nursing does not mean reduced contact, but contact of a different kind. Many older people will not go unnoticed and the impact of the 'Third Age' will become a considerable force within gerontological nursing itself. Older people may well have their own ministry and budget, consequently having a greater say in nursing. All these changes afford gerontological nursing greater diversity and varied approaches to care. To maximize on this potential, gerontological nursing must have a high expectation of itself. It must have strong achievable goals, with a clear sense of purpose. Standards of performance and outcomes of care must be set in conjunction with consumers (the older person's) preference. Boundary busting will not only benefit consumers but other professional groups, not only within health care. Future roles, for example consulting town planners, architects and travel companies, will be on the agenda of every gerontological nurse. The great advantage of being in a speciality that has new knowledge and language is the freedom it gives to develop an increasing maverick persona, therefore ensuring its survival.

CLINICAL DISCUSSION POINTS

Within your locality identify what patterns of informal care remain from before the introduction of the National Health Service.

Interview your clients to assess their perception of past and present nursing care.

Consider how far nursing development units have benefited gerantological nursing.

Keep a weekly diary of significant incidents that occur to you in practice. These may include clinical challenges and political changes. Discuss these with your manager at your performance review and include the most significant within your portfolio.

SUGGESTIONS FOR FURTHER READING

Texts on gerontological nursing and its development are few at present.

Dingwall, R., Rafferty, A. M. and Webster, C. (1988). **An Introduction to the Social History Of Nursing.** Routledge, London.
This book is a comprehensive analysis of the social history of nursing. Many of its themes give a voice to the ordinary person who provided care, as well as an indepth political critique of nursing politics.

Pelling, M. and Smith, R. (1991). **Life, Death and the Elderly**. Routledge, London.
This book uses a variety of primary sources to demonstrate the complex nature of ageing and provision of care from a historical perspective.

Webster, C. (1994). **Caring for Health: History and Diversity.** Open University Press, Milton Keynes.
The whole of this readable book has relevance for those interested in the development of gerontological nursing.

REFERENCES

Adams, J. (1991). Poor Law nursing in Northamptonshire from pauper to professional. **History of Nursing Society Journal 3** (5).

Adams, J. (1992). Master and matron work and marriage in the public assistance institution. **History of Nursing Society Journal 4** (3).

Audit Commission (1986). **Making a Reality of Community Care.** HMSO, London.

Butterworth, T. and Faugier, J. (1992). **Clinical Supervision and Mentorship in Nursing.** Chapman & Hall, London.

Benner, P. (1984). **From Novice to Expert.** Addison-Wesley, Wokingham, UK.

Black, M. (1993). **The Growth of Tameside Nursing Development Unit.** Kings Fund Centre, London.

Baker, D. (1978). Attitudes of Nurses to the Care of the Elderly. Unpublished PhD Thesis, University of Manchester.

Callahan, J. (1989). Case management for the elderly: A panacea? **Journal of Ageing and Social Policy 1** (2).

Dalley, G. (1988). **Ideologies of Caring.** MacMillan, London.

Davis, C. (1978). **Rewriting Nursing History.** Croom Helm, London.

Day Surgery Task Force (1993). **Day Surgery Report.** NHS Management Executive Baps, Publications Unit, Heywood Lancashire.

Dingwall, R., Rafferty, A. M. and Webster, C. (1988). **An Introduction to the Social History of Nursing.** Routledge, London.

Evers, H. K. (1984). Older women's self perception of dependency and some implications for service provision. **Journal of Epidemiology and Community Health 38,** 306–309.

Evers, H. K. (1990). The historical development of geriatric medicine as a speciality In: Johnson and Slater (Eds) **Ageing and Later Life,** pp. 102–110. Open University SAGE Publication, London.

Gormley, K. (1994). Self care and the elderly. **T.P.N. Update.** Issue No 2, September.

Goffman, E. (1961). **On the Characteristics of Total Institutions.** Essay on Asylums. Penguin, Harmondsworth.

Griffiths Report (1988). **Agenda for Action.** HMSO, London.

Himmelfarb, G. (1985). **The Idea of Poverty: England in the Early Industrial Age.** Faber, London.

Handy, C. (1990). **The Age of Unreason.** Arrow Books, London.

Harris, D. (1990). **Sociology of Ageing.** Harper & Row, New York.

Hockey, J. and James, A. (1993). **Growing Up and Growing Old.** Sage, London.

Home and Leisure Accident Research: Special Report on Accidents and Elderly People (1988). Consumer Safety Unit. Department For Enterprise.

Kitson, A. (1991). **Therapeutic Nursing and the Hospitalized Elderly.** Scutari Press, London.

Leonard, E. M. (1900). **The Early History of English Poor Relief.** Cambridge University Press, Cambridge.

MacLennon, W. J. (1993). The Future of Geriatric Medicine. **Hospital Update** (January).

Malby, R. (1992). Accredit where it's due. **Nursing Times 88** (43), 48–50.

McKee, P. and Kauppinen, H. (1987). **The Art of Ageing**. Insight Books, Human Science Press, New York.

Miller, A. (1979). A Study of Work Organisation by Nurses in Relation to Patient Outcomes in Geriatric Hospital Wards. Unpublished thesis. University of Manchester.

Norton, D., McLaren, R. and Exton Smith, A. W. (1962). **An Investigation Of Geriatric Nursing Problems in Hospital.** Churchill Livingstone, Edinburgh.

Orem, D. (1971). **Nursing: Concepts of Practice.** McGraw Hill, New York.

Øvretveit, J. (1993). **Co-ordinating Community Care.** Open University Press, Buckingham.

Pearson, A., Punton, S. and Durant, I. (1992). **Nursing Beds**. Royal College of Nursing Research Series. Scutari Press, London.

Pelling, M. and Smith, R. (Eds) (1991). **Life, Death and the Elderly.** Routledge, London.

Pelling, M. and Smith, R. (1992). **Life, Death and the Elderly.** Routledge, London.

Promoting Better Health (1987). White Paper, No 249, November 1987. HMSO, London.

Shaw, J. and Bosanquet, N. (1993). **A Way to Develop Nurses and Nursing-Development Units.** Kings Fund Centre, London.

Smith, J. E. (1986). Widowhood and ageing in traditional English society. **Ageing and Society 4** (4).

Summers, A. (1993). Hidden from history? The home care of the sick in the nineteenth century. **History Of Nursing Society Journal 4** (5), 227.

Thompson, D. (1983). The decline of social welfare: falling state support for the elderly since early Victorian times. **Ageing and Society 3** (1), 43–69.

Thompson, D. (1992). The welfare of the elderly in the past. In: M. Pelling and R. Smith (Eds) **Life, Death and the Elderly,** pp. 194–209. Routledge, London.

Thomson, P. (1990). Glimpses of a lost history In: J. Johnson and R. Slater (Eds) **Ageing and Later Life,** pp. 86.

Thompson, R. and Golding, G. (1975). **The Hospital: A Social and Architectural History.** Yale University Press, New Haven.

United Kingdom Central Council For Nurses, Midwives And Health Visitors (1992). **The Scope of Professional Practice.** UKCC, London.

Wade, L. (1992). The Impact of a Health Care Delivery System (Primary Nursing) on Older Women. Unpublished MA Thesis, Keele University.

Wear, A. (1986). Illness in strange places. **Paper Presented To The Welcome History Of Medicine Seminar,** January 29th.

Wells, T. (1980). **Problems in Geriatric Nursing Care.** Churchill Livingstone, Edinburgh.

White, R. (1978). **Social Change and the Development of the Nursing Profession: A Study of the Poor Law Nursing Service 1848/1948.** Henry Kimpton, London.

Wright, S. G. (1986). **Building and Using a Model of Nursing.** Edward Arnold, London.

Wright, S. J. (1992). The elderly and the bereaved in eighteenth century Ludlow. In: M. Pelling and R. Smith (Eds) **Life, Death and the Elderly,** pp. 102–114. Routledge, London.

Chapter Nine

Developing a Knowledge Base in Gerontological Nursing: A Critical Appraisal

Mike Nolan

Core Themes in Gerontological Nursing

Ageing Matters	New Social World	Lifespan Perspective	Health and Old People
Illness and Dependency	Quality Nursing Care	Therapeutic Intervention	Politicizing Gerontological Nursing

Key Words

Nursing Models • Knowledge Building • Mid-range Theory • Heterogeneity • Interdisciplinary Knowledge

INTRODUCTION

The central problem in geriatric nursing is the central problem in all of nursing: nurses do not know why they do what they do.
(Wells, 1980)

The above quotation, taken from an early and seminal study on the challenges facing nurses working with older people, highlights an enduring issue: what is the rationale underlying nursing care? Although the data on which Wells' conclusion is based are now 20 years old, her premise is as relevant today as it was then. The question, therefore, remains: is it still the case that most nurses 'do not know why they do what they do' or are nursing actions now underpinned by sound theoretical knowledge? This chapter reviews the development of theory in gerontological nursing, identifying both the progress that has been made and the work that has still to be undertaken. Such a review is both necessary and timely, as the context within which nursing operates is presently in a state of flux. In this rapidly evolving health care environment, the needs of older people are likely to become ever more prominent, both as a consequence of demography and the present policy emphasis on community care. The potential impact of such factors on nursing is significant and if the profession is to make an optimal contribution to the delivery of high quality care for older people, then there is an urgent need to take stock of the present position and to identify a way forward. The nature of such an undertaking, however, dictates that the exercise will raise more questions than it answers. Readers who approach this chapter looking for an 'off the shelf' model to apply to their practice will therefore be disappointed. No such model exists. Rather, it would be more accurate to say that models *do* exist, but these, as highlighted, are generally deficient and inadequate for the task in hand. The primary purpose of this chapter is to instil a questioning approach and hopefully to provide some pointers and likely directions for those who are inclined to follow them. This requires a constructively critical appraisal of the contribution of theory to nursing in general and to gerontological nursing in particular.

This Chapter aims to:

Provide a critical appraisal of the current knowledge base in gerontological nursing

Present a potential framework for building a more comprehensive knowledge base

Suggest a number of key concepts which might provide a focus for knowledge building in gerontological nursing.

NURSING THEORY: HELP OR HINDRANCE?

A number of authors have identified the considerable growth in the published literature describing the value of theory to the discipline of nursing (Walker and Avant, 1983; Meleis, 1991; Torres, 1990; Kenny, 1992). Such literature suggests that theory offers substantial benefits, which include an enhanced professional status, improved communication between practitioners, in addition to guiding practice, research and education (McFarlane, 1976; Craig, 1980; Torres, 1990; Draper, 1990; Chinn and Krammer, 1991; Meleis, 1991). However, despite such claimed advantages, a growing discontent is apparent, with many authors suggesting that theory has 'failed to deliver the goods' (Lewis, 1988; Moore, 1990; Girot, 1990; Ingram, 1991; Kenny, 1992). The tension between theory and practice stems in part from nursing's essentially vocational roots, with the antipathy towards theoretical knowledge being compounded by the often esoteric and abstract nature of much nursing theory (Meleis and Price, 1988). Miller (1985b) has argued that if experienced nurses cannot see the practical value of theory, then there is something wrong with either theory, practice, or both. However, debates as to the value of theory are not confined to nursing alone and are also apparent in other practice-based disciplines, such as social work (Lowenberg, 1984; Reay, 1986) and teaching (Carr, 1989; Elliot, 1991).

In suggesting a way forward, opinions tend to polarize, with some advocating that nursing should develop a unique body of knowledge that it can call its own (Draper, 1990; Torres, 1990), whereas others question both the desirability and possibility of achieving such an aim (McFarlane, 1976; Moore, 1990; Ingram, 1991). Discussions and disagreements are also apparent as to the type of theory that nursing should be striving to develop. Most of the better known nursing models (e.g. Orem, 1971; Roy, 1976; Roper et al., 1980), tend to operate at a very abstract level, often termed 'grand theory'. Such theories are broad in scope, supposedly offering an approach that is universally applicable. Meleis and Price (1988) term nurses using such models 'true believers', who 'attempt to fit all nursing knowledge, present and future, within this one theory...'. Recently, there has been considerable dissent amongst nurses, who question the usefulness of such highly abstract 'grand theories' suggesting that they are of limited value to nursing (Draper, 1990; Moore, 1990; Chinn and Krammer, 1991; Ingram, 1991; Kenny, 1992). The counter-argument is that the profession should seek to develop 'mid-range' theories that consider a smaller number of variables in particular situations (lower scope) and focus on practical problems (lower abstraction) (Clarke, 1986; Reed and Bond, 1991; Nolan and Grant, 1992). This divergence of opinion in the wider nursing literature is also reflected in the literature relating to the care of older people, which is equivocal as to the role and value of theory. In order further to develop the arguments outlined above and to place them in their current context, it is necessary to trace the historical development of nursing with older people.

WORKING WITH OLDER PEOPLE: THE NEED FOR A NURSING MODEL

The Royal College of Nursing (1993) contends that the health needs of older people are:

... among the most complex encountered within any health and social care setting, and nurses who work with older people have developed highly specialized understanding and skills to meet these needs.
(Royal College of Nursing, 1993)

Whilst few would argue with the first part of this statement, the latter half must be questioned and evidence provided that will sustain such a position. What are the 'specialized understanding and skills' that nurses possess and how are they developed and maintained? The contrast between what the Royal College of Nursing now believes to be the case and the situation described by Wells (1980) could not be starker, so which is closer to reality? Some of the most recent research (Armstrong-Esther *et al.*, 1994; Reed and Watson, 1994; Waters, 1994) belies the optimism reflected by the Royal College of Nursing and suggests that Wells' (1980) more pessimistic view is nearer the truth. On the basis of current research it seems that, despite some progress since Well's study, much of the nursing care received by older people today is still dominated by a routine approach that lacks a therapeutic and dynamic intention. Nolan (1994) contends that this situation is unlikely to improve until nurses working with older people clarify their sphere of activity and their role, both of which, he argues, are presently dominated by a pathological, illness-oriented model.

Evers (1991) believes that in order to understand how the nursing care of older people has evolved, reference must be made to the development of geriatric medicine as a distinct specialty. She contends that solutions to the problems faced by nurses working with older people will not be found until the relationship between medicine and nursing is explored fully and articulated clearly. From its inception in the 1930s and 1940s, geriatric medicine sought to create a new image and approach that would counter the pessimism surrounding the care of elderly patients that was prevalent at that time. Pioneering geriatricians illustrated what could be achieved in the former workhouses, rehabilitating long-stay clients and returning them to the community. However, as the specialty of geriatric medicine developed and entered the field of acute care, its continued growth and credibility depended upon demonstrating a turnover of clients (Wilkin and Hughes, 1986; Evers, 1991). Paradoxically therefore, long-term care which fostered and nurtured geriatric medicine in its early days is now an embarrassment (Evers, 1991), and geriatricians are increasingly distancing themselves from such a service. Today, long-term care of older people is in danger of disappearing from the National Health Service altogether (Age Concern, 1991).

The development of geriatric nursing (as it was then called) followed a similar path to medicine, focusing largely on the problems of care in hospital settings (Evers, 1991). The foundations of such an emphasis were laid in the first piece of gerontological nursing research in the UK (Norton *et al.*, 1962) and built upon by subsequent important studies (Baker, 1978; Wells, 1980). As a consequence, nurses working with older clients have tended to value 'cure', rather than 'care' and thereby failed to define appropriate goals for the 'non-cure patient who then suffered from aimless residual care' (Evers, 1991). Kitson (1984, 1986, 1988, 1991) believes that it is nursing's failure to value its caring role that is largely responsible for the poor care received by many older clients. She, together with other authors (Cormack, 1985; Wright, 1988), have argued for the need to develop an approach that is distinctly nursing and could differentiate the relative contributions of nursing and medicine.

This solution involved building a knowledge base for geriatric nursing centred upon nursing concepts in order to provide '... a dynamic and positive view of nursing care' (Cormack, 1985). The intention was that such concepts would '... relate less to patients' medical diagnosis and more to patients' nursing diagnosis and individual nursing needs' (Cormack, 1985). Taking a similar stance, Kitson (1984, 1991), argued for the development of a geriatric nursing model to 'organize, control and direct' the nursing care of older clients, a call reiterated by Wright (1988), who believed that such a model would identify and forge a 'common philosophy' and ensure a consistent approach to care. He states that:

> *Nurses therefore need nursing models that pull together their ideas in a coherent whole and guide them in what they do.*
> **(Wright, 1988)**

Reed and Robbins (1991) have highlighted the appeal of such an approach, suggesting that, as nursing is increasingly being required to describe and justify its actions, the use of models offers a way forward, providing a mechanism to both 'define and unify' nursing. However, whilst Reed and Robbins (1991) acknowledge the supposed advantages of abstract and generalized models, they are also highly critical, arguing that the models which have been developed to date have limited theoretical or empirical value. More often than not, such models are highly speculative and imprecisely stated so that key concepts are not adequately defined. Indeed, in analysing care plans based on the Roper *et al.* model (1980), Reed and Robbins (1991) discovered that 'prescribed care was so vaguely defined as to defy any evaluation'. If this is the case, it seems that Kitson (1984, 1991) was too optimistic in her belief that models would offer a mechanism to 'organize, control and direct' nursing care.

NURSING MODELS AND OLDER PEOPLE: A FAILURE WAITING TO HAPPEN?

If nursing models have generally failed to provide the hoped-for improvements to the care of older people, it is necessary to explore why. The roots of many of the ideas currently influencing the nursing care of older people can be traced to the early studies in this field (Norton *et al.*, 1962; Baker, 1978; Wells, 1980). Such studies highlighted the routine nature of most geriatric nursing, in which the care given was dominated by the need to 'get things done', rather than being designed to meet the individual needs of clients. Wells (1980) argued that nursing care addressed 'minimal universal needs', with Evers (1981) believing that nurses therefore 'warehoused' their clients, particularly those in non-acute settings where discharge was less likely. As a counter to such generally poor care, many authors heeded the call by Norton and colleagues (Norton *et al.*, 1962) to seek ways of individualizing nursing, so that the unique needs of each client could be identified and addressed.

Such a trend mirrored developments occurring in the wider profession, whereby individualized nursing care became universally approved (Reed, 1992). Allied to this aim was the introduction of a problem-solving approach to nursing, the nursing process, the benefits of which are widely extolled but have been little tested (Miller, 1984, 1985a,b). Therefore, largely as a reaction to poor care and the 'general gloom' which dominated many studies of older people from the 1960s onwards (Norton *et al.*, 1962, Baker, 1978; Wells, 1980; Evers, 1981; Miller, 1984, 1985a,b; Kitson, 1984, 1986), the touchstones of good care became characterized by the use of nursing models operating within the nursing process framework as a way of meeting the unique needs of individual clients (Cormack, 1985; Wright, 1988; Newtown, 1991; Kitson, 1991; Reed, 1992). Pursuing this line of reasoning, Wright (1988) contends that the universal themes underpinning high quality nursing for older people are individualized, personalized or client-centred nursing, linked with a problem-solving method of organizing care. He describes this in the following terms:

> *Essential to all nursing methods and nursing models, however, is the nursing process – a problem solving framework used to guide and direct a patient's care.*
> **(Wright, 1988)**

In this way, it is argued, problem-solving and care planning form the hallmarks of skilled professional nursing (Wright, 1988).

However, what has apparently escaped the attention of many are the striking parallels between such an approach and that adopted by geriatric medicine. This is illustrated by Kitson (1991), who describes the emergence of geriatric medicine in the following way:

> *A further guiding principle of the service (geriatric medicine) was that it was based on the acute medical model of care namely the problem solving approach to illness . . .*
> **(Kitson, 1991)**

Although some might argue that the nature of the problems to be solved in medicine and nursing are different, the guiding principles seem remarkably consistent. Herein lies one of the fundamental tensions and paradoxes in nursing's search for a theoretical and practical framework to shape the care of older people. For, while seeking to identify a distinct approach, nursing has none the less followed a path uncomfortably close to that of medicine. This may help to explain the relative failure of nursing models to deliver the hoped-for benefits, particularly in non-acute settings. A joint statement issued by the Royal College of Nursing, the British Geriatric Society and the Royal College of Psychiatrists in 1987 suggested that while the technical care received by older clients in hospital was frequently of the highest standards:

What is too often missing is a therapeutic approach which recognizes the personal, social and psychological implications of the illness.

It is just such an approach that nursing models were designed to promote, yet the latest research suggests that there has been only very limited progress (Waters, 1994; Armstrong-Esther *et al.*, 1994). Therefore, even in rehabilitation settings, it seems that 'a dependency-creating approach' is still all too apparent (Waters, 1994). Furthermore, despite placing a high value on interacting with their clients, nurses appear to spend very little time mixing with clients outside of routine care delivery. The fact remains that too often nursing in hospital settings still involves 'warehousing the elderly until they die' (Armstrong-Esther *et al.*, 1994).

As the best efforts to date have generally been less than successful in improving care, what is required is a re-evaluation of a number of key ideas so as to provide greater clarity and direction for nurses working with older people.

A POSITIVE ROLE FOR NURSING THEORY: A WAY FORWARD

Given the relative failure described above, a series of searching questions must be asked concerning the future role of nursing theory and strategies for knowledge generation in gerontological nursing. At the most fundamental level, our motives in seeking to develop nursing theory should be put under the spotlight and some soul searching is required in order to clarify what lies at the core of gerontological nursing.

The literature is fairly unequivocal in identifying that the drive to establish professional status for nursing was one of the primary factors motivating the development of nursing theory (Walker and Avant, 1983; Gruending, 1985; George, 1990; Torres, 1990; Girot, 1990; Ingram, 1991; Meleis, 1991). Meleis (1991), for example, states that '... theory is the goal of all scientific work ... and theoretical thinking is essential to all professional undertakings' and Torres (1990) considers that the development of a body of knowledge that can be applied to practice is a basic requirement for any professional discipline. In aspiring to professional status, nursing theorists therefore sought to develop a 'unique body of knowledge' that could be called 'nursing'. Moreover, being a relatively new scientific discipline, the early emphasis was placed on producing abstract and complex 'grand theories'. This presents something of a tension, however. For on the one hand, nursing claims to operate in an holistic fashion, providing individualized care, yet the vehicle for doing so has been through the use of models which focus more on the homogeneity of clients, rather than their heterogeneity. This contradiction has also been noted in other disciplines and was neatly summed up by Wilkin and Hughes (1986), who state:

... there is a basic conflict between the need for integrated health care which treats the whole person in his or her environment and the desire of the

professions to create a specialized knowledge base from which to exercise professional power and prestige.
(Wilkin and Hughes, 1986)

Recently, a number of nurses have questioned whether the professionalization of nursing should take precedence over the needs of clients (Gruending, 1985; Moore, 1990; Nolan, 1994), and such issues are not confined to nursing alone:

There is a need to begin a debate on the effectiveness of health care for the elderly and thus the sorts of service which might best achieve these. Central to this debate must be elderly people themselves and the health care professions other than medicine.
(Wilkin and Hughes, 1986)

Nolan (1994) has argued that the primary motivation for all service developments with older people *must* be a desire to improve the quality of the care they receive. This, he contends, will mean questioning nurses' role and function in working with older people. He postulates two main consequences of nursing's preoccupation with professionalization: *professional protectionism*: the tendency to defend that area of practice to which a discipline lays claim and *professional reductionism*; the tendency to reduce the focus of assessment or activity to a set of problems that are consistent with a particular professional paradigm.

In order to counter these tendencies, Nolan (1994) advocates that future efforts to develop a knowledge base to guide services for older people should abandon the search for 'the Holy Grail' of traditional scientific wisdom – the 'grand theory' – and focus instead on identifying and developing a range of concepts which, as Robinson (1992) suggests, will help nurses to 'understand and negotiate' their way around the health care world. Furthermore, in developing such concepts, the aim should not be to produce knowledge which is unique to nursing, but to build a core of practice which is of relevance to all those working with older people.

This stance is the opposite of that advocated by Kitson (1984, 1991) and these two differing perspectives reflect a debate that is still current in the nursing literature. For example, Bowser *et al.* (1993), in discussing the future agenda for nursing research involving frail older people, consider that:

If nursing is to take its place as a viable gerontological force, nursing research must be based in nursing theory. While the frameworks for other disciplines provide a valid theoretical base for research, the findings of studies conducted within non-nursing models do not contribute to the testing and development of nursing's theoretical base. For this reason, the knowledge base of gerontological nursing can only be extended through studies conducted within established nursing frameworks, or within thinking framed within a nursing perspective.
(Bowser et al., 1993)

In marked contrast is the position adopted by Phillips (1992), who differentiates between 'ageing research' and 'research on ageing'. She advocates that nursing should devote its time to the latter, which is 'designed to study the phenomenon of relevance to the experience of aging individuals'. This emphasis on the experience of older people themselves is consistent with a more holistic, less professionally reductionist approach. Furthermore, it also complements the current moves towards the application of consumerist principles in the Health Service.

It is suggested here that the way forward in building a more relevant knowledge base for nurses working with older people should be built upon three central premises:

- *knowledge building should begin from the perspectives of older people themselves;*
- *the search for a small number of 'grand theories' is not as useful as the definition and clarification of a wider range of less abstract, but more practice-relevant concepts;*
- *nursing should abandon its pursuit of a unique body of knowledge in favour of a more eclectic approach, which values and utilizes relevant knowledge no matter what its source.*

You may choose to disagree with one or all of these premises, but there is an emerging consensus in the literature, particularly with respect to the need to initiate knowledge building from the perspectives of older people (Redfern, 1991; Phillips, 1992; Dellasega, 1993; Royal College of Nursing, 1993). If this is accepted, then the other two premises become hard to deny.

STRATEGIES FOR BUILDING GERONTOLOGICAL KNOWLEDGE

If nurses working with older people have struggled to find a knowledge base to guide their practice, this is hardly surprising. As Redfern (1991) notes, society itself 'is still in the early stages of understanding and interpreting old age'. Furthermore, the whole notion of what constitutes nursing knowledge is still the subject of considerable debate, as are the methods that should be used to generate such knowledge (Rose and Parker, 1994).

Traditionally, there is seen to be a reciprocal link between research and theory (Meleis, 1991), yet despite the growth in gerontological nursing research, many of these studies lack an adequate theoretical basis (Murphy and Freston, 1991, Dellasega, 1993). Indeed, although national standards for gerontological nursing exist in the USA, these are not research based (Dellasega, 1993). Taking an opposing view, others would argue that nursing knowledge is not best derived from theory and research, but is a process of developing expertise by reflecting upon practice (Benner, 1984; Clarke, 1986; Dewing, 1990). If this is the case, then there would appear to be precious little in the way of such expert, reflective knowledge that has arisen from gerontological nursing practice.

A large number of strategies for the development and testing of knowledge have been suggested, but Meleis (1991) offers an approach that is readily comprehensible and can be applied in a variety of contexts. She rightly points out that there are no 'recipes' for knowledge building, 'no one way of doing it, nor is there a way by which the richness and haphazardness of the process can be fully captured'. She does, however, suggest seven stages, together with subprocesses, and these provide a useful framework. Meleis (1991) recognizes that knowledge building cannot be reduced to a simple linear process and that not all stages may occur and not necessarily in the order she provides. Nevertheless, there is a logic to her model which merits attention. The stages she describes are as follows:

- *taking in;*
- *description of phenomena;*
- *labelling;*
- *concept development;*
- *statement development;*
- *explicating assumptions;*
- *sharing and communicating.*

Taking In

Meleis (1991) defines taking in as 'a process for sizing up a situation that has attracted our attention for whatever reason'. The first stage of taking in is 'attention grabbing', when some event or subject commands our attention. This may often occur by chance or because of something that has been read or studied. Once something has 'grabbed' our attention, this is followed by a period of 'attention giving'. This is a more deliberate process of focusing on a particular subject or event.

Description

Meleis (1991) contends that the interest generated by the 'taking in' stage may 'gnaw' at someone over a period of time. During this period, the nurse asks a series of questions such as:

- *What is this event?*
- *When does it occur?*
- *What characteristics does it share with similar events?*
- *How does it differ from similar events?*

By asking such questions, the inquirer begins to build up a clearer picture of the subject of interest. Once this initial picture has been formulated, then a more precise description can be attempted. This may well lead to the stage of labelling.

Labelling

Meleis (1991) suggests that labelling always occurs at *some* stage in knowledge development, but that as the process unfolds, the label applied may change several times. The primary purpose of labelling is to produce a more precise and succinct description of the topic of interest, perhaps reducing a paragraph to a single statement or concept. Assuming that this label is now 'understood' by others, it makes ideas easier to convey and communicate. If appropriate, the label may also help to locate the subject of interest in a wider theoretical context.

Concept Development

According to Meleis (1991), a concept emerges once 'a complex constellation of impressions, perceptions and experiences' has become more organized and labelled. Several processes occur before a fully developed concept emerges and these include:

- *Defining – this is closely identified with labelling and helps to delineate the dimensions of a concept, clarify ambiguities and enable more precise definition.*
- *Differentiating – this involves the identification of the similarities and differences between the new concept and other similar ideas.*
- *Delineating antecedents – this involves identifying the factors which precede the concept.*
- *Delineating consequences – this involves identifying the results which follow from the concept.*

Building upon the above, Meleis (1991) also describes other processes which may occur in concept development, such as modelling, analogizing, and synthesizing, which help to lead to a more precise and clear understanding. Many would see the processes described so far as the *theory building* stage of knowledge development.

Statement Development

Once concepts have been developed and their antecedents and consequences identified, the stage of statement development is reached. This, according to Meleis (1991), is the further elaboration of the links between a concept, its antecedents and its consequences in order to explain, prescribe or predict events. This attempt to explain, prescribe and predict can be seen as the stage of *theory testing* and refinement.

Explicating Assumptions

Although formally presented by Meleis (1991) as the sixth process, she recognizes that explicating assumptions occurs at all stages. This involves pausing, reflecting and questioning the explicit and implicit assumptions underlying the developing theory, by 'reflection on and analysis of one's views, beliefs and theoretical underpinnings'. Ryan (1991) argues that explicating assumptions should be the first stage of knowledge building in gerontological nursing.

Sharing and Communicating

Meleis (1991) believes that this is a crucial stage and, indeed, that the whole process is incomplete without 'opportunities to share and communicate' knowledge with colleagues. This should not merely involve writing and publication, but rather should be 'defined as a daily happening in the lives of clinicians, theorists and researchers'.

Although the above description is a much condensed version of Meleis' persuasive arguments, it encapsulates the main ideas upon which her thinking is based.

APPLYING MELEIS' FRAMEWORK TO GERONTOLOGICAL NURSING

Applying Meleis' (1991) framework for knowledge development to the field of gerontological nursing provides a useful device to help map a way forward. At the present, it is clear that gerontological nursing practice remains poorly developed and lacks any real rationale. It is therefore legitimate to suggest that there is a need to rebuild the knowledge base so that it better reflects the needs and requirements of older people.

As Meleis (1991) suggested, her model was not intended to represent a linear progression, such that one step follows the preceding one, always in the same order. Nevertheless, there is a logic to the sequence she presents and this logic will be used to structure the next section – with one exception – that of explicating assumptions. Ryan (1991) believes that this should be the first stage in knowledge building, and this is a line with which the present author concurs. The basic premises upon which this chapter is built have already been stated, namely that:

- *there is a need to begin knowledge building from the older persons', rather than any professional, perspective;*
- *practice is best based upon a series of relevant concepts, rather than one or a few 'grand theories';*
- *knowledge is not the sole property of any given discipline: as Moody (1990) notes, 'knowledge has no surname'.*

Having stated these assumptions, the next consideration is to identify which factors nurses with older people should be 'taking in'. In other words, what is there to 'grab' our attention and to what areas should we subsequently 'give' our attention?

TAKING IN: GRABBING AND GIVING ATTENTION

If there is one central idea or concept that should be grabbing the attention of gerontological nursing, it is *heterogeneity*. That is, older people and the health care environments in which nursing operates are characterized more by the differences between people and contexts than the similarities.

Too often in the past, older people have been lumped together as a group – 'the elderly' (Wilkin and Hughes, 1986), suggesting that their needs and service responses to these needs are essentially similar. Certainly previous research and publications in the nursing care of older people reflects an obvious homogeneity, concerning itself largely with a hospital/illness orientated perspective. Two recent analyses of the published literature in gerontological nursing conducted independently in the USA (Dellasega, 1993) and the UK (Nolan, 1994) illustrate this point. Dellasega (1993) identifies an over-emphasis on institutionalized care in published literature and considers that mobility, cognition and incontinence account for the bulk of gerontological nursing studies in the USA. She is also of the opinion that gerontological nurses working in America are obsessed with their own attitudes. She advocates that nursing must move away from concepts such as self care and models such as that of Orem, towards concepts like empowerment, which are more holistic and less paternalistic.

Nolan (1994) similarly argues that nurses working with older people must expand their horizons. In analysing 1100 references from the International Nursing Index under the heading 'Geriatric Nursing', together with a more detailed consideration of 231 research studies on the computerized database Cinahl, he noted that:

> *52% of the studies had a hospital or institutional focus, compared to only 6% with any sort of community emphasis. Similarly, some 36% had a problem-orientated focus (21% physical problems, 15% relating to cognitive impairment), whereas only 6% had a psychological emphasis and 3% considered health ageing. Almost 4 out of 10 studies were orientated towards staff/professional issues such as attitudes, education, role and career development. This emphasis in recent published studies would not seem to reflect the commitment to holistic patient care that nursing espouses.*
> **(Nolan, 1994)**

These two analyses present a clear picture as to where nurse researchers and those publishing on the care of older people have focused their efforts. Relatively little has been published on issues outside of the hospital/institutional environment, with even less attention having been given to the role of nurses working with healthy older people. The role of the family with respect to older people has been similarly ignored.

Rempusheski (1991) contends that the gerontological nurse should not concentrate solely on nursing and health care, but must include social, political and economic factors also. If this is to happen, then we must widen the focus of the published literature and knowledge base.

Case Study: Attention grabbing

Accepting the need to broaden our conceptual horizons returns us to the notion of heterogeneity identified earlier. In applying this concept to the needs of older people, heterogeneity can be seen to apply in a number of contexts, including:

- *Demography. Older people span an age range of at least 40 years; however, various sections of the older population are increasing in number at different rates.*
- *Health needs. Health care is not restricted to the needs of the acutely ill older person. Healthy older people and those with chronic illnesses/disabilities have needs as well.*
- *The delivery and context of care. Care and services are delivered across a range of settings in both institutions and the community.*
- *The providers of care. The care needs of older people are met by informal carers, formal agencies and voluntary bodies, to name but a few. This constitutes the so-called 'mixed economy of care'.*
- *The organization of care. The care of older people crosses organization boundaries and divides. Even within individual agencies or authorities, the organization of care is becoming increasingly fragmented, a factor which tends to reinforce 'professional protectionism'.*
- *The philosophy of care. Political and economic factors are increasingly shaping the overall philosophy of care. Two major trends of particular relevance to older people are community care and consumerism.*

If the above constitute some of the main areas that should be 'grabbing' our attention at the moment, to which particular aspects should we be 'giving' attention?

GIVING ATTENTION: AREAS OF INTEREST TO GERONTOLOGICAL NURSING

Although the headings identified in the previous section will be used to provide a structure for what follows, this should be seen as a device to aid presentation. As will become apparent, many of the themes are interlinked and overlap.

Demography

As has been highlighted in an earlier chapter, the population of all countries of the world is ageing. This has significant implications for the delivery of health and nursing care.

In the UK, older people (those aged 65 and over) account for 41% of all NHS expenditure, making them not only the principal users of health services (Victor, 1991), but a major social and political issue in both organizational and humanitarian terms (Wilkin and Hughes, 1986). This challenge is not unique to the UK. While there is variation between countries and the rate of change is slower in some parts than others, the population of Europe is ageing. However, this ageing is not occurring consistently across differing age groups, with the most rapid and profound changes being amongst those aged 80+. This has a number of consequences, particularly the increase in the numbers and proportion of older people with dependency needs. Although definitions of dependency vary, approximately 10% of all people aged 65 or over have severe incapacity (Alber, 1993). However, between the ages of 60 and 69, this figure falls to about 5%, but rises to approximately 30% at the age of 80+ (Alber, 1993). The implications of this have not gone unnoticed:

> *The ageing of the population in Europe, especially the enormous increase in the very old, is a real challenge for all countries which want to provide security and well-being to the growing numbers of ageing individuals.*
> **(Dooghe, 1992)**

It is also a 'real challenge' for nurses working with older people.

Health Needs of Older People

As the previous discussion illustrated, the major emphasis among nurses working with older people has been placed on acute illness, within hospital settings. This has always been the most attractive area of work, providing the greatest job satisfaction for nurses, by enabling them to sustain a sense of 'therapeutic optimism' (Reed and Watson, 1994). Little attention has been given to work with both well older people and those with chronic conditions.

With the present Government emphasis on *The Health of the Nation* (DoH, 1991a), there is clear evidence that health promotion and allied concepts are increasingly being applied to older people. The Welsh Office (1993), in addressing the issue of health and social gain for older people, considers that there is a need:

> *To give explicit recognition to the fact that the well-being of older people involves more than simply physical, or even mental health, but extends to include their independence, self-fulfillment and dignity.*
> **(Welsh Office, 1993)**

Furthermore, concepts of health promotion and maintenance are not confined to currently healthy older people, but are increasingly seen as relevant to those with chronic conditions (Kaplun, 1992). Asvoll (1992) believes that chronic illnesses represent a major challenge for the health care systems of Europe and yet knowledge of chronic illness is not well developed, owing to the continued use of models of care designed for people with acute conditions (Pott, 1992). Nurses working with older people have not historically given chronic illness much attention (McBride, 1992), but there is growing recognition of the importance that such conditions play, with it being suggested that they are, or should be, at the 'heart of nursing' (Funk *et al.*, 1993).

Focusing attention on chronic illness returns us to the concept of *heterogeneity*. Unfortunately, health care disciplines, particularly medicine, tend to treat chronic conditions as being homogeneous (Rolland, 1988), yet nothing could be further from the truth. As Corbin and Strauss (1992) point out, what is required is an approach to nursing individuals with chronicity that recognizes the 'diversity, multiplicity and complexity of the problems that chronic conditions can bring'.

According to Woog (1992), nurses must engender a significant change in their attitudes towards chronic disease and the betterment of health. It is therefore useful to heed the advice of Verbrugge and Jette (1994), who assert that most people *live with*, rather than *die from* chronic conditions. Responding to needs of older people with chronic illness in order to help them *live with* their conditions is another challenge facing gerontological nurses.

The Context of Care

Heterogeneity extends to the contexts and settings in which care for older people is delivered. This has always posed something of a dilemma for both medicine and nursing. As discussed in the introduction to this chapter, the roots of geriatric medicine and nursing lie in long-stay environments. However, the search for professional status and recognition resulted in ever-greater attention and prestige being accorded to acute settings. Such developments now mean that continuing care environments in the Health Service are in danger of being abandoned altogether, and replaced by private sector provision. Furthermore, even in the acute sector, there is increasing integration of geriatric medicine with the acute medical services (Royal College of Physicians, 1994), a trend that will have obvious implications for nurses working in such settings.

The growth in the private nursing home sector has also not been without its problems, particularly the mounting concern about the standards of nursing care offered (UKCC, 1994).

The challenges such changes pose for gerontological nurses must not be underestimated. It is well established that most nurses, even those working in non-acute environments, value a curative orientation, even when this is inappropriate (Reed and Bond, 1991; Reed and Robbins, 1991; Reed and Watson, 1994). Such a value system is reinforced by the problem-solving emphasis within most nursing models. There is therefore a pressing need for nurses to clarify the values guiding the care of older people in *different* settings (Reed and Bond, 1991). Although there has been a general rejection of the 'medical model' as being reductionist, this approach is, in fact, quite appropriate where it meets the wishes and needs of patients (Reed and Watson, 1994). On the other hand, it is counter-productive in longer-term settings. Identifying relevant concepts for differing contexts and articulating them with clarity and precision must be another primary aim of any attempt to build a knowledge base for gerontological nursing.

The Providers of Care

There is no doubt that the majority of care received by older people is provided by so-called 'informal or lay carers', usually close family (Twigg and Atkin, 1994). The current UK government policy of community care has focused renewed attention on the needs of family carers, so that they are no longer the cinderellas of the policy arena (Twigg and Atkin, 1994). However, until fairly recently, nurses have tended to 'neglect' family carers (Nolan and Grant,

1989). This situation is slowly changing and there is an expanding literature on nursing interventions with families across the age span. While models and frameworks are emerging and being empirically tested, more work is still required in this area, particularly focusing on service outcomes for family carers (Nolan *et al.*, 1994).

Another important area to which gerontological nurses should be giving attention is the interface between primary and secondary care and between various professional groupings. One radical approach that has been suggested by Hollingberry (1993) is the creation of a new 'trans-disciplinary profession'. Although he does not deny the need for discipline-specific expertise, Hollingberry (1993) believes that much of the care of older people could be delivered by an appropriately trained and qualified but generic worker – *the Gerocomist*. If the phrase is somewhat clumsy and inelegant, the concept has much to commend it. Gerocomy is derived from 'old age tending', as opposed to geriatric (old age treatment) and is therefore a more appropriate basis for intervening with many older people. Hollingberry argues for the identification of 'shared core knowledge' necessary to deliver effective care to older people, that can be taught to all professionals wishing to work with such individuals. Upon qualification, practitioners could develop more specialist and expert roles, but always building on the same basic preparation. Such a development might be seen as too radical by many, but there is no doubt that the concept of joint training and learning at both pre- and post-qualification levels is one that merits further exploration.

The Organization of Care

Responsibility for the organization and delivery of care for older people has always been a 'grey' area, as it is difficult to disentangle the myriad of needs and to label them under either health or social care. If separation at this broad level poses difficulties, it is even more challenging and contentious to identify the role of nursing, physiotherapy, occupational therapy and so on. This is perhaps one reason why multidisciplinary teamwork has long been seen as essential to the delivery of good care (RCN, 1987). However, despite espousing the ideals of multidisciplinary working, its benefits in practice have rarely been demonstrated (Evers, 1981; Øvretveit, 1993).

Existing difficulties have been further compounded by the provisions of the Community Care Act (DoH, 1991b), which gave lead responsibility for the meeting of chronic needs to local authorities. Furthermore, even within the same organizations, the creation of purchaser/provider roles and the emergence of NHS Trusts have further fragmented previously established patterns of working. This represents another significant factor requiring the attention of nursing working with older people.

The Philosophy of Care

The pan-European dimension of the ageing population was alluded to earlier and it seems that policy responses to this challenge are consistent across Europe, with moves towards the community care of older people and the most cost-effective use of scarce health resources (Dooghe, 1992; Walker *et al.*, 1993). Mirroring these developments in many countries, there has been a widening health agenda based on strategies of health promotion and targets for health.

The push towards community care is based on both ethical/moral (older people would prefer to live at home) and economic (it's cheaper) arguments. It is also part of the political orthodoxy which asserts that responsibility for the dependent members of a society lies primarily with the family. This, in many ways, is consistent with Reed's (1992) critique of the idea of individualized nursing care which, she argues, ignores wider community and societal issues. Whatever the philosophical basis of such positions, there are obvious practical implications for those working with older people, particularly when it is remembered that the drive towards community care and the subsequent reduction in all forms of residential/institutional provision is occurring at the same time as the increase in the numbers of very frail older people, who are significantly more likely to require such placements.

Once consequence of these developments is that entry to an institutional environment will increasingly be viewed as a last resort and will not be considered until absolutely necessary. Admissions to care will therefore be increasingly made at a time of crisis, often from an acute hospital setting (Nolan, 1994). Patients and carers are more likely than ever to turn to nurses for advice and information – how well prepared are we to give it?

The above represent just some of the challenges currently facing gerontological nurses. However, they help to identify areas to which we must turn our attention if we are to develop a sufficient knowledge-base for us to respond effectively to the needs of older people and their carers.

DESCRIPTION, LABELLING AND CONCEPT DEVELOPMENT: PROGRESS AND PROSPECTS IN GERONTOLOGICAL NURSING

The lack of clarity with which the key concepts in nursing models have been defined has been highlighted as a major problem (Reed and Robbins, 1991), and Robinson (1992) believes that greater precision in identifying concepts is the best way forward for building a knowledge base for nursing care. To use Meleis' (1991) framework, this will require description, labelling and concept development. It is therefore encouraging to note that the nursing literature in general, and the gerontological nursing literature in particular, is giving greater attention to concept development. A quick trawl through just one journal (*Journal of Advanced Nursing*) revealed the following concepts in only a few months: dignity (Mairis, 1994); expert (Jasper, 1994); humour (Astedt-Kurki and Liukhonen, 1994); self-efficacy (Mowat and Laschinger, 1994); empowerment (Shelton, 1994); comfort (Morse *et al.* 1994); and failure to thrive (Newbern and Krowchuk, 1994).

It is interesting to note that the latter concept 'failure to thrive', usually associated with children, was in this case being applied to older people. This illustrates the value of the cross-fertilization of ideas. Other important concept that have particular relevance for work with older people include: rust out and therapeutic reciprocity (Nolan and Grant, 1992);

powerlessness and how to overcome it (Miller, 1992); pain (Closs, 1994); and hope (Forbes, 1994). However, probably one of the most significant concepts is that of rehabilitation.

Phipps and Kelly-Hayes (1991) suggest that rehabilitation is a 'philosophical theme' that underlies all aspects of care with older people regardless of the care setting. Certainly, issues surrounding rehabilitation in nursing have been the focus of considerable recent attention (Waters, 1994; Williams, 1994; Royal College of Nursing, 1994), and there is a growing awareness of the need to take a broader approach. Therefore, the key elements in the *Role of the Nurse in Rehabilitation of Elderly People* (Royal College of Nursing, 1991) as outlined by Waters (1994) include: intimate care; personal hygiene; care of the skin, including wound care; bowel and bladder function; provision of adequate nutritional intake; prevention of complications and promotion of self-medication. In just 3 years, however, thinking seems to have moved on considerably and in the latest document *Standards of Care: Rehabilitation Nursing* (Royal College of Nursing, 1994), it is acknowledged that previous definitions of the role of the nurse have been too limited and 'tended to focus on disability and illness, rather than health and wellness'. It is considered that such an approach is no longer appropriate and that there is a need to shift the focus away from disability and towards handicap (Royal College of Nursing, 1994). This, however, will pose its own problems, not least of which is the lack of agreement as to what the concepts of disability and handicap actually mean. Verbrugge and Jette (1994) contend that the literature on disability lacks a well-accepted conceptual scheme and, in fact, contains a 'bedlam vocabulary', in which terms have been invented and defined in numerous conflicting ways. They argue for the development of a conceptual scheme, which they define as:

... a rudimentary scientific model that guides terminology, measurement and hypothesis. It is the basic architecture on which research, policy and clinical care are built.
(Verbrugge and Jette, 1994)

Here then lies one of the major challenges for gerontological nursing – to define and clarify the meaning of rehabilitation. Returning to Hollingberry's (1993) arguments, this process should result in the generation of a 'shared core knowledge' with regards to rehabilitation. This means that the process of definition cannot successfully be undertaken by nurses alone. This is recognized by the Royal College of Nursing, who call for *interdisciplinary*, as opposed to simply *multidisciplinary* collaboration. Interdisciplinary working requires far closer collaboration and the breaking down of professional protectionism and professional reductionism.

Moving on from concepts, there are also some relevant models or conceptual schemes emerging, which might help to provide some of the 'basic architecture' for nurses working in a variety of contexts with older people and their carers. For example, Nolan *et al.* (1995) have extended the work of Bowers (1987, 1988), and present a typology of family caregiving. Bowers (1987, 1988) believed that definitions of family care used by professionals focused mainly on the *tasks* of care; that is, what carers actually do. She argued that the definition of care should focus on the *purpose* of care; that is, the motivation and reason behind carers' actions. Building on this work, Nolan *et al.* (1995) present eight different types of care given by family carers. They contend that if nurses and other service providers are not aware of the type of care that is being given, then their interventions can be counterproductive and are likely to be rejected. While not yet presented as a fully developed model or theory, typologies of this sort are a stage further on from concept development.

There are also some lesser-known but potentially very useful models of care available. The importance of responding adequately to the needs of older people with chronic illnesses has already been identified and Corbin and Strauss (1992) describe a model for this purpose. Although it is called the 'Corbin and Strauss nursing model' (Woog, 1992), it was, in fact, not developed as such. Indeed, the originators themselves argue that:

> *This research-based knowledge was never designed to be discipline bound; rather it was intended for use by any discipline in whatever manner might correspond to its purposes and functions.*
> **(Corbin and Strauss, 1991)**

They outline what they term a 'trajectory model' which, they suggest, will overcome the limitations of previous nursing interventions with chronic illness, namely that they have been too:

- *illness-specific; and*
- *focused on certain problems.*

The basic principle in their model is that any approach to chronic illness must take account of its variety and the way it changes over time. They believe that the purpose of intervening in chronic illness is to shape and manage the temporal dimension of illness. The model they outline is a potentially very useful one and they challenge nurses to adopt it and apply it to their practice. However, in doing so, Corbin and Strauss (1991) do not advocate that the model is seen as a static entity, but urge that nurses broaden it by 'adding new concepts and further developing and refining others'. This is sound advice with respect to any knowledge that gerontological nurses might use or develop.

CONCLUSIONS: NEW KNOWLEDGE: NEW DIRECTIONS

Johnson (1991) has argued that researchers working in gerontology in general have been guilty of perpetuating the myth that old age is a period of inevitable decline, because they have focused their research endeavours on the problems of ageing. The same could be said to be true of nursing. Acute illness will always be a significant part of health care, but there are wider issues, as this chapter has tried to illustrate.

The Royal College of Nursing (1993) have sought to highlight the value and skill of nurses working with older people, and there is no doubt that such work is amongst the most challenging and rewarding that nursing has to offer. For, although we cannot say with 'hand on heart' that nurses always know 'why they do what they do', there is enormous potential for further development. Nurses working with older people must continue to expand their knowledge and their role. We must be proactive in seeking better ways to deliver services and care. Norton *et al.* (1962) stated that the fundamental purpose of their study was to 'establish a new approach to the nursing care of the elderly patient'. New approaches are constantly required as we learn better to understand the needs of older people. The book is presented as a foundation text, and foundations are there to be built upon. It is hoped that this chapter has achieved its aims of instilling a questioning approach and providing some pointers and likely directions for building a knowledge base for gerontological nursing. Those of you who might be inclined to follow this path may not have an easy journey, but it will certainly be a stimulating and rewarding one.

CLINICAL DISCUSSION POINTS

Do you think that mid-range theories provide the most effective way to narrow the theory–practice gap in gerontological nursing?

'Nursing's search for a "unique body of knowledge" inhibits interdisciplinary collaboration and is not in the best interest of patient care'. Discuss this view with colleagues.

Consider whether chronic illnesses represents the greatest challenge to nurses working with older people.

SUGGESTIONS FOR FURTHER READING

Bowers, B. J. (1987). Inter-generational caregiving: adult caregivers and their aging parents. **Advances in Nursing Science 9**(2), 20–31.
An important paper highlighting both the usefulness of grounded theory methodology whilst also presenting an alternative view of the nature and meaning of family care.

Bowser, J., Bramlett, M., Burnside, I. M. and Gweldner, S. H. (1993). Methodological considerations in the study of frail elderly people. **Journal of Advanced Nursing 18**, 873–879.
Argues for the adoption of a rigorous and nursing-led approach to research and theory building in gerontological nursing.

Evers, H. K. (1981). Multi-disciplinary teams in geriatric wards: myth or reality? **Journal of Advanced Nursing 6**, 205–214.
An early and seminal paper looking at multidisciplinary working that is still very relevant today.

Meleis, A. I. (1991). **Theoretical Nursing: Developments and Progress**, 2nd edn. Lippincott, Philadelphia.
For an expanded version of the theory building model outlined in this chapter.

Nolan *et al.* (1995). Developing a typology of family care: implications for nurses and other service providers' **Journal of Advanced Nursing 21**(2), 256–265.
A paper which develops further the model of family caring suggested by Bowers (1987) and considers its implications for service development.

Reed and Watson (1994). The impact of the medical model on nursing practice and assessment. **International Journal of Nursing Studies 31**(1), 57–66.
An interesting and well-argued paper which considers the interface between nursing and medicine.

Rolland, J. S. (1988). A conceptual model of chronic and life threatening illness and its impact on families. In: C. S. Chilman, E. W. Nunnally and F. M. Cox (Eds) **Chronic Illness and Disabilities,** pp. 17–68. Families in Trouble Services, 2. Sage, Beverly Hills.
An excellent consideration of the nature of chronic illness which presents a comprehensive model of the disease process and identifies the implications of such a model for the development of better services. At 50+ pages it is a demanding but rewarding read.

Royal College of Nursing (1994). **Standards of Care: Rehabilitation Nursing.** Royal College of Nursing, London.
Worth a read to obtain an insight into the changing definition of rehabilitation. Read this reference in conjunction with the paper by Verbrugge and Jette and the need for a clear and unequivocal definition of rehabilitation soon becomes apparent.

Waters, K. (1994) Getting dressed in the morning: styles of staff/patient interaction on rehabilitation hospital wards for elderly people. **Journal of Advanced Nursing 19**, 239–248.
A telling account of how little actually seems to have changed in the past 30 years!

Wilkin, D. and Hughes, B. (1986). The elderly and the health services. In: C. Phillipson and A. Walker (Eds) **Ageing and Social Policy: A Continual Assessment,** pp. 163–183. Gower, Aldershot.
Traces the development of geriatric medicine from a sociological perspective and highlights the influence that the past can still exert on the present.

REFERENCES

Alber, J. (1993). Health and social services. In: A. Walker, J. Alber and A. M. Guillemard (Eds) **Older People in Europe: Social and Economic Policies,** pp. 100–133. The 1993 Report of the European Observatory, Commission of the European Communities.

Age Concern (1991). **Under Sentence: Continuing Care Units for Older People Within the National Health Service.** Age Concern, London.

Armstrong-Esther, C. A., Browne, K. D. and McAfee, J. G. (1994). Elderly patients; still clean and sitting quietly. **Journal of Advanced Nursing 19**, 264–271.

Astedt-Kurki, P. and Liukhonen, A. (1994). Humour in nursing care. **Journal of Advanced Nursing 20**(1), 183–188.

Asvoll, J. E. (1992). Foreword. In: A. Kaplun (Ed.) **Health Promotion and Chronic Illness: Discovering a New Quality of Health,** IX–X. WHO (Europe), Copenhagen.

Baker, D. E. (1978). Attitudes of Nurses to the Care of Elderly People. Unpublished PhD Thesis, University of Manchester.

Benner, P. (1984). **From Novice to Expert: Excellence and Power in Clinical Nursing Practice.** Addison-Wesley, Menlo Park, California.

Bowers, B. J. (1987). Inter-generational caregiving: adult caregivers and their aging parents. **Advances in Nursing Science 9**(2), 20–31.

Bowers, B. J. (1988). Family perceptions of care in a nursing home. **Gerontologist 28**(3), 361–367.

Bowser, J., Bramlett, M., Burnside, I. M. and Gweldner, S. H. (1993). Methodological considerations in the study of frail elderly people. **Journal of Advanced Nursing 18,** 873–879.

Carr, W. (1989). Action research: ten years on. **Curriculum Studies 21**(1), 85–90.

Chinn, P. L. and Krammer, M. K. (1991). **Theory and Nursing: A Systematic Approach,** 3rd edn. Mosby Year Book, St Louis.

Clarke, M. (1986). Action and reflection: practice and theory in nursing. **Journal of Advanced Nursing 11,** 3–11.

Closs, S. J. (1994). Pain in elderly people: a neglected phenomenon. **Journal of Advanced Nursing 19**(6), 1072–1081.

Corbin, J. M. and Strauss, A. (1992). A nursing model for chronic illness management based upon the trajectory framework. In: P. Woog, (Ed.) **The Chronic Illness Trajectory Framework,** pp. 9–28. Springer, New York.

Cormack, D. (Ed.) (1985). **Geriatric Nursing: A Conceptual Approach.** Blackwell Scientific, Oxford.

Craig, S. L. (1980). Theory development and its relevance for nursing. **Journal of Advanced Nursing 5,** 349–355.

Dellasega, C. (1993). Nursing research on older adults: a transatlantic perspective. International Network Conference, Jonkoping, December 1993.

Department of Health (DoH) (1991a). **Health of the Nation: A Consultative Document for Health in England.** HMSO, London.

Department of Health (1991b). **NHS and Community Care Act.** HMSO, London.

Dewing, J. (1990) What a relief. **Nursing Times 86**(8), 43–45.

Dooghe, G. (1992). The ageing of the population in Europe: socio-economic characteristics of the elderly people. Commission of the European Communities, Brussels.

Draper, P. (1990). The development of theory in British nursing: current position and future prospects. **Journal of Advanced Nursing 15**, 12–15.

Elliot, J. (1991). **Action Research for Educational Change.** Open University Press, Milton Keynes.

Evers, H. K. (1981). Multi-disciplinary teams in geriatric wards: myth or reality? **Journal of Advanced Nursing 6**, 205–214.

Evers, H. K. (1991). Care of the elderly sick in the UK. In: S. J. Redfern (Ed.) **Nursing Elderly People,** pp. 417–436. Churchill Livingstone, Edinburgh.

Forbes, J. (1994). Hope: an essential human need in the elderly. **Journal of Gerontological Nursing 20**(6), 5–10.

Funk, S. G., Tornquist, E. M., Champagne, M. T. and Wiese, R. A. (1993). **Key Aspects of Caring for the Chronically Ill.** Springer, New York.

George J. B. (Ed.) (1990). **Nursing Theories: The Base of Professional Practice,** 3rd edn. Prentice Hall, New Jersey.

Girot, E. (1990). Discussing nursing theory. **Senior Nurse 10**(6), 16–19.

Gruending, D. C. (1985). Nursing theory: a vehicle for professionalization. **Journal of Advanced Nursing 10**, 553–558.

Hollingberry, R. (1993). Gerocomist – a new trans-disciplinary profession. Paper given at the British Society of Gerontology Conference, Norwich, 1993.

Ingram, R. (1991). Why does nursing need theory? **Journal of Advanced Nursing 16**, 350–353.

Jasper, M. A. (1994). Expert: a discussion of the implications of the concept as used in nursing. **Journal of Advanced Nursing 20**(4), 769–776.

Johnson, M. L. (1991). The meaning of old age. In: S. J. Redfern (Ed.) **Nursing Elderly People,** 2nd edn., pp. 3–18. Churchill Livingstone, Edinburgh.

Kaplun, A. (1992). **Health Promotion and Chronic Illness: Discovering a New Quality of Health.** WHO (Europe), Copenhagen.

Kenny, T. (1992). Nursing models fail in practice. **British Journal of Nursing 2**(2), 133–136.

Kitson, A. L. (1984). Steps Towards the Identification and Development of Nursing's Therapeutic Function in the Care of the Hospitalised Elderly. Unpublished DPhil Thesis. University of Ulster, Belfast.

Kitson, A. L. (1986). Indicators of quality in nursing care: an alternative approach. **Journal of Advanced Nursing 11**: 133–144.

Kitson, A. L. (1988). Something special. **Geriatric Nursing and Home Care 8**(6), 20–22.

Kitson, A. L. (1991). **Therapeutic Nursing and the Hospitalized Elderly.** Scutari Press, London.

Lewis, T. (1988). Leaping the chasm between theory and practice. **Journal of Advanced Nursing 13**, 345–351.

Lowenberg, F. M. (1984). Professional ideology, middle range theories and knowledge building for social work practice. **British Journal of Social Work 14**, 309–322.

McBride, A. B. (1992). Managing chronicity: the heart of health care. In: S. G. Funk *et al.* (Eds) **Key Aspects of Caring for the Chronically Ill,** pp. 8–20. Springer, New York.

McFarlane, J. K. (1976). The role of research and the development of nursing theory. **Journal of Advanced Nursing 1**, 443–451.

Mairis, E. D. (1994). Concept clarification in professional practice. **Journal of Advanced Nursing 19**(5), 947–953.

Meleis, A. L. (1991). **Theoretical Nursing: Developments and Progress,** 2nd edn. Lippincott, Philadelphia.

Meleis, A. I. and Price, M. J. (1988). Strategies and conditions for teaching theoretical nursing: an international perspective. **Journal of Advanced Nursing 13**, 592–604.

Miller, A. (1984). The nursing process and patient care. **Nursing Times (Occasional Papers) 179**(25), 56–58.

Miller, A. (1985a). A study of the dependency of elderly patients in wards using different methods of nursing care. **Age and Ageing 14**, 132–138.

Miller, A. (1985b) Nurse/patient dependency: is it iatrogenic? **Journal of Advanced Nursing 10**, 63–69.

Miller, J. F. (1992). Concept development of powerlessness: a nursing diagnosis. In: J. F. Miller (Ed.) **Coping with Chronic Illness: Overcoming Powerlessness,** pp. 50–82. F. A. Davis, Philadelphia.

Moody, L. E. (1990). **Advancing Nursing Science Throughout Research,** Vol 1. Sage, Newbury Park, California.

Moore, S. (1990). Thoughts on the discipline of nursing as we approach the year 2000. **Journal of Advanced Nursing 15**, 825–828.

Morse, J. M, Botroff, J. L. and Hutchison, S. (1994). The phenomenology of comfort. **Journal of Advanced Nursing, 20**(1), 189–195.

Mowat, J. and Laschinger, H. K. S. (1994). Self-efficacy in caregivers of cognitively impaired elderly people: a concept analysis. **Journal of Advanced Nursing 19**(6), 1105–1113.

Murphy, E. and Freston, M. (1991). An analysis of theory–research linkages in published gerontologic nursing studies. **Advances in Nursing Science 13**(4), 1–13.

Newbern, V. B. and Krowchuk, H. U. (1994). Failure to thrive in elderly people: a conceptual analysis. **Journal of Advanced Nursing 99**(5), 840–849.

Newtown, C. (1991). **The Roper, Logan and Tierney Model in Action,** Macmillan, Basingstoke.

Nolan, M. R. (1994). Geriatric Nursing: an idea whose time has gone: a polemic. **Journal of Advanced Nursing 20**, 989–996.

Nolan, M. R. and Grant, G. (1989). Addressing the needs of informal carers: a neglected area of nursing practice. **Journal of Advanced Nursing 14**, 950–961.

Nolan, M. R. and Grant, G. (1992). Mid-range theory building and the nursing theory practice gap: a respite care case study. **Journal of Advanced Nursing 17**, 217–223.

Nolan, M. R. Grant, G. Caldock, K. and Keady, J. (1994). **A Framework for Assessing the Needs of Family Carers: a Multi-disciplinary Guide.** BASE Publications, Stoke-on-Trent.

Nolan, M. R., Keady, J. and Grant, G. (1995). Developing a typology of family care: implications for nurses and other service providers' **Journal of Advanced Nursing 21**(2), 256–265.

Norton, D., McClaren, R. and Exton-Smith, A. N. (1962). **An Investigation of Geriatric Nursing Problems in Hospital.** Research Report NCCOP, Reprinted 1979. Churchill Livingstone, Edinburgh.

Orem, D. E. (1971). **Concepts of Practice.** McGraw Hill, New York.

Øvretveit, J. (1993). **Co-ordinating Community Care: Multidisciplinary Teams and Care Management.** Open University Press, Buckingham.

Phillips, L. R. (1992). Challenges of nursing research with the frail elderly. **Western Journal of Nursing Research 14**(6), 721–730.

Phipps, M. A. and Kelly-Hayes, M. (1991). Rehabilitation of older adults. In: E. M. Baines (Ed.) **Perspectives on Gerontological Nursing,** pp. 357–372. Sage, Newbury Park, California.

Pott, E. (1992). Preface. In: A. Kaplun (Ed.) **Health Promotion and Chronic Illness: Discovering a New Quality of Health,** XI–XV. WHO (Europe), Copenhagen.

Reay, R. (1986). Bridging the gap: a model for integrating theory and practice. **British Journal of Social Work 16**, 49–64.

Redfern, S. J. (1991). **Nursing Elderly People,** 2nd edn. Churchill Livingstone, New York.

Reed, J. (1992). Individualised nursing care: some implications. **Journal of Clinical Nursing** 1(1), 7–12.

Reed, J. and Bond, S. (1991). Nurses' assessment of elderly patients in hospital. **International Journal of Nursing Studies 28**(1), 55–64.

Reed, J. and Robbins, I. (1991). Models of nursing: their relevance to the care of elderly people. **Journal of Advanced Nursing 16,** 1350–1357.

Reed, J. and Watson, D. (1994). The impact of the medical model on nursing practice and assessment. **International Journal of Nursing Studies 31**(1), 57–66.

Rempusheski, V. F. (1991). Historical and futuristic perspectives on aging and the gerontological nurse. In: E. M. Baines (Ed.) **Perspectives on Gerontological Nursing,** pp. 3–28. Sage, Newbury Park, California.

Robinson, J. J. A. (1992). Problems with paradigms in the caring profession. **Journal of Advanced Nursing 17,** 632–638.

Rolland, J. S. (1988). A conceptual model of chronic and life threatening illness and its impact on families. In: C. S. Chilman, E. W. Nunnally and F. M. Cox (Eds) **Chronic Illness and Disabilities,** pp. 17–68. Families in Trouble Services, 2. Sage, Beverly Hills.

Roper, N., Logan, W. and Tierney, A. (1980). **The Elements of Nursing.** Churchill Livingstone, Edinburgh.

Rose, P. and Parker, D. (1994). Nursing: an integration of the art and science within the experience of the practitioner. **Journal of Advanced Nursing 20,** 1004–1010.

Roy, C. (1976). **Introduction to Nursing: An Adaptation Model.** Prentice Hall, New Jersey.

Royal College of Nursing, British Geriatric Society & Royal College of Psychiatrists (1987). **Improving Care of Elderly People in Hospital.** Royal College of Nursing, London.

Royal College of Nursing (1991). **The Role of the Nurse in Rehabilitation of Elderly People.** Scutari Press, London.

Royal College of Nursing (1993). **The Value and Skill of Nurses Working with Older People.** Royal College of Nursing, London.

Royal College of Nursing (1994). **Standards of Care: Rehabilitation Nursing.** Royal College of Nursing, London.

Royal College of Physicians (1994). **Ensuring Equity and Quality of Care for Elderly People.** Royal College of Physicians, London.

Ryan, J. E. (1991). Building theory for gerontological nursing. In: E. M. Baines (Ed.) **Perspectives on Gerontological Nursing,** pp. 29–40. Sage, Newbury Park, California.

Shelton, R. (1994). Nursing and empowerment: concepts and strategies. **Journal of Advanced Nursing 19**(3), 415–423.

Torres, G. (1990). The place of concepts and theories within nursing. In: J. B. George (Ed.) **Nursing Theories: The Base for Professional Nursing Practice,** 3rd edn, pp. 1–12. Prentice Hall International, Englewood Cliffs.

Twigg, J. and Atkin, K. (1994) **Carers Perceived: Policy and Practice in Informal Care.** Open University Press, Buckingham.

UKCC (1994). **The Future of Professional Practice – the Council's Standards for Education and Practice Following Registration.** UKCC, London.

Verbrugge, L. M. and Jette, A. M. (1994). The disablement process. **Social Science and Medicine 38**(1), 1–14.

Victor, C. R. (1991). **Health and Health Care in Later Life.** Open University Press, Milton Keynes.

Walker, L. O. and Avant, K. C. (1983). **Strategies for Theory Construction in Nursing.** Appleton-Century-Crofts, Norwalk, Connecticut.

Walker, A., Alber, J. and Guillemard, A. M. (1993). **Older People in Europe: Social and Economic Policies.** The 1993 Report of the European Observatory, Commission of the European Communities, Brussels.

Waters, K. (1994). Getting dressed in the morning: styles of staff/patient interaction on rehabilitation hospital wards for elderly people. **Journal of Advanced Nursing 19**, 239–248.

Wells, T. J. (1980). **Problems in Geriatric Nursing.** Churchill Livingstone, Edinburgh.

Welsh Office (Welsh Health Care Planning Forum) (1993). **Health and Social Gain for Older People.** Welsh Office, Cardiff.

Wilkin, D. and Hughes, B. (1986). The elderly and the health services. In: C. Phillipson and A. Walker (Eds.) **Ageing and Social Policy: A Continual Assessment,** pp. 163–183. Gower, Aldershot.

Williams, J. (1994). The rehabilitation process for older people and their carers. **Nursing Times 90**(29), 33–34.

Woog, P. (1992). **The Chronic Illness Trajectory Framework: The Corbin and Strauss Nursing Model.** Springer, New York.

Wright, S. (1988). **Nursing the Older Patient.** Harper & Row, London.

Chapter Ten

Rehabilitation

Karen Waters

INTRODUCTION

The need for highly skilled intervention for older people in hospital is likely to continue to increase, given demographic trends in combination with the committment to transferring resources from hospital to the community. Shorter stays in hospital following acute illness means that hospital-based rehabilitation services for older people will have to be more responsive to the needs of their clients.

This chapter traces the history of rehabilitation nursing with older people, analogous with geriatric nursing, considering the predominance of 'routine' care and questioning the *status quo*. Recent research into the role of the nurse in rehabilitation settings with older people is presented and finally some suggestions are made for future practice.

Throughout this chapter you will be asked to think about situations you have experienced which may illustrate the points raised in the text.

This Chapter aims to enable you to:

Trace the development of rehabilitation nursing for older people

---

Examine critically the practice of rehabilitation nursing for older people and apply this to your own situation.

THE DEVELOPMENT OF REHABILITATION NURSING FOR OLDER PEOPLE

In the mid 1950s chronic sick wards were staffed by unqualified staff, either nursing assistants or student nurses, working in wards which tended to be poorly equipped and maintained. Changing the name from chronic sick wards to 'geriatric', was underpinned by an assumption that it was good to get older patients out of bed. Norton (1988) described how this resulted in geriatrics being seen as 'nothing more than an exchange of the (said) evils of the bed for the evils of the chair' (Norton's parentheses).

Baker (1978) highlighted the links between the development of geriatric medicine and geriatric nursing, and suggested that the dominance of the traditional medical model within geriatric medicine led to the devaluation of care which did not effect cure, and reinforced nursing's dependency on medicine for leadership. Rehabilitation wards fall between two stools in this analysis since, whilst they effect discharge from hospital, they do not do so by medical treatment, but rather by the use of various therapies.

Norton (1988), in summarizing the development of geriatric nursing towards the end of six articles tracing the history of the care of older people, resumes:

Collectively ... the story of geriatric nursing has been one of ignorance and educational neglect by the profession, based on a false premise either that it is 'only basic nursing' or that the preponderance of elderly patients in general nursing situations itself engenders enlightened attitudes to their care and welfare.

HOSPITAL CARE OF OLDER PEOPLE

It has been suggested that sometimes a stay in hopsital can be detrimental to older people (Roberts, 1975; Bowling and Betts, 1984; Waters, 1987). The way in which hosptial wards are run, with many services provided, can sometimes mean that old people are likely to be deskilled in certain activities of daily living, such as preparation for washing and dressing, meal preparation, and going to the bathroom for washing and toilet purposes. A study by the author found that many older people felt less independent after a short hospital stay. The implication is that hospital care does not always enable the regaining of function and may even disable its recipients (Waters, 1987).

There are several possible explanations for the decrease in independence after hospitalization. The most likely is that the acute illness itself may lead to decreased functioning. Second, the emphasis on high turnover from geriatric departments increases the probability that full recovery is not made before discharge. Finally, the nature of hospital care itself may play a significant role in a loss of independence. This last possibility will be explored in more detail.

Nursing care may contribute to the fostering of dependence in hospital, through such factors as prescribed rising and retiring times, set meal times and the discouragement of risktaking (Miller, 1985). Perceptions of older people as stigmatized and expectations that they will be dependent may lead to a custodial rather than a rehabilitative approach to care (Baker, 1983). Baker describes this custodial care as 'routine geriatric style', which is founded on the belief that older people have less than adult status. The characteristics of this style are:

- *emphasis on physical activities of daily living at the expense of psychosocial needs;*
- *a lower standard of care than was normally expected;*
- *tidiness was afforded a higher priority than were clients' needs;*
- *importance was attached to the expectations of nurse managers and medical staff and these were met before the needs of the clients.*

Baker summarizes, 'The organization of work according to the routine geriatric style was geared to getting the work done with the maximum economy of human resources'.

Over the past 15 years there has been an increasing number of studies into the nursing care of older people in hospital and while a number have included rehabilitation wards in their samples (Baker, 1983; Wells, 1980; Evers, 1981a), there has been a tendency to discuss geriatric nursing as an entity or to focus on long-stay care, thus it is difficult to discern what characterized rehabilitation nursing in the settings observed.

One notable exception is the work of Fairhurst (1978) whose thesis was entirely devoted to the study of rehabilitation in geriatric wards from a sociological perspective. Although this work was carried out a long time ago, the findings are echoed by both Reed (1989) and Waters (1994). Fairhurst presented a 'fly on the wall' view of rehabilitation in an urban hospital. She painted a picture reminiscent of the 'routine geriatric style' described earlier. The same pervasive organizational routines were evident; she reports that in the 'taken for granted aspects of every day life', little choice or control was afforded to clients; choice of food was limited, toileting was routinized and early retiring times were imposed by nurses on 'those being rehabilitated'. Conversing with patients was secondary to the routine and could be fitted in when the work had been done.

Fairhurst also observed differences between the practice of rehabilitation in the day and night time. She reported a greater emphasis on client safety at night, to the extent that clients regaining independence could pose problems for the night staff. Night routines were geared to the expectation of the next day shift and certain activities had to be completed within the timespan of the night shift, irrespective of any unusual night time occurrences. Rehabilitation should be a 24-hour process, not delimited by nursing staffing patterns.

Fairhurst's study suggests that the rehabilitation setting she studied showed similarities with the routinized care reported in previous studies, rather than characteristics of a particular rehabilitative style of ward practice.

The lack of a clear distinction between long stay care and rehabilitation is of great concern since the studies cited suggest that a preponderance of 'routine geriatric style' care exists in long stay care. In this style of nursing, clients are afforded a less than adult status and great value is placed on 'getting the work done' (Baker, 1983).

REHABILITATION

The notion of regaining independence for discharge is generally considered to be the purpose of rehabilitation (Brocklehurst, 1978; Turner, 1981; Hawker, 1974; Walley, 1986). The term 'rehabilitation' has become such a frequently used word in the vocabulary of carers for older people, that sometimes writers omit to define their own understanding of it. For example, in Redfern's (1991) comprehensive textbook on nursing older people, the term is used in several places, but never explored in depth or given any kind of definition. Similarly, medical writers assume shared meaning with the reader (e.g. Hall, 1988). This may be because rehabilitation straddles the boundaries of both acute and long stay care for older people and therefore it is problematic to define the process accurately. This is apparent in the way in which departments of geriatric medicine are structured. In a survey of the geriatric departments in England, Brocklehurst and Andrews (1985) found that over three-quarters had rehabilitative facilities combined with either acute or long stay care. This may lend support to the argument that rehabilitation is something which underpins the whole of geriatric medicine, but alternatively it could indicate the complexity of identifying the meaning of rehabilitation.

It is acknowledged within medical and nursing literature that the term rehabilitation is difficult to define. The Piercy Report (1956) states that rehabilitation 'signifies the whole process of restoring a disabled person to a condition in which he is able, as early as possible, to resume a normal life'. Jackson (1984) described three kinds of activity which might be carried out under the guise of rehabilitation:

- *Reactivation: the encouragement of patients to be active within their surroundings.*
- *Resocialization: encouragement of physical and/or verbal contact by patients with peers, families and others.*
- *Reintegration: restoration of the patient to society and the regaining of status as a person.*

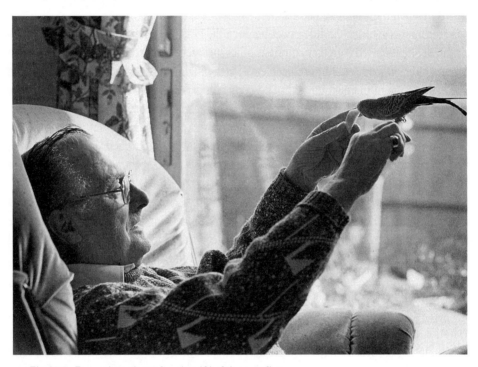

Fig. 10.1   *Encouraging patients to be active within their surroundings*

In this chapter rehabilitation is taken to mean the whole process of enabling and facilitating the restoration of a disabled person to regain optimal functioning (physically, socially and psychologically) to the level they are able or motivated to achieve.

THE MULTIDISCIPLINARY TEAM

The notion of multidisciplinary teamwork is central to the policy and practice of the care of older people and is identified as one of the ways in which it can be distinguished from other specialities (Fairhurst, 1981). The multidisciplinary team fits into the category of 'complex team', a term used by Webb and Hobdell (1980) to describe a group of people working together whose tasks and skills are of differing types and levels. Nurses and doctors are the personnel who are involved in the care of the most clients in geriatric wards, but the team members normally include physiotherapists, occupational therapists and social workers. Other more peripheral team members may be consulted for particular patients only, for example speech therapists or clinical psychologists. The client and his or her relatives have been identified as being of central importance in the team (RCN/BGS/RCP, 1975) but this is not always supported in texts of geriatric medicine and/or nursing, nor is it borne out in practice (Fairhurst, 1977; National Corporation for the Care of Old People, 1979). Evers (1981b) suggested that clients and relatives were deliberately excluded from the team because taking on board their perspectives would result in uncertainty and conflict for the team.

The nursing role in the rehabilitation team is often viewed as one of co-ordinator of the multidisciplinary team and manager of the nursing team. The nurse can be seen as the lynch-pin of the team. The business of nurses has been seen as the maintenance of daily living activities and general wellbeing and comfort of the client. Specialized functions have been ascribed to nurses in older people care settings, such as tissue viability and continence promotion. In a multidisciplinary setting, where clients are having treatment with a number of different disciplines, the nurse may assume a 'carry-on' role, carrying on the work of therapists in their absence, for example walking and dressing practice. This role is very important in the facilitation of independence in older people as therapists are not present in ward settings for over 50% of the clients' waking time.

The RCN document *The Role of the Nurse in the Rehabilitation of Elderly People*, itemizes the following elements of the nursing role within the multidisciplinary team:

- *liaison with relatives and carers;*
- *initiating contact with other team members;*
- *giving and receiving information;*
- *administering prescribed therapy;*
- *monitoring effects of other therapies;*
- *reporting back;*
- *taking part in evaluation;*
- *assessing clients;*
- *giving encouragement and support to clients and carers.*

A more recent document, RCN (1994), emphasizes the nurse's role in health promotion with rehabilitation clients.

REHABILITATION NURSING RESEARCH

The following sections draw heavily on research conducted into the nursing role in rehabilitation with older people (Waters, 1991; Booth, 1994; Ellul *et al.*, 1993; O'Connor, 1993).

The Concept of Rehabilitation

This section uses findings from a study of staff working in rehabilitation settings with older people. Information was collected by interviews conducted by the author with 56 staff in one centre of excellence.

Rehabilitation was seen in essence as the process which returned clients to their former or improved state of health. This was illustrated by one interviewee: 'It's getting the patient back to be as well as they possibly can be ... getting them to do as much for themselves as possible'. The ultimate aim of rehabilitation was to enable clients to return home if possible or, failing that, to alternative residence in the community.

The relearning of lost skills and the regaining of independence, seemed to have become subsumed into the actions of staff working with clients on rehabilitation wards; thus, a number of respondents used the word as a verb in the following manner: 'We're not always rehabbing people just for going home ...' and 'You learn how to rehab someone'. Staff were using the word to describe what they did, not the process which clients go through to become independent.

How Do You Use the Word Rehabilitation?

The onus for rehabilitation lay predominantly with staff, and the impression was given that it was something was done by staff to clients and which resulted in physical improvement. Several staff used expressions such as 'facilitate', 'build up' and 'encourage' which might denote a more participative approach to rehabilitation but in general the clients were seen to be the recipients of rehabilitation.

The staff perceptions of rehabilitation were largely confined to physical functioning. Little reference was made to social activities, or to the social implications of the clients' conditions. The focus was mainly on clients' abilities in physical activities of daily living, and in particular transferring, walking, dressing and kitchen skills. While these skills may be important for survival at home; they may be insufficient to sustain any quality of life. In the hospital it seems that the *social world* of older people can be forgotten.

Factors Influencing the Process of Rehabilitation

Resources

Two kinds of resources are reviewed here: resources in the community and the resources of the individual. The structure of community resources and/or the personal resources of an older person can indirectly affect the nature of hospital care itself.

The interplay and effect of these two resources are admirably illustrated by the cases of Hannah and Lizzie. Both these clients were considered to be 'at risk' in terms of living alone in the community, but the outcomes were very different. Read through the two stories of Lizzie and Hannah and consider the following questions as you do:

- *How are decisions made about whether old people are safe to live alone?*
- *Who makes these decisions?*

- *What is the purpose of home visits?*
- *What do you think were the differences between the two women and why did one achieve her goal and other not?*

Case Study: Hannah S.

Hannah was a 94-year-old woman admitted to hospital after falling in her own home. After 13 days on the acute ward, she was transferred to the rehabilitation ward. During her stay on the ward, she was seen four times for dressing practice and had a kitchen assessment. She was seen nine times for walking practice and had a home visit after 18 days on the rehabilitation ward.

At the home visit she performed adequately in most tasks but was not able to make a hot drink, because she was unable to light the cooker, and left the gas tap in the 'on' position. Her daughter, who had been a non-resident main carer prior to Hannah's admission, was present during the visit to the house. During the time there, she spoke with the occupational therapist about her mother's future. She felt that her mother would not be able to manage at home any more and she herself felt unable to provide the level of help she had previously offered. Her own daughter was expecting a second baby and Hannah's daughter wanted to be able to offer help to her. She expressed feelings of being torn between her mother and her daughter and of guilt. Hannah was in the same room during this conversation, but did not comment. In the home visit report, it was stated 'Mrs S. appears passive and did not particularly express an opinion to be discharged home'. At the next case conference, the home visit was reported as 'no go'. It was stated by the senior house officer, that Hannah could not go home, because 'Her daughter feels she can't cope any more.' A brief discussion followed this statement, but no-one challenged this perspective. Just before Hannah came into the ward round, the senior registrar announced 'We know what we're going to do with her, it's just a question of persuading her.'

The social worker was detailed to discuss the future with Hannah. Details of the conversation during the ward round were not recorded, but Hannah did not object to their suggestions.

She was discharged within 2 weeks of the home visit to a residential home, near to where her daughter lived and not in her previous locale. She seemed content when interviewed, but did refer to her own home – 'Well, I used to like my house…They took me to see it and they decided, I couldn't go back because I turn the taps on wrong.'

She expressed two main concerns during the interview: first, she was worried about having to relocate again in the future and this was linked to financial concern – 'The only thing I'm worried about is can I afford to stay here. I'm frightened of changes.' Her daughter, who was present during the interview, reassured her that the finances were taken care of and she did not need to worry about that. Some difficulty had been experienced by her daughter in finding a home which charged only the rate available from the Department of Social Security. The residential home had agreed to charge Hannah this rate, although their prices were normally higher.

Hannah did not voice any strong desire to go home, and in the ward round it was the daughter's perspective which seemed to sway the decision-making. The information from the home visit was presented in a way which left little room for discussion and only one likely outcome.

Again this raises questions, not so much about the execution of the home visit, but about the way in which the home visit report is presented in the ward round. In Hannah's case, in the absence of dissent in the team the way the report was presented was likely to pre-empt the decision that Hannah needed residential care.

Case Study: The triumph of Lizzie S.

Lizzie was a 97-year-old woman, admitted to hospital after falling at home. Prior to hospitalization, she mainly occupied the downstairs living room of a council house. She spent 1 week on the acute ward and was then transferred to a rehabilitation ward.

During the first week on Marsh Ward, she was seen by the physiotherapist five times for muscle strengthening exercises and walking practice, and by the occupational therapist once for dressing practice and once to join in group activities in the occupational therapy department. The possibility of a home visit was raised at a ward round and a date arranged for the following week. In an interim ward round when Lizzie came up for discussion the consultant ventured:

> **'A jolly prospect. In last month, out and in again. What are we doing, trying to get this lady home? We haven't decided we're going home – we'd better be clear. This is problematic. Better ask her in and see if she's ever had thoughts of residential accommodation. The home visit is only to confirm she can't go home.'**

The home visit was duly carried out 2 days after this ward round. Two inexperienced therapists were responsible; one had only just qualified and the other was a final year student awaiting results. The author was present in a research capacity on the visit, and the consultant's view of the purpose of the home visit was realized. Lizzie was given only one opportunity to try each activity and at the first sign of difficulty she was told she could not manage. The visit did not run its full course. After she had ostensibly 'failed' at transferring on and off the bed and chair, the occupational therapist told her the visit was being stopped. At interview Lizzie told me she felt she had performed badly on the visit, because she had just started with a cold that morning and felt they could not have picked a worse morning.

The home visit report stated that residential care was felt to be essential, because of potential danger with the cooker, her poor transfer techniques and her instability. At the next ward round, the home visit report was given and the consultant's response to it was 'How are we going to persuade her we are right?'

The patient was brought into the room and the following conversation took place between the consultant (AA) and Lizzie, (LT):

AA: 'I want you to think very carefully about going to live in supervised accommodation, where there are skilled staff – you might be better off.'

LT: 'I want to stay at home, doctor.'

AA: (To social worker) 'Would you like to help us look...don't worry too much about the niceties, put it to her and see if she'll go.'

No further conversation took place with Lizzie at this ward round but at the next, when her name was introduced, Dr A said to the team in general:

'Another lady who keeps asking to go home. If she went home, she wouldn't have a home help. She's not fit to be at home at all...we put it to her and she just refuses.'

The patient was then brought in and was helped to sit down by the physiotherapist, and the following conversation ensued:

AA: 'Good morning.'

LT: 'Good morning.'

AA: 'How are you?'

LT: 'Bit better than I was.'

AA: 'How old are you?'

LT: '97, 98 in August.'

AA: 'Think about your situation, when you go home what do you think your main problems will be?'

LT: 'Getting up, getting the fire lit and the rest of the work, I have a daily help.'

AA: 'Any risk of falling?'

LT: 'Not if I'm careful.'

AA: 'Have we suggested that you might go into a home for older people?'

LT: 'If that is so, I'll choose my own.'

AA: 'Are you willing to think about it?'

LT: 'No, I haven't thought about it, it doesn't appeal to me.'

AA: '(Aside) Technically certifiable, but no one would dream of doing so.'

A week later, when her name was introduced, the consultant retorted:

'Oh dear, must we. Her nephew came and he insists.'

The social worker added:

'I've spoken to her and she's insistent on going home.'

The consultant conceded to Lizzie's wishes and said to the team:

'Well, let's get it organized and off she goes.'

When she came into the room, he said to her:

'Well it looks as if you'll be going home.'

She replied:

'Alright, I shall be very pleased.'

She left hospital 3 days later, and appeared to be managing well when she was interviewed in her own home a week later. Ironically, the services arranged by the hospital had not materialized, and while she was being interviewed some of her family arrived and complained that the hospital 'dumped' her. Considering the battle she had fought to come home the family's perspective was surprising.

The decision Lizzie took was being interpreted almost as 'discharging oneself against medical advice', with the hospital then seemingly abdicating responsibility for any subsequent outcomes. In spite of being aware of the risks Lizzie chose to be at home and was assertive in stating her case. She won the day against the better judgement of the team.

Two kinds of resources impinged on this process, the community resources, but also the hospital resources, the need to clear the beds. For older people considered to be at risk, the exercising of their autonomy is conditional on their personal situation; the poor and the isolated are, in the current climate precluded from exercising their autonomy.

Physical Environment

The physical environment in which rehabilitation is expected to occur is not conducive to the regaining of independence. As discussed, being a hospital patient is likely to mean some loss of autonomy. In addition, it has long been suggested that there can also be a loss of identity (Goffman, 1961). In rehabilitation wards it is common practice that clients get dressed; indeed dressing itself is part of the assessment and treatment programme and so is an integral part of life in rehabilitation wards for older people. However, this is not to underestimate the effect of being a *patient* on an older person. Some of the clients in my study felt that they had had no treatment while in hospital, treatment referring to medicines and physical manipulation by the doctor. Some clients of the rehabilitation experience stated that 'nothing was done for them'. The traditional idea of going into hospital is that you go to be made better by the doctors; this of course does not happen in a rehabilitation ward. While the physical environment may be identical to every other ward, the expectations of what clients are supposed to do may be different. But it seems that the client is not informed of this leading to expectations of treatment that do not materialize and consternation by clients about the sheer hard work of rehabilitation.

While the purpose of rehabilitation is the regaining of independence, within the hospital ward there are many practices which militate against this, for example:

- *beds made and linen laundered;*
- *meals cooked and distributed;*
- *drinks made and distributed;*
- *lockers tidied;*
- *floor cleaned;*
- *lights swithced on and off;*
- *day structured by others.*

It could be argued that these are hotel services, but the majority of these clients are not going to live in a hotel, and so the hospital environment constrains the achievement of independence. Is it possible for an older person to achieve and exercise autonomy as a hospital inpatient? It is likely that an older person is subject to double jeopardy; being old in itself can threaten autonomy, being an old client in hospital is potentially a much more vulnerable position.

Nursing Role

We turn now to the process of caregiving and examine the way in which the organization of nursing care influences rehabilitation.

THE NURSING ROLE IN REHABILITATION

This section is drawn from the author's research into the role of the nurse in rehabilitation with older people, which finds support in other work (e.g. Gibbon, 1992; Ellul *et al.*, 1993; Booth, 1994). Interviews with and observation of staff in a rehabilitation setting provided the data.

Sometimes nurses are not perceived as making a major contribution to the rehabilitation process. This is not to say that they are considered to be unimportant; on the contrary, their work is seen as vital for rehabilitation to take place, but they are not viewed as the driving force within the process. The terms 'maintaining' and 'carrying on' were most frequently used in describing the nurse's role. This suggests that nurses are seen to have a secondary, rather than primary, function in rehabilitation.

The nursing role in rehabilitation was difficult for many staff, including nurses themselves, to elucidate but it fell broadly into three categories – general maintenance work, specialist functions and the 'carry-on' role.

General Maintenance Work

General maintenance work; often referred to as 'general or basic nursing care' has been described as '... all the things we take for granted ... and all the little bits of your everyday routine such as hairdressing, oral hygiene and cleaning spectacles'. The function of general maintenance work was described by one physiotherapist: 'They (nurses) get the body able to function so that I can get at it'. Thus general maintenance work occupied a lot of time and seemed to take priority.

Specialist Functions

Two specialist functions of nurses were identified by staff respondents: continence promotion and the prevention and treatment of pressure sores.

Continence Promotion

While continence promotion is viewed as a specialist function, part of which it could be argued might be assisting patients to the toilet, sometimes it is viewed predominantly as a task.

> *I think the toileting is a problem, because often there aren't enough of us. I mean we all do it constantly, 'just a minute, I'll be back in a minute'...That's somewhere that we do fall down, not because we don't care or we can't be bothered, there just isn't the time (enrolled nurse).*

Toileting was viewed as one of the morning tasks:

> *Mostly in the mornings, it's mundane tasks like bed-making and breakfasts, to and from the tables and to the toilet.*

Post-basic education relating to continence promotion may have assisted these nurses to view continence promotion more positively.

Prevention and Management of Pressure Sores

Various factors were identified during the study which indicated that it was difficult for nurses to discharge this specialist role. These were: absence of pressure sore risk calculation during nursing assessment; lack of suitable equipment for pressure sore prevention; and disagreement between one of the consultants and trained staff about responsibility for and the prescription of treatment for pressure sores.

These findings illustrate the rocky foundation on which the claim to a specialist nursing function was built. It appears from the findings that neither of the specialist roles in rehabilitation ascribed to nurses was fulfilled. Reasons for this are explored in the discussion.

The Carry-on Role

In the study unit there was a policy of ward-based therapy practice, one of the consultants believed that rehabilitation was a 24-hour process and explained that:

> *It's very important that the nursing staff know what techniques are being used for an individual patient, what piece of equipment might be needed for a disabled person and what the risks for an individual patient are because of their disability. So it is important that they all work very closely together and that's why we have a lot of our rehabilitation that's actually done on the ward rather than patients going to a separate rehabilitation area, because it's educational for the nurses and it's also educational for the therapists because they get feedback for the nurses as to what the patients can manage when they are not with them.*

The rationale of ward-based therapy practice then is to effect two-way communication between therapists and nurses so that rehabilitation can be a continual process. This suggests that the practice of rehabilitation may be dependent upon the nature of the interrelations between nurses, physiotherapists and occupational therapists.

'Carry-on' work refers to the work of physiotherapists and occupational therapists which nurses were expected to continue in the absence of the therapists. All respondents described this function in one way or another. The following typify the statements made.

A nursing auxiliary on Marsh ward commented:

> *You take over from the physios when they are not there and it's the same over the weekend when the OTs are not there, you are still carrying on what the OTs and the physios are laying down.*

A staff nurse of Fern Ward described nurses as:

Carrying out all those things that everyone's prescribed, to carry on the physiotherapy when the physios aren't there and use the aids the OTs give them.

Those things which nurses were expected to 'carry on' were helping patients to wash and dress and continuing walking practice during the absence of physiotherapists. It might be suggested that nurses should be able to assess a client's ability to dress and/or undress and their level of mobility, but this skill was not conveyed by the majority of the nurses interviewed. In general, the impression was given that occupational therapists and physiotherapists were the experts in these activities of daily living. Each of the ward sisters subscribed to this belief. One sister stated:

We work very closely together with the OT and physio. and they'll come and say 'Oh they can do this now'. We find out from them what the patient is doing at the time and just keep encouraging them to do what they've been doing with other members of the team.

The sister of another ward explained that:

We're just sort of filling in from what the physios and OTs have started, we just go by what they say, they're the experts really aren't they? They are the ones that know what the patient is actually capable of from the movement point of view or dressing themselves.

The majority of the staff of each ward echoed the sisters' views. It seems that, on the whole, nurses and therapists alike considered that nurses were dependent on therapists for information concerning dressing and movement.

In the observation study of early morning care, a routinized form of nursing care was observed. Between the hours of 6 a.m. and 7.30 a.m. the 'routine' began at 6 a.m. when the night staff began to get the clients up. It fell to them to have all the clients washed and out of bed before the day staff came on duty. At weekends this meant dressing all the clients as well, but on weekdays, those clients having dressing practice with the OT were only washed. As a rule there were two night staff on duty, and this meant that there was less than 10 minutes per client in which to accomplish morning care. Getting through the work took precedence over the rehabilitative needs of the client and the result for the client was either being 'left to get on with it' or being dressed completely by the nurse. The goal of getting the clients up, meant that the nurses often worked against the work of the therapists much less 'carried it on'.

There appear to be no advantages for clients in this routine and dissatisfaction was expressed. Many clients felt it was too early to get up and even if it wasn't, would have liked a cup of tea before getting washed and/or dressed. In the study unit there was a policy of ward-based therapy practice, which meant that as much physiotherapy and occupational therapy as possible was actually carried out on the rehabilitation ward. Many staff stated that clients had to be 'ready' for when the therapists came on the ward. The irony of this is that 'getting ready' for the therapists may actually undo some of their work, rather than facilitate it.

Developing the Nursing Role in Rehabilitation

The framework for care delivery is likely to improve both the process and outcome of rehabilitation. It is postulated that, in the absence of medically prescribed care on the rehabilitation wards, the nurses were uncertain about their input, and therefore fell back into a more traditional nursing role of compensating for disability, rather than promoting independence. The development of an accepted nursing rehabilitation model would greatly assist this.

It is evident that certain structural elements can impinge on the nurse's role and, consequently, the client's experience. In order to facilitate a more significant nursing role in the rehabilitation of older people in hospital, such elements would have to be altered. The early morning rising system, in particular, seemed to result in undesirable outcomes for its main participants and also for staff. Where different getting up patterns have been described (Wright, 1989; Pearson, 1987; Booth and Davies, 1991) they have been on nursing development units where special effort has been made to facilitate the implementation of individualized client care, usually within a primary nursing framework.

It appears that the early morning rising system in the study unit was a default system, which operated in the absence of any other. Tentatively, it may be suggested that 'routine' is nursing's default mechanism and so, on a rehabilitation ward where there have been few role models, the default system operates, hence the picture of routinized care observed in this study.

The nursing role in the rehabilitation of older people is multifaceted. Besides the management and custodial functions with which all ward nurses are charged, there are specific functions which the nurse carries out in rehabilitation settings. What makes this role unique is not the separate activities but the combination of them in this setting.

Nursing role	Patient education	Health promotion	Tissue viability	Continence	Dressing	Mobility	Personal hygiene
General maintenance							
Specialist							
Carry on							

Fig. 10.2 *Conceptualization of nursing role*

CONCLUSIONS: THE FUTURE

Urgent consideration needs to be given to the whole milieu of the rehabilitation wards. The study suggested that the structure was dependency-creating; alternative models of rehabilitative services need to be explored. Admission policies, physical environment, shift patterns and working hours could all be manipulated to effect maximization of available resources. The current focus on shifting care from the secondary to the primary sector provides opportunity to examine the efficacy of secondary versus primary sector rehabilitation.

Professional education of nursing staff relating to rehabilitation is a high priority and this is being developed in this country. However, we are woefully behind the USA, where all rehabilitation nurses have to gain certification in rehabilitaiton nursing prior to praticising.

The relationship between therapist and nurse needs to be explored so that maximum use of resources can be made. Turf wars about what's your job and what's mine will find little sympathy with the current management ethos. Consideration should be given to the style of nursing intervention, which was not always appropriate to the needs of the client. Support for nurses in the implementation of rehabilitative practice is needed, so that they are enabled to take on a primary role in rehabilitation.

CLINICAL DISCUSSION QUESTIONS

What do you think the nurses' role in the multidisciplinary team in a rehabilitation setting should be?

What is the nurses' role in rehabilitation in your clinical area? Is it how you think it should be? How could it be changed for client benefit?

How do members of the multidisciplinary team communicate with each other where you work? Think about different forms of communication – oral, written, electronic?

Is there a difference in the practices during the day and night in your clinical area? Can you identify good reasons for this?

SUGGESTIONS FOR FURTHER READING

Andrews, K. (1987) **Rehabilitation of the Older Adult**. Edward Arnold, London. *Useful overview.*

RCN (1991). **The Role of the Nurse in the Rehabilitation of Older People.** Royal College of Nursing, London. *Focuses specifically on rehabilitation with older people. Useful to compare with RCN (1994).*

RCN (1994). **Rehabilitation Nursing: Standards of Care.** Royal College of Nursing, London. *A useful overview of rehabilitation nursing.*

Swain *et al.* (1993). **Disabling Barriers, Enabling Environments.** Sage publications in association with OUP, London. *Excellent review of some issues for rehabilitation of disabled people.*

REFERENCES

Andrews, K. and Brocklehurst, J. C. (1985). A profile of geriatric rehabilitation units. **Journal of the Royal College of Physicians of London 19**(4), 240–242.

Baker, D. E. (1978). Attitudes of Nurses to the Care of the Elderly. Unpublished PhD Thesis, University of Manchester.

Baker, D. E. (1983). 'Care' in the geriatric ward: an account of two styles of nursing. In Wilson-Barnett (Ed) **Nursing Research: Ten Studies in Patient Care**, pp. 101–117. John Wiley, Chichester.

Bowling, A. and Betts, G. (1984). Communication on discharge. **Nursing Times 81**, 26–28.

Booth, J. (1994). The nursing role in geriatric day hospitals. **Journal of Advanced Nursing**, in press.

Booth, J. and Davies C. (1991). Happy to be home: A discharge planning package for elderly people. **Professional Nurse 6**(6), 330–332.

Brocklehurst, J. C. (1978). **Textbook of Geriatric Medicine and Gerontolgy,** 2nd edn. Churchill Livingstone, Edinburgh.

Brocklehurst, J. and Andrews, K. (1985). Geriatric medicine – the style of the practice. **Age and Ageing 14,** 1–7.

Ellul, J., Watkins, C., Ferguson, N., Barer, D. and Rowe, J. (1993). Increasing patient engagement in rehabilitation activities. **Clinical Rehabilitation 7**(4), 297–302.

Evers, H. K. (1981a). Tender loving care? Patients and nurses in geriatric wards. In: L. A. Copp (Ed.) **Care of the Aging,** Edinburgh: Churchill Livingstone.

Evers, H. K. (1981b). Multidisciplinary teams in geriatric wards: myth or reality? **Journal of Advanced Nursing 6,** 205–214.

Fairhurst, E. (1977). **Teamwork as Panacea: Some Underlying Assumptions.** Unpublished Paper read at Annual Conference of the Medical Sociology Group of the British Sociological Association, University of Warwick.

Fairhurst, E. (1978). A Sociological Study of the Rehabilitation of Elderly People in an Urban Hospital. Unpublished PhD thesis. University of Leeds.

Fairhurst, E. (1981). 'What do you do?': multiple realities in occupational therapy and rehabilitation. In: P. Atkinson and C. Heath (Eds) **Medical Work: Realities and Routines,** pp. 171–187. Gower, Farnborough.

Gibbon, B. (1992). The role of the nurse in rehabilitation. **Nursing standard 6**(36), 32–35.

Gibbon, B. and Littlewood, V. (1993). Improving Strole Care Through Action Research. Unpublished report, University of Liverpool.

Goffman, E. (1961). **Asylums.** Doubleday Anchor, New York.

Hall, M. (1988). Geriatric medicine today. In: N. Wells and C. Frear (Eds) **The Ageing Population: Burden or Challenge,** pp. 65–86. MacMillan, Hampshire.

Hawker, M. (1974). **Geriatrics for Physiotherapists and the Allied Professions.** Faber & Faber, London.

Jackson, M. (1984). Geriatric rehabilitation on an acute medical unit. **Journal of Advanced Nursing 9,** 441–448.

Miller, A. (1985). A study of the dependency of elderly patients in wards using different methods of nursing care. **Age and Ageing 14,** 132–138.

National Corporation for the Care of Old People (1979). **Organizing Aftercare: Continuing Care Project.** NCCOP, London.

Norton, D. (1988). Wartime and the beginnings of geriatric nursing, part 4 **Geriatric Nursing and Home Care 8**(4), 26–28.

O'Connor, S. (1993). Nursing and rehabilitation; the perceived role of the nurse in the medical and nursing literature. **Journal of Clinical Nursing 2,** 29–34.

Pearson, A. (Ed) (1987). **Primary Nursing – Nursing in the Burford and Oxford Nursing Development Units.** Croom Helm, London.

Piercy Report (1956) **DHSS Report of the Committee of Enquiry on the Rehabilitation, Training and Resettlement of Disabled Persons.** HMSO, London.

RCN (1991). **Role of the Nurse in the Rehabilitation of Elderly People.** Scutari Press, Harrow.

RCN (1994). **Standards of Care: Rehabilitation Nursing.** Scutari Press, Harrow.

Redfern S. (1991). (Ed.) **Nursing Elderly People.** Churchill Livingstone, Edinburgh.

Reed, J. (1989). All Dressed up and Nowhere to Go: Nursing Assessment in Geriatric Care. Unpublished PhD Thesis, Newcastle-upon-Tyne Polytechnic.

Roberts, I. (1975). **Discharge From Hospital.** Royal College of Nursing, London.

Royal College of Nursing/British Geriatric Society/Royal College of Psychiatrists (1975). **Improving Geriatric Care in Hospital.** Royal College of Nursing, London.

Royal College of Nursing/British Geriatric Society/Royal College of Psychiatrists (1987). **Improving Care of Elderly People in Hospital** Royal College of Nursing, London.

Swain, J., Finkelstein, V., French, S. and Oliver, M. (1993). **Disabling Barriers – Enabling Environments.** Sage publications in association with the Open University Press, London.

Turner, A. (Ed.) (1981). *The Principles of the Activities of Daily Living in the Practice of Occupational Therapy.* Churchill Livingstone, Edinburgh.

Walley, H.M.L. (1986). Ward Sisters' Concept of Rehabilitation. Unpublished dissertation submitted in part fulfilment of MSc thesis, University of Southampton.

Waters, K. R. (1987). Outcomes of discharge from hospital. **Journal of Advanced Nursing 12,** 347–355.

Waters, K. R. (1991). The Nurse's Role in the Rehabilitation of Elderly People in Hospital. Unpublished PhD thesis, University of Manchester.

Waters, K. R. (1994). Getting dressed in the early morning: styles of staff/patient interaction on rehabilitation hospital wards for elderly people. **Journal of Advanced Nursing 19,** 239–248.

Webb, A. L. and Hobdell, M. (1980). Co-ordination and teamwork in the health and personal social services. In S. Lonsdale, A. L. Webb, and T. L. Briggs (Eds) **Teamwork in the Personal Services and Health Care.** Croom Helm, London.

Wells, T. (1980). **Problems in Geriatric Nursing Care.** Churchill Livingstone, Edinburgh.

Wright, S. G. (1989). **Changing Nursing Practice.** Edward Arnold, London.

Chapter Eleven

Advanced Practice:
The Case of Leg Ulcers

Yvonne Awenat

Core Themes in Gerontological Nursing

Ageing Matters	*New Social World*	*Lifespan Perspective*	Health and Old People
Illness and Dependency	Quality Nursing Care	Therapeutic Intervention	*Politicizing Gerontological Nursing*

Key Words

Leg ulcers • Advanced Nursing Practice • Assessment • Effective Treatment

INTRODUCTION

Many people with leg ulcers currently receive a less than satisfactory service from health care providers. This situation arises from professional ignorance, the lay public's acceptance, and in many cases is led by the absence of a clearly defined strategy for care of clients with this condition.

However, although there exists a misguided perception that work with leg ulcer clients is demoralizing, uninteresting and trying, my own experience suggests that this field is challenging and rewarding, calling into use the full range of skills possessed by a competent nurse. In fact far from being an area devoid of opportunities, the possibility for advancement of nursing practice are abundant.

This chapter presents a comprehensive account of the nursing treatment of leg ulcers. This is an example of seizing the window of opportunity in rehabilitation nursing. The chapter is very clinically oriented, to illustrate the diverse nature of the differing nursing roles in gerontological nursing.

The aims of this Chapter are to:

Give a brief background of the incidence of leg ulcers

Explore why the treatment of leg ulcers has, until recently, not been a high profile activity

---

Consider the opportunities for advancing nursing practice in this field

PRESENT DAY EPIDEMIOLOGY

Today it is estimated that around 1% of the general adult population are affected by leg ulcers (Callum *et al.*, 1985). Additionally, there exists a strong relationship between increasing age and higher prevalence. Henry (1986) found that 4.7% of people aged over 65 years old had experienced leg ulceration. So although the incidence and prevalence has decreased over the past few centuries, the work of treating people with this condition still remains a high volume activity.

Callum *et al.*, (1985) discovered that one-third of all ulcers occur before the age of 50, and the rest occur before the age of 65. This raises some interesting questions for it would appear that ulcers mainly occur prior to old age, and yet undoubtedly the majority of sufferers are old. This point will be returned to later in this chapter.

Ulcers presenting in people under the age of 30 are mainly caused by trauma with equal sex distribution. Between 30 and 80 there are more than twice as many females affected and this trend increases still further for those aged over 80 when it rises to 7:1 (Dale and Gibson, 1986). The predominance of older females affected is partially explained by their overall dominance of the older population, but also because of the occurrence of deep vein thrombosis during pregnancy. Although this still occurs today, it occurred far more frequently when present-day octogenarians had their babies, and this may be attributed to maternity care practices many years ago when women spent several weeks 'lying-in' following childbirth. Deep vein thrombosis is a well recognized complication of immobility and remains the most likely cause of later development of a venous leg ulcer (Dale and Gibson, 1986).

TYPES OF ULCERS

The main causes of leg ulceration are venous hypertension, arterial insufficiency or a combination of both these factors. Cornwall *et al.* (1986) found that in 75% of clients with venous ulceration the underlying cause was either deep or superficial vein incompetence. In the remaining 25%, the cause was either arterial insufficiency alone or in combination with venous pathology. There are other causes of ulcers but these are quite rare, for example tuberculosis, syphilis, pyoderma gangrenosum, pretibial myxoedema, drug-induced (ergot, cytotoxics) pressure necrosis, lymphoedema, burns, self-inflicted and malignant (Dale and Gibson, 1986).

Venous Ulcers

A venous ulcer is the visible sign of underlying chronic venous disease. In normal health, vein valves prevent backflow of blood in the legs, as it travels upwards against gravity to the heart, and this is assisted by calf muscle pump action. However, when a vein valve has been damaged by a previous thrombosis, backflow of blood occurs from the deep to the communicating and superficial veins. This produces a situation where high pressures develop in the veins which then become engorged and tortuous. Research conducted in Scandinavia in 1942 found that 79% of clients who had experienced continued swelling following deep vein thrombosis developed ulcers in the next 20 years (Bauer, 1942). The presence of unrelieved chronic venous hypertension leads to increased permeability in the capillaries allowing leakage of blood components from the circulation to the surrounding interstitial tissue. This fluid leakage causes oedema, and skin irritation occurs due to the presence of proteolytic enzymes (e.g. fibrinogen) in the tissues. A characteristic brown pigmentation occurs due to leakage of red blood cells which decompose leaving deposits of haemosiderin behind causing permanent skin staining (Blair *et al.*, 1988b; Dale, 1990). This process upsets the normal balance of tissue perfusion and at this stage ulceration is imminent. Often a minor injury such as a knock or even superficial scratches caused by the client in an attempt to relieve itching may then develop into an ulcer.

Unless these underlying pathological changes of the venous disease process are understood, health care professionals and clients may falsely believe the ulcer itself to be the sole problem, when in fact it is only a sign of hidden disease.

Arterial Ulcers

Peripheral vascular disease is the main causative factor for arterial (or ischaemic) ulcers. The lumen of the artery becomes narrowed due to the build up of yellow plaque deposits of atherosclerosis. This leads to thickening and calcification of the wall of the artery accounting for its lay terminology 'hardening of the arteries' (Horton, 1980).

Other causes of ischaemic ulceration include the presence of autoimmune type diseases such as rheumatoid arthritis, scleroderma, systemic lupus erythromatosus and diabetes. Here the problem lies mainly in the smaller arterioles.

In all cases the limb is deprived of adequate tissue perfusion and ischaemia and necrosis develop.

THE RELATIONSHIP BETWEEN ULCERS AND AGEING

There is no doubt that leg ulcers are found far more frequently in older people. In Ireland, Henry (1986) identified a venous ulcer prevalence of 4.7% in persons of 65 years and over, while others estimate a slightly lower figure of 3.6% (Callum et al., 1987). Therefore, although exact figures may vary, it is clear that increasing age is associated with a higher prevalence of ulcers. Ebersole and Hess (1981) state that in the absence of disease, venous circulatory changes are not a normal part of the ageing process. In one study of 600 clients the peak age of onset of ulceration was between the ages of 50 and 69 years. In the same study, analysis of information concerning the duration of ulceration reveals that almost half of the sample had suffered from ulceration for over 10 years (Callum et al., 1987a). It is therefore likely that this chronicity factor rather than the effects of physiological ageing may explain why a large number of older people are affected. Likewise, arterial disease is no longer thought to be solely due to advancing age, although some loss of elasticity within the arteries usually ensues with old age (Rose, 1991).

Immobility in older people, irrespective of its cause, can lead to deep vein thrombosis (DVT) which, as explained above, increases the risk of future ulcer formation. Furthermore, acute illness in older people is frequently compounded by dehydration, the haemoconcentration of which makes DVT more likely (Hodkinson, 1976). DVT is not always recognized and many cases remain undiagnosed. Often this is because there are no clear clinical signs, the circulation may not be completely obstructed, as the thrombosis may only have a small area of attachment to the vein with the main bulk of it 'floating like an eel' in the blood (Horton, 1980).

The aetiology of venous and arterial ulcers may be described as two entirely separate issues, but in practice clients can be unlucky enough to have elements of both diseases occurring simultaneously. These are referred to as 'mixed' ulcers. In the Harrow Health Authority study, Cornwall (1991) found that 22% of the leg ulcer clients had mixed ulcers and that older people were those most affected.

NURSING WORKLOAD

Nurses employed in a variety of different settings can expect to come in contact with clients who have leg ulcers. Callum *et al.* (1985) found that 87% of all leg ulcer clients were being cared for in the community, with the remaining 13% identified as either hospital inpatients or outpatients. Therefore, community nurses are those most likely to be looking after clients with this condition. Bosanquet (1991) found that 75% of district nurses in the Riverside area spent at least a quarter of their time in this way. Others have estimated that as much as 50% of district nursing time is utilized treating leg ulcers (Cherry and Ryan, 1989). Undoubtedly then, much nursing time is spent in this activity. However, sadly, much of the present-day input is misguided and ineffective. This sorry state of affairs arises from a number of interrelated issues.

Professional Lack of Knowledge

The aetiology, pathophysiology, diagnosis and management of leg ulceration is conspicuous by its absence in most nursing and medical education courses. This in itself is probably indicative of the general low status of this topic. Leg ulceration is a classic condition and most chronic illnesses are associated with old age. Could the lack of professional interest in leg ulceration therefore be attributed to ageist beliefs? At the strategic level of planning, is the low priority usually ascribed to leg ulcer care related to the common age of this client population? Since the treatment workload falls mainly on nurses rather than doctors, issues concerning status and gender may also be involved. Leg ulcers are not life threatening, they are not dramatic, exciting events, consequently they do not inspire widespread public sympathy and interest.

The medical model of care favours illnesses that are exciting, technologically demanding and likely to proceed to full cure as rapidly as possible. Leg ulcers do not fulfil this criteria, although they are by no means quite as difficult to heal as some badly informed health workers believe.

This professional ignorance is actually very damaging to clients, who absorb the negative attitudes projected and become pessimistic. It is not unusual to come across clients who have been unsuccessfully treated by a number of hospital and community health care agencies. Clients become depressed when constantly faced with failure and eventually lose all hope of their ulcer healing. As consumers, older people are not always very assertive when dealing with health care professionals and sometimes their expectations of health care are low and therefore easily satisfied.

Lack of Availability of Diagnostic Aids

Approximately 75% of all ulcers are venous with 25% containing some amount of arterial component. Because some clients have mixed aetiology ulcers it is essential to utilize objective tests to determine the quality of arterial supply to the limb. If this is not done there is a real risk of the client receiving inappropriate treatment. Callum *et al.* (1987b) surveyed 154 surgical consultants regarding the number of clients seen with compression-induced necrosis. They found that 40% of surgeons had seen a total of 147 cases of such damage in a 5-year period, seven patients had required arterial reconstruction surgery and 12 had undergone amputation. This is avoidable if the correct test is carried out as part of the general assessment of each client. The simplest test used is called the ankle-brachial pressure index (ABPI) and involves comparing the systolic blood pressure of the arm with that at the foot (see Appendix 1 at the end of this chapter for a detailed explanation of what is involved).

It is generally accepted that an index of 1 reflects normal health (Negus, 1991). Any figure of less than 1 indicates a degree of arterial insufficiency; the lower the index the higher the degree of arterial insufficiency. For clients with mixed ulcers, most authorities take an index of 0.8 to be the lowest acceptable for use of compression bandaging. Even so, in these situations great care and close observation of the effects of compression must be instigated.

Experience has shown that it is fairly common for nursing and medical practitioners to misjudge the presence of arterial insufficiency, combined with what appears to be an uncomplicated venous ulcer. It is for this reason that routine testing with doppler ultrasound is advocated. The equipment can be purchased for under £300, and requires no maintenance other than periodic replacement of batteries. Qualified nurses can be trained to use it effectively, following instruction and supervised practice. However, in some areas availability of this equipment is severely restricted by managers' unwillingness to allocate the relatively small amount of funding necessary for its purchase. Although this is undoubtedly due to ignorance, it is nevertheless inexcusable. The pressure placed on managers to allocate funding for too many competing causes is understood, but this is a situation when a small investment is guaranteed to do a lot of good.

Lack of Availability of Effective Treatment Products

While an adequate range of primary dressings is available in hospital, and on prescription in the community for the treatment of arterial ulcers, the essential component of effective treatment of venous ulceration is compression bandaging. There are certain bandages classified under the Drug Tariff as 'compression' but many have not demonstrated their efficiency in clinical trials of sufficient rigour. Conversely, the four-layer system of bandaging, which has undergone extension research and has shown excellent results demonstrating that 74% of clients with venous ulceration can be treated within 12 weeks (Blair et al. 1988), is not available to community practitioners because it is not on prescription. Most hospitals are able to obtain supplies from their Regional Warehouse, but some have to do this through special order procedures which are time consuming and therefore prohibitive. The fact that each single component of the four-layer system is manufactured by a different company further complicates the procurement and handling of supplies. The four-layer system is extremely cost effective as the average cost per leg is only £4.60 per week. There are few situations where the system needs to be reapplied more frequently than weekly. Another product, the Granuflex hydrocolloid compression bandage, which although it has not received as extensive testing, nevertheless has demonstrated its efficiency, is likewise difficult to obtain in the community, as it is not on prescription (Sockalingham *et al.*, 1990; Cherry *et al.*, 1990).

Experience suggests that while the four-layer system is generally the method of choice, it is useful to be able to offer clients an alternative.

Lack of Co-ordinated Strategy

The scale of the 'leg ulcer problem' and its consumption of NHS resources in terms of manpower and supplies indicate that this issue should be on the agenda at the highest level of management. In practice this does not happen. Even the huge cost savings waiting to be realized fail to command the attention deserved. Matters associated with leg ulcers suffer from the influence of negative feelings which seem to prevent people from realizing the potential for improving client care and saving money. The leg ulcer issue is just crying out to be tackled and promises nothing but gains all round. Contrary to popular opinion, it is an extremely rewarding and often challenging area to work in. There is so much that can be done to help people with this condition by enlightened and innovative practitioners. The sad thing is that clients are so grateful for effective help which brings improvement to their condition, when in fact they should be angry that this has not happened sooner thus preventing them from the unnecessary experience of years of ulceration.

Callum *et al.* (1987a) found that almost half of the clients surveyed in their research reported leg ulceration spanning over 10 years. Indeed, most nurses working in this field will know clients who have had ulcers for 20 and 30 years. However, consider for a moment the possibilities already identified as achievable – most venous ulcer clients can expect to have their ulcer healed with the four-layer bandage in less than 12 weeks (Blair *et al.*, 1988).

Individual nurses, irrespective of how interested and dedicated they may be in this area, cannot tackle these issues on their own. Strong managerial and clinical support is necessary in order to identify the health care needs of the local population and design a strategy suitable for meeting them. Health care purchasers, whether they be local GP fundholders or health authorities, have been slow to act on this issue. This has led to a situation where health care providers are often isolated in their attempts to stimulate interest and battle against obstacles in attempts to secure appropriate care for clients. The first point on the Patient's Charter states that each client has the right to receive care on the basis of clinical need. Quite simply, this is not happening. Undoubtedly there are scattered pockets of excellence such as the Charing Cross Venous Ulcer project, Withington Hospital Venous Research Department, and some others, but the best practice possible should be available to all clients wherever they live.

The way forward is for community managers, general practitioners and specialist hospital departments to get together and formulate an effective comprehensive approach. In most instances this will be operationalized through the establishment of community clinics supported by an outreach service for those clients unable to travel to a clinic (Moffatt and Franks, 1990; Awenat, 1992)

Recurrence of Healed Ulcers

Once healing has taken place, often despite and not because of treatment, an unacceptably high number of clients suffer recurrence of ulceration. Callum *et al.* (1987a) identified recurrence in 67% of clients. This is solely due to deficits in staff and client knowledge, and is symbolic of the misconception of believing the ulcer to be 'the problem' rather than merely a visible sign of the underlying problem, which is venous hypertension. It is understandable that clients may assume that once the ulcer has healed the problem is over, but in fact unless correctly fitted compression hosiery is worn, venous pressures will return increasing the likelihood of subsequent ulceration. This is demoralizing and frustrating for all concerned, yet it is avoidable. The best way of preventing recurrence is to ensure that adequate aftercare is provided. This involves measuring and fitting suitable compression hosiery which has been chosen by the client and arranging for periodic review.

Dinn and Henry (1988) demonstrated the value of 3-monthly review clinics for clients with previous ulcers. They found a recurrence rate of 14.7% in a sample of 122 clients studied, which compares very favourably with the alternative of 67% (Callum *et al.*, 1987a).

Review or Prevention of Recurrence Clinics are an opportunity to check that clients are satisfied with their choice of compression hose, are wearing it correctly, understand how to care for their legs and hosiery, how and when to obtain replacements, and know the signs and symptoms of imminent re-ulceration. The legs should be periodically remeasured as their size can and does alter over time. Clients known to have had mixed ulcers should have at least an annual check on their ankle/brachial pressure index, as the possibility of insidious advancement of arterial disease needs monitoring. If the index is found to be decreasing, then decisions need to be made concerning the advisability of continuing to wear compression hose; sometimes this may indicate a change to a lower strength of compression.

Understandably, most people would prefer not to have to wear compression garments, especially during warm weather, but for ex-leg ulcer sufferers who wish to avoid further ulcers this is not an option. Coming to terms with any enforced lifestyle change is never easy, feelings of dependence can create frustration and resentment. It is important that professional carers acknowledge these issues and allow clients the opportunity to talk about their feelings.

An approach that can help to give clients feelings of control over the situation is to ensure that they are able to make an informed choice of the exact type and style of compression hose to be worn. This can only be accomplished if the client is able to see and handle samples of garments available. Most manufacturers are willing to provide clinics with samples from their range. Clients can then choose the kind of product which they feel they will be able to live with. Styles available vary and include below-knee, thigh length, tights, and men's compression socks. Colours are numerous and include flesh, black, brown and navy; men generally preferred the darker colours.

Small chemists and hospital appliance departments may be unwilling to stock a large range of products, and this can be detrimental to client choice and ultimately compliance. However, there are companies such as Credenhill in Derbyshire who will obtain virtually anything for clients. In this situation the client sends the prescription to them and the product is returned by post. Such companies are also an important source of advice for clients and health care professionals. An excellent article by Dale and Gibson (1990) provides further information about compression hosiery.

Another important reason why ulcers recur is particularly evident in older people living alone, who due to problems with manual dexterity, immobility or confusion may be unable to apply and remove their compression hose. The Community Care Act (1990) heralded the introduction of comprehensive health and social care assessments designed to identify problems and needs leading to the construction of an individualized package of community care. A key principle of the Act is the promotion of user responsive seamless care. Once again leg ulcer sufferers have missed out! When leg ulceration is present, the highly qualified district nurse will attend. However, when it is healed district nurses feel overqualified to attend 'merely' for the application and removal of hosiery. Home helps and sheltered housing wardens do not accept this to be part of their remit. So while everyone argues about whose job it is, venous hypertension is gradually creeping back and just a slight knock to the leg produces the next ulcer, followed by the next visit by the district nurse.

Innovative schemes need to be established to ensure that health education and preventative care is provided. An idea being considered locally is for education community auxiliaries, home helps, wardens and other grades of unqualified staff to be able to integrate simple, but essential, assistive and monitoring measures into their job. Such an approach, however, would not negate the need for periodic review by professional staff.

Public Awareness

Many studies acknowledge that their figures of incidence and prevalence are, at best, an underestimation owing to the unknown numbers of people who are treating their own ulcers without any professional support. Because clients do not realize that effective treatment is possible they rarely assert demands for better care. A small number of clients positively 'opt out' of the health care system with which they are frustrated and self-treat. Nurses regularly come across people who have been self-treating for months or years. Treatments used are invariably topical applications, often quite inappropriate and sometimes potentially harmful. Compression bandaging or hosiery are seldom used by the lay public without professional advice. Therefore, the main treatment agent is usually missing and ulcers fail to respond owing to this and the effects of local applications which can include lanolin, steroid and antibiotic creams, all of which are not recommended. There is now an abundance of support groups and organizations for many other diseases such as diabetes, psoriasis, etc., but at the present time this is lacking for leg ulcer clients.

ADVANCING NURSING PRACTICE

Having now explored some deficiencies in the current system, let us now consider the opportunities presented for advancing nursing practice.

Nursing Assessment

Whenever leg ulcer clients are encountered, whether in the community or in hospital, a full assessment exploring the biological, psychological and social aspects of the clients' health status is necessary. The particular model of nursing used will be influenced by personal preference and local practice. Experience suggests that an activities of living framework modified to include extra sections for leg and wound assessment and pain with scope for special health education, works well (Roper *et al.*, 1980; Awenat, 1992). The 'fix-it-quick' superficial approach, which deals mainly with the legs, thereby ignoring all other aspects of health, is unsatisfactory, and often proves more costly in time and effort later on.

As already identified clients may have lived with a leg ulcer for many years, and inevitably the effects of this become integrated into each person's lifestyle. Distressing symptoms such as pain cause anxiety, frustration, anger and eventually a sense of hopelessness that this unremitting drain on life's energy will ever leave them. Lifestyle patterns that have been dictated by 'waiting-in' for the nurse to visit to renew dressings become restricted. Social contacts are sometimes lost and the paraphernalia of boxes of pads and dressings, etc. takes over the house. Before long, the home becomes a shrine to the leg ulcer with daily worshipful ceremonies performed by visiting professionals! Because life seems to revolve around treatment for the ulcer and consideration of restrictions caused by it, clients appear to be obsessed with it. This preoccupation becomes a source of annoyance and irritation for some nurses. Leg ulcer clients are frequently labelled as non-compliant and unpopular. Often they are victims of the processes and circumstances they have found themselves in along the course of seeking a cure for the ulcer.

Clients' previous experiences of treatment inevitably influence the present. They frequently relate long lists of different wound care products, matched only by the variety of nurses and doctors consulted. In one health district, Murray (1990) found that 65 different wound care products or combinations were being used to treat leg ulcers.

Blair (1988a) conducted a randomized comparative study of healing rates of venous ulcers using either a simple non-adherent dressing, a hydrocolloid or an antimicrobial agent, all with the four-lay bandages. They found no differences in healing rates and concluded that it is the graduated compression and not the dressing that is influential, thereby recommending the use of the simple cheap non-adherent dressing.

Professional Attitude

The attitude of health care professionals is vitally important, as this can be contagious to clients who, having been led to believe that their venous ulcer will never heal, naturally acquire a sense of pessimism. Equally, it is obvious that clients will lose confidence in staff who frequently substitute one treatment for another in a 'trial or error' approach.

From the outset, it is crucial to display an open and honest approach for until assessment is completed, ulcer aetiology remains unknown and therefore the nurse is not in a position to discuss the issue of likely prognosis. Once the causative factor is identified, an indication of expected outcome can be made. The situation is very optimistic for those with venous ulcers, but less so for mixed or arterial ulcers.

Older Clients

The older client frequently presents with multipathology where a number of co-existing illnesses affect and are affected by the ulcer. For example, osteoarthritis may limit the individual's ability to walk and exercise the calf muscles. Anaemia will hinder wound healing, as will consumption of steroids taken for a chest or joint condition. A history of diabetes or rheumatoid arthritis increases the likelihood of small vessel arterial disease (arteritis) (Dale and Gibson, 1986).

Health Education

Baseline information of the client's existing knowledge and beliefs about the ulcer is needed for use in planning to meet health education needs. Clients sometimes have rather strange ideas about why they have an ulcer. It is not unknown today to encounter almost medieval ideas about the ulcer being an escape route for badness, etc.

Invariably, people think that the ulcer is caused solely by the relatively minor traumatic injury which often precedes its appearance. This misconception is understandable as it is frequently shared by nurses, but it needs correcting otherwise it is unlikely that the client will understand the rationale for compression treatment. As the venous disease process is largely invisible, occurring beneath the skin, it is useful to use diagrams to illustrate what is happening.

Lewin's theory of change, which maps out the driving forces and the restraining forces in any situation where a change is aimed for, is a useful framework when considering each client's unique situation (Pearson and Vaughan, 1984).

Becker's Health Belief Model is another useful tool that aids understanding of sick role behaviour and likelihood of treatment compliance. Becker (1974) explains that to achieve compliance clients must believe in the diagnosis, and the prescribed treatment; they must also believe in the likelihood of serious consequences of untreated disease. There must be more gains than losses in complying with treatment and there needs to be a cue for action.

This can be applied not only to the local treatment of compression bandaging, but also to other factors such as smoking cigarettes which is known to be detrimental to wound healing and health in general.

The best results are obtained when the client is abled to participate in a full discussion of the scientific facts with the nurse helping to point out areas of particular relevance. However, clients have the right to reject information and suggestions made, and the nurse's role does not involve dictating and imposing his or her own standards and beliefs upon the client. A heavy handed autocratic approach tends to limit the acceptability of information given and may serve to alienate clients from the desired course of action.

Psychosocial Assessment

Clients' feelings about the ulcer, and their expectation of whether it will heal or not are often suppressed, as questions concerning these issues are rarely asked. Yet when such matters are explored they often release considerable pent-up anger and sadness. Discussion with the consequent exploration of previously unspoken feelings is often therapeutic in its own right.

In the past such discussions have revealed the existence of depression, relationship problems and other serious psychosocial consequences of leg ulceration. The odour caused by one man's ulcer caused his wife to move out of their bedroom to the spare room, as it made her nauseated. This caused the patient to feel rejected and unclean, and their relationship became strained. Happily this man, who had also suffered much pain for the 12 years of his ulcer's duration, was completely healed within 12 weeks and has remained so ever since.

Many more couples separate at night owing to the partner's fear of banging the ulcer when turning over in bed, or worry about exudate leakage from dressings. To have knowledge of the particular worries and fears of an individual client is very useful in planning their care in order to utilize the motivating forces necessary for compliance with treatment.

Alternatively, there are sometimes restraining forces present; that is, reasons why an individual feels that overall he or she will not benefit if the ulcer heals. Undoubtedly, a very small number of people do 'need' their ulcers psychologically, but this will only be identified by sensitive exploration of their feelings during the psychosocial aspect of assessment. When this is apparent, a non-judgemental approach is of paramount importance in order to engage the client in a plan of action.

Leg ulcer clients are frequently labelled non-compliant by district nurses, yet experience suggests that situations where this truly occurs are uncommon. Sometimes this may manifest when clients feel they have very little to gain if the ulcer heals. For example, it has been known to occur in an older person who lived in a deprived inner city area where the only friendly person encountered was the nurse who came to do her dressings. Unless such needs for social contact and stimulation can be met by other more appropriate agencies the problem could remain unsolved indefinitely.

Occasionally patients may need their ulcer for the sick role status it gives them, sometimes clients can become institutionalized not by a building, but by a system that invokes passivity and dependence. A graduated long-term plan to empower such clients and help them regain control over their own lives is required.

Pain

During assessment particular attention should be paid to any history of pain, the type, intensity, location, precipitating factors along with measures commonly employed by the client to manage the problem. Severe cramp-like pain which occurs when the limb is elevated, for example in bed at night, or which occurs during exercise is highly suggestive of arterial insufficiency. Rest pain eventually occurs in advances states of arterial disease (Negus, 1991).

Again, merely having the chance to talk about the problem of pain and feel that this is being taken seriously by the nurse, is in itself therapeutic. This is especially so when talking leads to a plan of action for either more indepth investigation or treatment. In situations where the picture is unclear, it sometimes helps to ask the client to complete a pain chart listing details of where and when the pain occurs, how strong it is, and any measures that either reduce or increase the pain. When this is reviewed with the client, simple measures such as altering the timing of analgesia consumption may help. Attempts to quantify the subjective experience of pain are necessary in order to be able to determine clear goal statements and evaluate progress. For this purpose it is useful to ask clients to rate their pain by scoring it on a scale of 0–10 (Hayward, 1975).

Clients with venous ulcers treated with the four-layer compression bandages usually find that any pain diminishes and then ceases completely within a few weeks. One such client had lost several months working time owing to his painful ulcer and was so desperate that he was begging for admission to hospital on presentation to the leg ulcer clinic; within 1 week of bandaging he was pain free.

The ability to reduce pain was demonstrated in a sample of 168 clients treated with the four-layer system (Franks *et al.*, 1992).

Examination of the Legs

Examination of the legs is carried out following general health assessment. Particular attention is paid to the presence of pedal pulses (dorsalis pedis and posterior tibial), brown skin staining, ankle flare (visible five network of venules around the medial malleolus) and tissue induration, all of which are characteristic of a venous aetiology. Signs of arterial insufficiency include a cold white hairless limb, sluggish capillary refill, and weak or absent pedal pulses. The ankle/brachial pressure index of each limb is then identified using the doppler ultrasound instrument. If there is any difficulty in obtaining a conclusive result, the client may need to be referred to the clinical physiology department for more extensive tests.

The nature and characteristics of the ulcer itself are also important in judging its aetiology. Venous ulcers are typically situated around the ankle area. They are shallow with sloping edges, often sloughy and progress slowly. Arterial ulcers may be situated anywhere on the leg or foot, are often deep and described as 'sharply punched out'. The wound edges are very defined and the ulcer may be necrotic. Deep ulcers may expose tendons or even bone. Venous ulcers are never found on the toes or heels or other parts of the foot, so when this situation presents an arterial cause must be suspected. These lesions are particularly found in patients with diabetes (Elkeles and Wolfe, 1991)

Unusual Ulcers

Rarities such as malignant ulcers should be suspected if overgrowth of tissue occurs at the base or edges of the ulcer, or if the edges have a rolled appearance. Surgical biopsy should be requested as a matter of urgency (Negus, 1991).

Another unusual type of ulcer is that caused by pyoderma gangrenosum. Here the ulcer appears to burrow under the skin edges which are a bluish\purple colour. Progression is rapid and the condition is associated with a history of rheumatoid arthritis or inflammatory bowel disease. Medical referral is essential as steroids are necessary (Kingston, 1992).

Nursing Practice Development

A sound knowledge base is essential preparation for nurses working in environments where they are developing autonomy in caring for patients with leg ulceration. The UKCC (1992) document *The Scope of Professional Practice* supports such roles provided that education underpins professional development. Thankfully, the system of 'extended roles' so engulfed in bureaucracy, which restricted rather than extended professional practice, is now behind us. Nurses have tremendous potential to help clients with leg ulceration provided that matters are approached sensibly. Innovative nurse-led schemes must be developed in full consultation with managers and medical staff. There is usually little if any resistance to nurses wishing to develop advanced clinical skills, as doctors are generally happy to withdraw from extensive input to leg ulcers. Barriers, when they do occur, are invariably due to difficulties in securing funding for the purchase of the four-layer bandage system, which is still not on community prescription. Schemes that allow the nurse easy and rapid access to medical consultants, especially vascular specialists for support when needed, are important. Regular contact with such staff promotes mutual understanding and develops effective interdisciplinary relationships crucial for teamwork.

MANCHESTER ROYAL INFIRMARY LEG ULCER CLINIC

In my own clinic, which was set up in January 1991, considerable efforts have been invested into creating the right atmosphere for clients. Attempts have been made to move away from the standard outpatient clinic model where clients feel they are processed along a conveyor belt. A more individualized humanistic approach which facilitates the development of therapeutic relationships and environments is adopted. It is pleasing that these initiatives were recognized by the Secretary of State and have been included in the Quality Compendium (DoH, 1993).

Care Plan Contracts

New clients are seen by one of two specialist nurses for a full assessment of their problems and needs. Older clients with leg ulcers invariably have other coexisting problems that affect and are affected by the ulcer; immobility, and nutritional deficiencies are fairly common. The first visit usually takes at least 1 hour by which time both nurse and client should be able to agree on the next course of action. This is documented in the form of a nurse–client care plan contract which is set out in columns so that the problem, desired outcome, nursing interventions and client's role can be clearly stated. Both nurse and client sign and keep a copy of the completed care plan contract. This approach was arrived at because we were aware that clients were required to absorb considerable amounts of new information about their ulcer, including how they could help themselves by following certain instructions. We also knew that clients often presented to us in a fairly anxious state, because of the effects of their ulcer, combined with anticipation surrounding attending a hospital clinic and meeting new staff.

Anxiety is a well-recognized barrier to learning; studies suggest that as much as 40% of what is said during consultations may be forgotten by clients. Use of learning contracts aims to reduce the pressure felt by clients relating to the need to retain verbal information. Also important is the potential to individualize suggested approaches for each client, and to offer clients the opportunity to be fully participant in their own care. Learning about their condition and its treatment is a necessity for empowering clients so that they can exercise their rights of choice and involvement in care by informed decision making.

Learning contracts are now used extensively in nurse education programmes following increasing frustration with traditional methods (Keyzer, 1986; Richardson, S., 1987; Richardson, M., 1988). However, their use in client care situations is equally appropriate but less frequently practised. 'Nursing contracts' may also be used with clients, having advantages for clarification of treatment objectives and client participation in health-giving activities.

Use of purpose designed nurse–client contracts has confirmed their usefulness in providing clients with clear written information which acts as an *aide-mémoire* for instructions given; can be used as a tool for negotiating mutually shared goals and treatment plans; and encourages investment in and ownership of the treatment programme.

Evaluation

Evaluation of care follows similar principles of a shared and participative approach and specific documentation has been designed to record this. Accurate evaluation is achieved by use of objective measurements of the progress of ulcer healing such as wound tracing, and polaroid photographs. Serial photographs are particularly helpful for clients to be able to visualize the improvements in the size and nature of their ulcers. They are also useful for clients to take home with them in order to show progress to a spouse. Access to photographs helps them to stay in touch with progress and prevents feelings of exclusion.

Treatment for Venous Ulcers

The mainstay of treatment for venous ulcers in graduated compression bandaging, the four-layer system, is the main treatment used in the Manchester Royal Infirmary clinic. However, some clients, who wish to receive compression but feel unable to compromise regarding continued use of fashionable footwear, choose a single layer hydrocolloid compression bandage (Frank *et al.*, 1990). Whilst this product cannot compete with the extensively researched four-layer system, experience suggests that it is effective and can produce excellent results for some clients. An inner layer of tubular stockinette is applied over the primary dressing and under the hydrocolloid bandage leaving a few centimetres exposed at the toes and below the knee to ensure good adhesive contact of the hydrocolloid bandage. Like the four-layer, this is applied once each week. Another similarity is that this also is not on prescription!

There are training implications for the application of compression bandages, which need to be addressed by all nurses prior to attempting this treatment. Dale (1990) identifies the decline of practical instruction in nurse training programmes and the upsurge in popularity of tubular bandages as reasons why the art and skill of compression bandaging has been overlooked. The technique needs to be learnt in clinical practice under the supervision of an experienced practitioner. Straight tubular bandages are totally unsuitable for treatment of leg ulcers as, when fitted to apply even minimal pressure at the ankle, they will be too tight around the calf, and conversely if comfortable at the calf will be useless, supplying no compression to the ankle. Shaped tubular bandages are available but difficult to obtain as they are not usually stocked in regional warehouses owing to their increased cost, and are not on prescription.

Moffatt (1992) reviews the literature on the technical aspects of compression bandages and highlights the importance of measurement of the ankle when using the four-layer system. Such considerations relate to the underlying principles of the laws of physics (Laplace's Law) (Moffatt, 1992). Most clients' ankle measurements fall within the 18–25 cm range indicating the suitability of the standard four-layer components. However, measurements outside of this range indicate the need for modification to this regime. Cornwall (1988) describes practical techniques for application of compression bandages and some companies supply instructional videos, or will sponsor training sessions by paying for the costs of organizing training workshops facilitated by visiting specialists.

Allergy

The problems associated with allergy and irritation known to occur with paste bandages (Moffatt, 1992) and clients' reported distaste for those products mean that they are not used in our clinic. Cameron (1990) advocates routine skin patch testing for clients with leg ulcers, although having visited specialist skin centres our opinion is that the techniques are expensive, can only be successfully performed and interpreted by experienced specialists in dermatology, and that this is unnecessary when only bland non-irritant products are used in treatment.

Ulcer Cleansing

Ulcers, and indeed all wounds, heal best when there is minimal disturbance to the natural environment of the wound surface. Weekly cleansing with plain warm tap water is followed by application of a simple non-adherent dressing and compression bandaging. Like many other centres we previously cleansed with sterile normal saline solution, but found this appeared to have no advantages in practice over tap water. A clean plastic bag is used to contain the water irrigated over the client's leg. This approach is supported by experts in this field (Gibson, 1990; Moffatt; 1992). Use of a plastic bag avoids the need to use a bowl or leg bath which could be a source of cross-infection. Since using tap water we have noticed that our wound infection rate has been much reduced, and we feel that this may be due to the effects of the entire leg and foot receiving a wash. Another advantage of this approach is that there is no need for dressing packs and cotton wool balls, which have been implicated in the problem of depositing microscopic filaments of wool into the wound bed, causing inflammation, sepsis and delaying healing (Thomas, 1990).

Infection vs. Contamination

Experience suggests that acute infection of leg ulcers does not occur as frequently as some nurses believe. All leg ulcers become colonized with bacteria, but this does not necessarily cause a problem or interfere with the progress of wound healing. Blair *et al.* (1988a) studied the bacteriology swabs of 120 venous ulcers at fortnightly intervals for 12 weeks and concluded that bacterial contamination did not prevent healing. The differences between contamination and acute infection are that in the latter the wound may have a purulent exudate, smells offensive, is painful, appears reddened and inflamed and the surrounding skin, or even the whole leg may feel hot to touch. In severe infection the client may feel generally unwell and have a pyrexia. When this situation presents a bacteriology swab should be taken, but otherwise routine swabbing is unnecessary and a waste of money. When an acute wound infection is suspected medical referral is mandatory as oral antibiotics will be needed.

There is no place for topical antibiotics in the form of creams or impregnated tulles in the management of leg ulcers. They are likely to be ineffective at controlling any infection present, may provoke development of allergic responses and can lead to resistant strains of the organism developing.

General Health

Assessment of the client's general health may reveal the need for advice about nutrition, particularly in relation to the need for adequate amounts of protein, vitamins and minerals. Exercise should be encouraged as walking uses the calf muscle pump which aids venous return. However, avoidance of gravitational posture such as standing inactively or sitting for long periods with the legs dependent should be stressed. Diagrammatic exercise sheets can be given to assist calf muscle pump action and maintain ankle joint mobility. Clients with a stiff ankle joint may need referral to a physiotherapist for more specialized help.

Arterial Ulcers

Clients who are found to have arterial or mixed aetiology ulcers should be referred to a vascular surgeon for consideration of operative measures. For those clients for whom these procedures are unsuitable the treatment objectives may well be confined to control of pain, maintenance of general health and local wound care, which should aim to prevent infection and promote healing. Each wound should be individually assessed and an appropriate dressing selected to meet the needs of the wound at that time.

Skin Grafting

Large surface area wounds benefit from skin grafting. Millard *et al.* (1977) reported success rates of 50 and 70% for venous and arterial ulcers, respectively, 2 years following pinch skin grafting. This is a technique which is now being performed by some specialist nurses (Freak, 1992), and this demonstrates yet another area into which nurses are willing to move to help clients.

Professional Networking

Requests to visit our clinic by nurses from other areas identified a great deal if interest in the nursing care for clients with leg ulcers, and this stimulated formation of a special interest group named the North West Nurses Leg Ulcer Special Interest Group. In its first year of existence membership reached around 150 and is steadily growing. The aims of the group are essentially to provide a forum for the exchange of ideas and innovations in this field, and to offer support to nurses. Meetings are held quarterly and a guest speaker presents a session on a topic of relevance. Plans are now underway to support the establishment of similar linked groups nationwide.

CONCLUSIONS

The low status of leg ulcers and work involving the care of such clients who are predominantly older has mitigated against widespread activity to develop more effective treatments.

While a few centres of excellence are transcending barriers to effective care and striving ahead with research and innovative methods of care, far too many others are lagging behind using outdated practices. The situation is remediable with good management and education, and it is pleasing to note the support and interest of Mrs Yvonne Moores (present day Chief Nurse for the Department of Health of England) who has promised to explore ways of championing these issues from the highest level of government (Moores, 1993).

The prospect of cure and prevention of recurrence is within the reach of the vast majority of clients with venous ulcers. Denial of the basic requirements to achieve this is intolerable and reflective of ageism. Until this problem is dealt with effectively nurses must continue to practice client advocacy by raising this matter with policy makers.

The day when a venous leg ulcer would be considered an acute wound could occur within a few years if managers and practitioners would devise effective strategies for change.

CLINICAL DISCUSSION POINTS

How are leg ulcers treated in your clinical area? Do clients have access to a specialist clinic? In clinical practice, is the distinction made between venous and arterial ulcers?

Try to arrange a visit to a specialist clinic. Discuss with the nurses there how they see their role.

Find out if there are any specialist interest groups or support networks for nurses working with older people in your area. Discuss setting one up for your area with your colleagues.

SUGGESTIONS FOR FURTHER READING

Louden, I. (1981). Leg ulcers in the 18th and early 19th Century. **Journal of the Royal College of General Practitioners 31**, 263–273.

Ryan, T. J. (1983). **The Management of Leg Ulcers.** Oxford University Press, Oxford.

REFERENCES

Awenat, Y. (1992). Leg ulcer clinic: Advanced nursing. **Nursing Standard** 7(7), 4–7.

Bale, S. (1987). Dressing leg ulcers. **Journal of District Nursing** 5(9), 9–13.

Bauer, G. (1942). A roentological and clinical study of the sequels of thrombosis. **Acton Chirurgica, Scandinavia 86** (Suppl 74), 104.

Becker, M. (1974). The health belief model and sick role behaviour. **Health Education Monograph 2**, 409–419.

Blair, S., Backhouse, C., Wright, D., Riddle, E. and McCollum, C. (1988a). Do dressings influence the healing of chronic venous ulcers?

Blair, S., Wright, D. Backhouse, C., Riddle, E. and McCollum, C. (1988b). Sustained compression and healing of chronic venous ulcers. **British Medical Journal 297**, 1159–1161.

Bosanquet, N. (1991). Venous ulcers. Treatment, costs and benefits. **Charing Cross Study Day Papers.** London

Callum, M., Ruckley, C., Harper, D. and Dale, J. (1985). Chronic ulceration of the leg: extent of the problem and provision of care. **British Medical Journal 290**, 1855–1856.

Callum, M., Harper, D., Dale, J. and Ruckley, C. (1987a). Chronic ulcer of the leg: clinical history. **British Medical Journal 294**, 1389–1391.

Callum, M., Ruckley, C., Dale, J. and Harper, D. (1987b). Hazards of compression treatment of the leg: an estimate from Scottish surgeons. **British Medical Journal 295**, 1382.

Cameron, J. (1990). Patch testing for leg ulcer patients. **Nursing Times. Journal of the Wound Care Society Supplement 86**, 63–64.

Cherry, G. and Ryan, T. (1989). **Blueprint for the Treatment of Leg Ulcers and Prevention of Recurrence.** Squibb Surgical, Middlesex.

Cherry, G., Cameron, J., Cherry, C. and Ryan, T. (1990). Clinical comparison of a new adhesive compression bandage with other treatments. **Care Science and Practice 8**(2), 80–82.

Cornwall, J. (1988). Venous ulcers and compression. **Journal of District Nursing** (September), 4–6.

Cornwall, J. (1991). Managing venous leg ulcers. **Community Outlook** (May), 36–38.

Cornwall, J., Dore, C. and Lewis, J. (1986). Leg ulcers: epidemiology and aetiology. **British Journal of Surgery 73**, 693–696.

Dale, J. (1990). Compression – how and why? **Care Science and Practice 8**(2), 63–66.

Dale, J. and Gibson, B. (1986a). Leg ulcers: a disease affecting all ages. **Professional Nurse May**, 213–214.

Dale, J. and Gibson, B. (1986b). Leg ulcers: the nursing assessment. **Professional Nurse June**, 236–238.

Dale, J. and Gibson, D. (1990). Back-up for the venous pump. Compression hosiery. **Professional Nurse,** 481–486.

Department of Health (1993). **A–Z of quality, a guide to quality initiatives in the NHS.** NHS Management Executive, Leeds.

Dinn, E. and Henry, M. (1988). The effectiveness of graduated compression stockings with regular follow-up in prevention of venous ulcer recurrence. **Swiss Medicine, 10**, 127–128.

Ebersole, P. and Hess, P. (1981). **Toward Healthy Ageing.** CV Mosby, London

Elkeles, R. and Wolfe, J. (1991). The diabetic foot. **British Medical Journal 303**, 1053–1055.

Frank, M., Sharik, C. and Queen, D. (1990). Granuflex hydrocolloid compression bandage, a new practical treatment for leg ulcers. **Care Science and Practice 8**(2), 89–90.

Franks, P., Moffatt, C. Connolly, M., Bosanquet, N., Oldroyd, M., Greenhalgh, R. and McCollum, C. (1992). Quality of life during leg ulcer treatment. **Phlebologie 92**, 275–277.

Freak, L. (1992). Personal Communication. Vascular Research Sister, Withington Hospital, Manchester.

Gibson, B. (1990). Use of compression in the treatment of leg ulcers. **Care Science and Practice 8**(2), 67–69.

Hayward, J. (1975). **Information – A Prescription Against Pain.** Royal College of Nursing, London.

Henry, M. (1986). Incidence of varicose ulcers in Ireland. **Irish Medical Journal 79**(3), 65–67.

Hodkinson, H. (1976). **Common Symptoms of Disease in the Elderly.** Blackwell Scientific, Oxford.

Horton, R. (1980). **Vascular Surgery.** Hodder & Stoughton, London.

Keyzer, D. (1986). Using learning contracts to support change in nursing organisations. **Nurse Education Today 6**, 103–108.

Kingston, R. (1992). Personal Communication. Paper presented at Withington Hospital Leg Ulcer Study Day. Dr R Kingston, Consultant Dermatologist, Stepping Hill Hospital.

Langford, T. (1983). Establishing a nursing contract. **Nursing Outlook June**, 386–388.

Millard, L., Roberts, M. and Gatecliffe, M. (1977). Chronic leg ulcers treated by the pinch graft method. **British Journal of Dermatology 97**, 289–295.

Moffatt, C. (1992a). Personal Communication. Presentation to the North West Nurses Leg Ulcer Special Interest Group, Preston.

Moffatt, C. (1992b). Compression bandaging – the state of the art. **Journal of Wound Care 1**(1), 45–50.

Moffatt, C. and Franks, P. (1990). A new approach. **Community Outlook July**, 35–36.

Moores, Y. (1993). Personal Communication. North Western Regional Health Authority, Manchester.

Murray, Y. (1990). **A Description and Discussion of the Diagnosis and Management of Leg Ulcers Treated by Staff Working in Stockport Health Authority** Unpublished Document. Stockport Health Authority.

Negus, D. (1991). **Leg Ulcers – A Practical Approach to Management**. Butterworth, Heinemann, Oxford.

Pearson, A. and Vaughan, B. (1984). Introducing change into nursing practice. Module 7 in the Open University – **A Systematic Approach to Nursing Care.** Open University Press, Milton Keynes.

Richardson, M. (1988). Innovating androgogy in a basic nursing course. **Nurse Education Today 8**, 315–324.

Richardson, S. (1987). Implementing contract learning in a senior nursing practicum. **Journal of Advanced Nursing 12**, 201–206.

Roper, N., Logan, W. and Tierney, A. (1980). **The Elements of Nursing.** Churchill Livingstone, Edinburgh.

Rose, G. (1991). Epidemiology of atherosclerosis. **British Medical Journal 303**, 1537–1539.

Sockalingham, S., Barberel, J. and Queen, D. (1990). **Care Science and Practice 8**(2), 75–78.

Thomas, S. (1990). **Wound Management**. Pharmaceutical Press, Cardiff.

UKCC (1992). **The Scope of Professional Practice.** UKCC, London.

APPENDIX: ANKLE/BRACHIAL PRESSURE INDEX TEST

This test is performed as part of a comprehensive patient assessment, and will indicate the quality of arterial blood supply to the leg. Nurses wishing to use this test should ensure that adequate educational preparation is received before attempting it alone.

A hand-held portable doppler ultrasound unit with an 8 megahertz transducer and conducting gel are required.

The patient should have had both legs elevated for at least 15 min prior to the test.

A blood pressure cuff of appropriate size is applied to the upper arm with the tubes extending upwards. It is important to ensure that the inflatable bladder inside the cuff is positioned directly over the medial area where the brachial artery will be.

The brachial artery position is identified by manual palpation and conducting gel applied to this area. The doppler is then switched on and the transducer is positioned at an angle of around 45° over this area. The characteristic rhymthic beat of the arterial pulse will then be heard. It is helpful to gently rest your hand on the client's arm in order to secure your position, as this is easily lost with any slight movement.

With your other hand you now need to inflate the BP cuff to about 20 mmHg above the part where the beat disappears. Slowly deflate the cuff carefully noticing when the sound of the pulse returns and make a note of this reading.

The procedure is then repeated in the leg with the cuff being applied to the lower leg with the bladder covering the medical aspect of the leg and the tubes again extending upwards.

Consideration of means of prevention of cross-infection via the equipment is necessary. The ulcer should be covered with a dressing and the BP cuff should be waterproof, thus allowing decontamination with an alcohol wipe in between patients. If the ulcer extends across the areas near to the position of the artery to be examined it may be necessary to protect the transducer by means of an examination glove finger.

For the leg pressure recording either the dorsalis pedis, posterior tibial or peroneal artery may be used. Manual palpation should be attempted to locate the position of the artery, but if unsuccessful the gel and transducer are applied over the likely area.

It is important that both you and the patient are positioned sitting comfortably, as this sometimes takes several minutes when performed by an inexperienced person or when arterial insufficiency is present.

The readings obtained are arranged as a formula $\dfrac{\text{ankle pressure}}{\text{brachial pressure}}$ and divided out, e.g. $\dfrac{165}{150} = 1.1$

Arterial characteristics	*Venous characteristics*
Weak or absent foot pulses	Foot pulses present
Ankle pressure index less than 1	Ankle pressure index of 1 or more
Pale/whitish limb	Tissue induration
Sluggish capillary refill	Brown staining
Cool skin temperature	Dry skin scale
Pain at night/on exercise	Normal skin warmth
Deep punctured ulcer	Ankle flare sign
Ulcer situated anywhere	Shallow ulcer
	Ulcer around gaiter area

STEPS FOR ANKLE PRESSURE INDEX

- *Elevate both legs for 15 min.*
- *Record brachial systolic BP using doppler transducer.*
- *Record ankle systolic BP using doppler transducer.*
- *Calculate index:* $\dfrac{ankle\ BP}{brachial} = ?$
- *Index of 1 or more indicates normal arterial supply*.*
- *Index of below 1 indicates arterial insufficiency.*

*NB: Spuriously high readings may be obtained in older clients with atherosclerosis, as calcified deposits in the artery walls prevent occlusion of the artery with the sphygmomanometer cuff.

Chapter Twelve

The Challenge of Advocacy: A Moral Response

Kevin Kendrick

Core Themes in Gerontological Nursing

Ageing Matters	*New Social World*	*Lifespan Perspective*	*Health and Old People*
Illness and Dependency	*Quality Nursing Care*	*Therapeutic Intervention*	*Politicizing Gerontological Nursing*

Key Words

Advocacy • Best Interests • Power • Parentalism • Consent • Autonomy

INTRODUCTION

In recent times, it has become fashionable to use the term 'patient advocate' to describe the way that nurses represent, safeguard and promote the interests of clients during all aspects of care delivery. The central thrust of this chapter will be to explore critically the concept of patient advocacy with particular reference to care of older people.

This Chapter aims to provide an opportunity for the reader to:

Identify reasons why advocacy is required in health care

Critically explore the relationship between advocacy and the dominance of medicine

---

Analyse the term 'best interests' in relation to advocacy

Examine the usefulness of advocacy when seeking client consent.

'CARE TO ADVOCATE'

Nurses have always been expected to represent the best interests of clients. This theme is intrinsically reflected by the following edict from the UKCC (1992) *Code of Professional Conduct*:

Each registered nurse, midwife and health visitor shall act at all times, in such a manner as to safeguard and promote the interests of individual patients and clients.

The central purpose of the *Code of Professional Conduct* is to make clients' best interests a focal point for the nursing endeavour; this reflects the very essence of the professional creed. There is a clear link between the UKCC's directive to 'promote the interests of individual patients and clients' and the main elements of advocacy. Such themes have been embraced by nurses as a key aspect of their professional role; in terms of logical sequence, this involves becoming an 'active voice' when clients feel unable, for whatever reason, to articulate or represent their own best interests. Commenting upon the end point and purpose of patient advocacy, Brown (1985) states it is a 'means of transferring power back to the patient, to enable him to control his own affairs'.

What we have seen, so far, is that advocacy appears to fit comfortably as a feature of the nurse's role. The notion of the nurse as client advocate brings with it images of nurturing and caring which are firmly rooted in the professional ethos. Not to represent the client's best interests seems anathema to all that is sacred to nursing traditions and values. Yet we seem to be missing a fundamental question which should be at the very heart of our enquiry, namely, why should a nurse ever have to act as an advocate for the client? The earlier quote from Brown offers a starting point for beginning to answer this question when reference is made to 'transferring power back to the patient'. If clients are seen as autonomous equals in the delivery of health care, then why should there ever be a need to transfer 'power back'? What this reveals is that the process of delivering health care is based upon a power-laden scenario where client vulnerability and disempowerment become the validating themes for the role of the nurse as advocate. This is powerfully supported and echoed by Abrams (1978) who states 'The need for advocacy is the result of the failure of the health care structure to function as it should'. Thus, advocacy's shining veneer covers a lack-lustre concept that is a response to the health care system's own inadequacies.

We are beginning to challenge a concept which holds centre place in much of nursing's contemporary rhetoric. If advocacy is to hold real meaning, focus and direction for nurses then it must be viewed with a critical and enquiring gaze. Our next step will be to examine the power structures that give credence and reason to the existence of advocacy in health care.

DOCTOR KNOWS BEST

Nurses and doctors are undoubtedly key players in the delivery and practice of health care. However, the traditional association between each of these professional groups has centred upon the nurse giving prescribed care based upon the doctor's orders. Research indicates that doctors and lay public continue to see nurses as passive, acquiescent and servile (Mackay, 1989, 1993; Kendrick, 1994a). Such images are further reinforced by media representations which tend to fit nurses into a subservient role to doctors; such themes are graphically illustrated by Mackay (1989) who states:

> *Greater respect is bestowed on doctors because they can 'cure' people. Doctors can postpone death, therefore they command both authority and respect. Stereotypes in the mass media appear to enhance the status of doctors at the expense of nurses. Nurses are presented in the media as less helpful and less empathetic to the needs of patients and doctors. Yet when the reality of nurses' work is considered the stereotype is revealed for what it is: a put down of nurses and of women.*

The net result of these influences upon relationships between doctors, nurses and patients is presented by Chadwick and Tadd (1992, p. 49) in the following way:

Characteristically the doctor has been portrayed as 'all knowing' and powerful; the nurse as caring, unselfish, obedient and submissive; and the patient as helpless and utterly trusting.

In seeking to clarify reasons for this inequality between doctors and nurses, Turner (1986) argues that the servile themes traditionally associated with nursing has given doctors *carte blanche* to delegate and prescribe the activities of care-giving. This image of the nurse as subservient is placed in the medical student's psyche very early in the educational process, as Kendrick (1995, p. 245) states:

Medical students see themselves as scientists with a clear clinical mandate to use these skills to diagnose, treat and cure disease. This level of objectivity is absent in student nurses who value more highly the elements of caring as opposed to curing. However, not only do medical students view their work as having more intrinsic value than nursing, but they also have negative role models who propagate the view that nurses are essentially a pair of 'helping hands'. These two disparate levels of initiation set the tone for future relationships which doctors and nurses experience in their clinical work; it is a scenario borne out by tradition and is a prominent feature in the status quo of ward-based reality.

The nurse is often depicted as the 'victim' in professional dealings with doctors. Yet the question must be asked 'what has nursing done to confront and reduce medicine's often patriarchal and dominant stance?' The short answer is 'not very much'. Such accusations are vividly supported by research in care of older people settings; Kitson (1991, p. 23) comments upon the lack of distinction between nursing and medical frameworks by stating:

When one considers the corresponding nursing care model, which could have served as the theoretical framework for the geriatric nursing care model, a major problem arises, namely that nursing does not have an operational model independent of the medical model.

What this indicates is that nursing has seldom stood collectively against the affront of medical dominance and influence; Kitson (1991, p. 220) takes this further and asserts:

Nursing practice seemed content to follow in the wake of medical innovation and change. In consequence, nursing was unable to consider seriously the complexities involved in providing care. Nursing also failed to build a framework that would ensure the goal of care was achieved in the practice setting.

So often doctors are portrayed as power-crazed demagogues who purposively dwarf the position of nurses in health care; Kitson's research is so refreshing because it asks us to reflect critically on our own passivity in allowing such a position to exist and be propagated for so long. If accountability and responsibility are to be more than just 'buzz words' we need to be able to explain why such situations exist. At the centre of Kitson's research is a call for nurses to accept some culpability for the profession's inferior standing to medicine.

The tone of this section has been written in a deliberately challenging way. If we are to explore the reasons why nurses are expected to pick up the mantle of advocacy then we must be familiar with those themes which inform, create and maintain power and the *status quo*. Rather than argue it is all 'the doctor's fault', it would be more critical, reflective and, ultimately, more creative, to accept that part of the problem has been nursing's lack of impetus or collective vision to create change and address the balance of power.

What our enquiry has revealed, so far, is that nurses are collectively less powerful than their medical colleagues. Despite this unequal position, nurses have willingly grasped the role of advocate and argue that they are ideally placed to represent patients' best interests (Penn, 1994). To clarify the validity of this claim, we shall consider briefly the notion of advocacy within the legal profession.

When somebody is accused of a criminal charge, he or she has a legal right to be represented by a lawyer. An onus rests upon the lawyer to represent the interests of the accused during the course of the legal process – in this way the role of advocate is fulfilled. The person accused of an alleged crime would feel that justice and due process was compromised if a lawyer was perceived as inferior or shackled by a tradition of subservience to other officers of the court. Applying these themes to a parallel scenario, how can nurses effectively fulfil the role of advocate when they hold unequal power in relation to doctors? This holds tremendous implications for the notion of 'best interests' and how they are defined.

IN WHOSE BEST INTERESTS?

We have discovered that health care delivery is heavily laden with issues of power. The very need for advocacy arises from the client entering a milieu which is both unfamiliar and disempowering; commenting upon this, Kendrick (1994b, p. 827) states:

> *The dual effect of illness and being cast into a clinical environment which is full of hidden rules and agendas places the patient in the centre of an alien and confusing quagmire of uncertainty.*

Clients are fully aware of the power which doctors hold and are reticent about challenging the established 'norms' of client behaviour. These themes are further reflected by Mackay (1993, p. 153) who states:

> *Patients are well aware of their role as the audience and as performer: they know what is expected of them. They know to be deferential when the 'great consultant' visits them and deigns to chat. They have been prepared for this great visit by the nursing staff.*

This creates an environment where the client is expected to acquiesce passively to treatment without question – the whole ambience of the clinical theme discourages notions of client participation or active enquiry; as Penn (1994) states:

Patients are frequently reluctant to discuss their feelings with doctors and rarely challenge doctor's decisions.

What we have is a position where clients feel vulnerable, disempowered and disenfranchized. Against this background, it is perfectly understandable that clients feel the need to have someone who can represent their best interests in a scenario which is dwarfing and threatening. The great paradox about lay perceptions is that, whilst they see nurses as subservient to doctors, they still feel they can ask the nurse to represent their best interests. This phenomena is made more poignant by clients tending to seek advocacy from the most junior of staff – often student nurses; Thompson *et al.* (1988, p. 24) give this parody great resonance when they draw parallels between the process of becoming, a nurse with that of becoming a client:

The process of becoming a nurse is in some ways similar to that of becoming a patient. The loss of a certain amount of identity, taking on a generalised role and behaving accordingly, are experiences common to nurses and patients ... New nurses often feel that they are in a rigid hierarchy which relies upon rank and punitive measures rather than rationality and reason.

Given the themes we have discovered about the relation between doctors, nurses, clients and power, it seems increasingly dubious to argue that nurses can play a credible and effective role as advocates. This gains further cogency when related to terms such as 'empowerment', which are often used to describe a process which has seen the best interests of the client realized in practice. Some commentators have taken this further and write about a utopian world where clients freely prescribe their best interests, unshackled by the constraints of vulnerability and disempowerment which we have already discussed. Reflecting this tendency, Murphy and Hunter (1984, p. 95) state:

The professional, while obligated to act in the patient's best interests, is not permitted to define that interest in any way contrary to the patient's definition; it is not the professional but the patient that shall define what 'best interests' shall mean.

Thus, if we, as nurses, are supposed to represent the themes of 'best interests' as the patient defines them, what should our responses be in the following scenarios?

- *Bill is a 79-year-old alcoholic. He is being treated on a surgical ward for varicose veins. The surgery has been successful and the postoperative period uneventful. However, the surgical registrar had noticed a bottle of whisky behind Bill's locker and confiscated it saying 'You can have it on discharge but your not drinking while in my care'. Bill is distraught and pleads with a nurse saying 'Look, please get my whisky back, if I start to get the "shakes" all hell will break loose – I need that whisky'.*

- *Julie is 64 and has been sectioned in an acute mental health unit. She has been suffering with depression and tried to commit suicide by jumping in front of a train. This is her thirtieth admission for similar problems. Each time she receives a course of electroconvulsive therapy and is then sent into the community where she is visited monthly by a community psychiatric nurse who gives her an injection. She is constantly depressed and even after treatment she pleads to be allowed to die. One evening she is talking to Neil, a student nurse and says 'why won't they let me do what I want, I just do not want to live, why won't anybody listen to me?'.*

In these scenarios it would be highly unlikely that the nurses involved would actively advocate for the clients in a way that mirrored their subjectively defined, best interests. These themes are eloquently supported by Allmark and Klarzynski (1992, p. 34) who argue:

> **An advocate should plead someone's cause as the person, and not the advocate, sees it. If a liberal lawyer pleads the cause of a neo-Nazi group to have freedom of speech then this is true advocacy. A nurse is unable to provide the alcoholic with a drink, plead for the overdose not to be treated, and for the sectioned patient to be allowed to leave.**

Part of the underlying trend which propagates such themes is a preoccupation among health professionals to treat patients in a way which is directly analogous to the way parents deal with a child. This forms the focus of our next section and is a sobering indictment against the effectiveness of nurses as client advocates.

'THE PATIENT CHILD'

As we have already discovered, the combined impact of illness and being in hospital can leave clients feeling exposed and vulnerable. This situation is made worse when health professionals deal with clients in a manner which is both demeaning and patronizing. When women engage in this sort of behaviour it is sometimes called matriarchy, and patriarchy in men. If these traits are intrinsic to the delivery of care, they can reinforce the power equation between doctors, nurses and clients (Lewin, 1977). Commenting upon the nature of this dynamic, Kendrick (1994b, p. 828) states

> **The combined influence of patriarchy and matriarchy is sometimes refered to as parentalism. Emerging from this is an image of a 'pseudo-family',**

*where the disempowered patient (child) conforms to the dominant wishes of
the doctor (father) and nurse (mother).*

These themes are graphically reflected in the following example based upon a real life
incident; all names used are fictitious:

Case Study: Mrs Smith's companion

*Mrs Irene Smith is 82-years-old and has advanced Parkinson's disease. A widow of some
25 years, Mrs Smith has lived a full and varied life, working as a nurse in many of the
developing countries before, in her early forties, training to be a teacher – finally retiring at
60 as the head of an infant's school.*

*The progressive nature of Parkinson's disease had slowly chiselled at Mrs Smith's
lifestyle; now she was completely immobile and unable to do the simplest of things for herself.
Talking was becoming increasingly difficult and it was with great regret that Mrs Smith
agreed to go into a gerontological unit.*

*Always a realist, she knew she would never see her home again and made
arrangements with her solicitor for the house and its contents to be sold. There was one
overriding problem which Mrs Smith did not know how to handle – what was to become of
Sam, a close companion who had shared her life for the past 10 years.*

*Sam also had poor health, severe arthritis had severely restricted his movements and
he would spend much of his life closely huddled on Mrs Smith's lap – he was a most
cherished cat and dearly loved by his owner.*

*Mrs Smith broached her concern's about Sam with Dr Simpson, the consultant
overseeing her medical care. With a rigid, staccato voice she pleaded that Sam be allowed to
come into the unit with her. The consultant's reply was minimal and patronising:*

**Now, now my dear, that would be quite out of the question – you don't
seem to appreciate the infections which cats can bring; no! it simply
would not do.**

*Pauline Geer, a staff nurse accompanying the consultant, knelt at Mrs Smith's side
and reinforced what had already been said 'Dr Simpson is right, cats carry all sorts of germs
and we couldn't risk this harming other patients – I'm sure with the money from the sale of
your house you will be able to pay for a lovely place for your cat to stay'.*

Mrs Smith weeps quietly and feels so very alone.

As this scenario reveals, the combined elements of power and parentalism can form a
potent cocktail which limits the framework in which clients can voice their own best
interests. In a part of her research which deals with power and advocacy, Makay (1993,
p. 153) states:

Quite a number of nurses were concerned simply to do what the senior doctor told them to do. They seemed to have no interest in a patient's advocate role. For these nurses, what was important was to obey the instructions of the doctor. For the less assertive nurse, there is little chance of being heard, and, if heard, of being attended to. These obedient nurses may serve the medical profession but they do not serve the patient.

Such language throws down a gauntlet to all of us who feel that clients should not be threatened or inhibited by the barbs of parentalism. There is little doubt that Mrs Smith has been treated in a demeaning fashion by both her doctor and nurse. Commenting upon this sort of behaviour, Kendrick (1995, p. 248) states:

This triangular relationship is based upon inequality and power: it should have no place in contemporary health care and is a moral anathema to those who feel client empowerment should be the focus of skills and care giving.

The way Mrs Smith was dealt with by the staff nurse makes a stark comment about the effectiveness of nurses as client advocates. Quite simply, if nurses are so steeped and embroiled within the confines of the health care system, with its inhibiting themes and threatening conventions, how can they possibly hope to represent the best interests of clients? Taking this to its logical conclusion, Allmark and Klarzynski (1992, p. 34) make the following, penetrative comment:

To suggest that a patient has an advocate when it is that very person who may be involved in the treatment that patient is trying to resist is analogous to suggesting that the police can act as advocates for people in custody.

The nature of this enquiry is concerned with a logical and systematic exploration of the central themes surrounding the notion of the nurse as the client's advocate. It is not sufficient that nurses merely claim ownership of the advocate role; such assertions should be supported with a cogent rationale which clearly displays the power and position needed to give such themes depth, focus and direction. What has emerged from our discussion, so far, is that the balance of power is weighed heavily against nurses having any real impact as client advocates in the delivery of care. The next section takes this further and considers some of the central issues surrounding advocacy and informed consent.

ADVOCACY AND FREEDOM TO CHOOSE

By its very nature, the term 'informed consent' demands that clients be given all of the necessary information to make an informed decision about whatever intervention is being offered to them. This should include an explanation of the potential risks and benefits involved and the possible ramifications if the treatment does not take place. These themes are echoed by Gillon (1986, p. 113) who argues that consent is:

A voluntary and uncoerced decision made by a sufficiently competent or autonomous person, on the basis of adequate information and deliberation, to accept rather than reject some proposed course of action that will affect him or her.

A question which logically follows from such thinking is: how much information should be given to patients before informed consent can be given to the treatment or intervention offered?

This question is both complex and controversial and different perspectives are held about possible answers. In seeking to clarify this situation, Kendrick (1991, p. 4) states:

There are two opposing views concerning informed consent: at one end of the spectrum there are those who believe that the patient should have access to every conceivable issue involved in their treatment or care. This is based on the understanding that a patient who is privy to both negative and positive aspects of treatment or care will be able to make an informed and valid consent. In contrast to this perspective is the paternalistic view that a nurse has the necessary insight and professional knowledge to judge when the giving of certain information would be harmful to the patient.

Arguments in favour of informed consent are usually based upon a respect for the client's autonomy. In its most fundamental form, autonomy simply refers to the level of an individual's self-government. Broadening this, Faulder (1985, p. 23) states that autonomy is essentially concerned with 'the individual's freedom to decide her or his goals and to act according to these goals'.

Linking all these themes to the notion of advocacy, a nurse should be able to represent the best interests of the client, as the client defines the term, throughout the process of gaining an informed consent. This is where we meet a conceptual schism between the well-meaning rhetoric of abstract concepts and their practical application in the delivery of care. Taking this further, talk of informed consent and advocacy fits comfortably in simple scenarios where, for example, a nurse asks a doctor to describe a procedure again, because the client did not understand the original explanation. The parameters surrounding such themes become much more blared and difficult to define when the clients autonomy is impaired or even absent; as Henry and Pashley (1990, p. 33) state:

Full autonomy is an ideal notion and we can only approximate to it. It is obvious that, in reality, some situations, states and circumstances will diminish a person's autonomy (such as the ability to control his or her action) through being restrictive in some e.g. illness, psychological impairment, physical or mental disability.

Consider the implications of what we have said when reading the following scenario. Once again, it is based upon a real life event – all names used are fictitious.

Case Study: Advocating consent

Mrs Josephine Douglas has lived in a long-stay gerontological unit for the past 5 years. She has advanced Alzheimer's disease and all of her relatives are now dead. In recent times, Mrs Douglas has become increasingly agitated whenever nursing staff try to attend to any of her needs. She is now very weak, confused and unable to do anything for herself.

Jolene is Mrs Douglas's primary nurse and has cared for her since admission. It has saddened Jolene to slowly watch Mrs Douglas ravaged by the nature of the disease; she remembers the early days when Mrs Douglas still had the vestiges of dignity which gave her demeanour such presence. One day remains poignantly vivid in Jolene's memory, when Mrs Douglas said 'I don't mind you calling me Josephine, but these young girls can have a bit of respect – I'm old enough to be their grandmother; so they can call me "Mrs Douglas" and nothing else'. This had endeared Jolene to Josephine and set seal to their relationship.

Josephine had becoming increasingly agitated over the course of the last 2 weeks; Jolene also noticed that Josephine had not had her bowels open for almost 5 days – quite out of keeping with her normal pattern. This was mentioned to the senior registrar who said she wanted to do a rectal examination. Jolene was surprised by the doctor's choice of action and gently suggested 'Mrs Douglas wouldn't like that, why don't we try some medication first?'

The registrar gave a terse reply, 'Yes! well before I make a decision about the medication I'd like to substantiate my position with facts – that's what clinical decisions are about!'

Jolene tries to explain to Josephine what the doctor wants to do. All through the examination, Josephine kicked out at the doctor continually screaming 'No, no'. This was not the first time that Jolene had been through this sort of thing with Josephine, and it caused her real anguish to see the reaction it caused.

Jolene was riddled with guilt at not being able to persuade the doctor to try medication before such an invasive procedure; running through her mind were questions such as:

- *'What if Josephine does have some inkling about her outside world and felt humiliated and affronted by the examination? She may have found the examination unbearable'.*
- *'How can I advocate for Josephine when the doctors don't act upon what I say and try and support their position by calling them 'clinical decisions'? After all, medicine is not an absolute science and we can only say, beyond reasonable doubt, that Alice does not know what is going on around her'.*

This example from practice bears a crushing testimony to the ineffectual base from which nurses try to act as client advocates. The very essence of the interaction between the doctor and nurse is wrapped in the politics of power. What emerged, during this scenario, are a number of themes which cogently reflect the impotence of the advocate role for nurses:

- *The doctor refers to her position with the scientific weight of a 'clinical decision'; this mirrors the traditional image of medicine as an objective process where clients passively submit to the laws of scientific enquiry.*
- *The thrust of this scenario draws an intense difference between the respective values which underpin medicine and nursing. Even though Josephine will not be cured, the methods of medicine are still seen, by doctors, as having much more worth than the intrinsic themes of caring associated with nursing.*

The doctor and the staff nurse disagreed about what would be the best way of dealing with Mrs Douglas's problem; often disagreements take place as a natural element in the process of achieving consensus. It is not the disagreement that causes a problem but the way in which the doctor dismisses Jolene's suggestion in such a patronizing manner. This is not to say that all interaction between doctors and nurses follow the pattern of this example. However, the incident is based upon a real event from practice and serves as a cogent example of how power can infringe upon the nurse's effectiveness to act as an advocate in the process of obtaining consent. In a chapter which explores why doctors and nurses disagree, Adshead and Dickenson (1993, p. 167) state:

> **If nursing is defined as being about caring, and medicine about curing, medicine will continue to be seen as more important. If the role of the female paradigm profession of nursing is seen as caring, the old stereotype of the nurse as doctor's 'helpmeet' will be revived. Caring is likely to be seen as less important than curing because we fear death and wrongly attribute to medicine the power to cure us of mortality.**

CONCLUSIONS: THE LIMITS OF ADVOCACY

At the very core of this chapter has been a plea for nurses to reflect critically on the themes and issues surrounding advocacy in relation to their own practice. It is not enough to act as advocates when we feel it is safe to do so. To represent the client's best interests in a way which is counter to the dominant themes of medicine's influence and power demands careful consideration, insight and understanding. Indeed, the overwhelming weight of this chapter strongly stands against the notion that nurses can effectively act as client advocates. Ask yourself the following questions:

- *Would you give an alcoholic client a drink of whisky?*
- *Would you actively advocate for the patient dying of cancer who wants a lethal injection to 'die with dignity'?*

Few of us would stand up and do what these clients request; indeed, there are strong moral and legal precedents which prevent us doing so. What we have then, is a form of advocacy which is relative to context and circumstance – it is fine to advocate in some situations but not in others. Explaining this further, you would advocate for the client who wants a bed bath, but would be unlikely to do so if a client posed one of the questions raised above. Commenting upon the precarious nature of the themes surrounding patient advocacy, Kendrick (1994b, p. 829) states:

> **When patients realise their best interests are not represented as a mirror of their own wishes, it can conflict with the trust placed in the health care team. What emerges from this is the realisation that care which was supposed to be delivered with a velvet glove carries with it a fist of steel.**

Once we lose the client's trust, any basis for care becomes violently and, often irredeemably, crushed. If advocacy carries with it the potential to achieve such an explosive end, we should openly question the moral basis for nursing's involvement with it. The purpose of this chapter is to make a small contribution towards this contentious, but vital debate.

Case Study: A dilemma in dying

Joe is 68 years of age and in the advanced stages of acquired immune deficiency syndrome (AIDS). He has succumbed to various opportunistic infections over the past 2 years and is currently being treated for pneumonia. He is terribly weak, finds it difficult to breathe and is confined to bed by the debilitating nature of the syndrome.

Recently Joe has become increasingly depressed; he is daunted and overwhelmed by the advancement of the illness and just cannot take the thought of spending the rest of his life being continually sick. There had been a little hope for a while with AZT but the periods between setbacks are getting shorter and shorter. However, what frightens Joe most is the fact that he is becoming increasingly forgetful and has noticed that his moods change without any rhyme or reason. Open discussion with the nurses and doctors emphasize Joe's most primal of fears – the possibility that the syndrome can lead to a form of dementia. Despite reassurances from the medical and nursing staff that Joe's state of mind would reflect that of anybody undergoing such a series of crisis – he remains absolutely petrified of dying in a demented state.

During his frequent periods in hospital, Joe has developed a warm relationship with the staff nurse – Daniel. When in conversation, Joe feels able to share with Daniel his hopes and worst fears about his illness and future. It has not all been 'doom and gloom' and many positive aspects have emerged during their time of sharing. However, one afternoon Joe seems particularly burdened and asks Daniel if he can be completely 'up front' with him.

Daniel tells Joe that he is glad that he feels able to be so open to which Joe replies 'I just cannot take it anymore Daniel...never knowing what illness is going to "throttle" me next. Last night I . . . I . . . wet the bed. There is no way that I'm going to spend the rest of my days like that. My mind is going – I know it is. Listen Dan, I'm telling you this because we've had some special moments that have helped me a lot . . . I've got some tablets and tonight it's going to be the old brandy and barbiturates. I'm not asking you to do anything to help me, but please be there when I take them; I can't carry on living like this; but I can't stand the thought of dying alone'.

CLINICAL DISCUSSION POINTS

Do you think it is possible for Daniel to advocate for Joe in this scenario? Give reasons for your answer.

What do you think this case study tells us about the role of the nurse as client advocate?

As a group, do you think the concept of advocacy should be a part of the nurse's role? Support your answers with reasoned argument.

REFERENCES

Abrams, N. A. (1978). A contrary view of the nurse as patient advocate. **Nursing Forum 17**(1), 260–266.

Adshead, G. and Dickenson, D. (1993). Why do doctors and nurses disagree? In: D. Dickenson and M. Johnson (Eds) **Death, Dying and Bereavement,** pp. 161–168. Sage, London.

Allmark, P. and Klarzynski, R. (1992). The case against nurse advocacy. **British Journal of Nursing 2**(1), 33–37.

Brown, M. (1985). Matter of commitment. **Nursing Times 81**(18), 26–27.

Chadwick, R. and Tadd, W. (1992). **Ethics and Nursing Practice: a Case Study Approach.** Macmillan, London.

Faulder, C. (1985). **Whose Body Is It? The Troubling Issue of Informed Consent.** Virago Press, London.

Gillon, R. (1986). **Philosophical Medical Ethics.** Wiley, Chichester.

Henry, C. and Pashley, G. (1990). **Health Ethics.** Quay, Lancaster.

Kendrick, K. (1991). Ethics: a baseline for practice. **Nursing 4**(34), 17–19.

Kendrick, K. (1994a). Towards professional parity. **Journal of Reviews in Clinical Gerontology 4**(4), 277–279.

Kendrick, K. (1994b). An advocate for whom – doctor or patient? How far can a nurse be a patient's advocate? **Professional Nurse 9**(12), 826–829.

Kendrick, K. (1995). Nurses and doctors: a problem of partnership. In: K. Soothill, L. Mackay and C. Webb (Eds) **Interprofessional Relations in Health Care,** pp. 239–252. Edward Arnold. London.

Kitson, A. L. (1991). **Therapeutic Nursing and the Hospitalised Elderly.** Scutari Press. Harrow.

Lewin, E. (1977). Feminist ideology and the meaning of work: the case of nursing. **Catalyst 10**(11), 78–103.

Mackay, L. (1989). **Nursing a Problem.** Open University Press, Milton Keynes.

Mackay, L. (1993). **Conflicts in Care: Medicine and Nursing.** Chapman & Hall, London.

Murphy, C. and Hunter, H. (1984). **Ethical Problems in the Nurse–Patient Relationship.** Allwin & Bacon, Boston.

Penn, K. (1994). Patient advocacy in palliative care. **British Journal of Nursing 3**(1), 40–42.

Thompson, I. E., Melia, K. M. and Boyd, K. M. (1988). **Nursing Ethics.** Churchill Livingstone, Edinburgh.

Turner, B. S. (1986). **Medical Power and Social Knowledge.** Sage, London.

United Kingdom Central Council for Nursing, Midwifery and Health Visiting (1992) **Code of Professional Conduct for the Nurse, Midwife and Health Visitor.** UKCC, London.

Section 4

European Perspectives

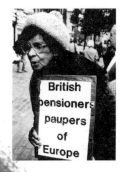

European Perspectives
Tom Keighley

*"For each age is a dream that is dying,
Or one that is coming to birth"*

Arthur O'Shaughnessy, 1844-1881

Chapter Thirteen

European Perspectives

Tom Keighley

Core Themes in Gerontological Nursing

Ageing Matters	*New Social World*	*Lifespan Perspective*	*Health and Old People*
Illness and Dependency	*Quality Nursing Care*	*Therapeutic Intervention*	*Politicizing Gerontological Nursing*

Key Words

Europe • Cost of Caring • Health Service Reforms • Elderly • Empowerment

INTRODUCTION

As we have seen in earlier chapters, there is an amazing mythology about old age. It is based on assumptions rather than tested reality. For example, many believe that old age is associated with illness and disability. The fact is that in the under 85 age group in the Western world, the vast majority of people live a full active and independent life (Bond and Carstairs, 1982; Feller, 1986; Finch, 1986; OPCS, 1989a; Stone *et al.*, 1987; Van Mannen, 1988; Ory and Bond, 1989; Smith and Jacobson 1991). Another myth is that old age is associated with loneliness. In reality, it is only when considering the over 85-year olds that this becomes an issue. It is fascinating to see that myths like this are common across the European Community (EC). Equally interesting are the common approaches chosen to address the care needs of people who are elderly.

In exploring this, a number of themes will be addressed:

The cost of caring: demography; contributing to the care cost; role of the state

---

Reforming care services: commissioners and providers; social service reforms; care groups; primary health care; the private and voluntary sector

---

Empowerment: notions of old age; role of the media; postretirement education; social contribution; creativity; the role of family/partner.

While addressing these issues there will also be consideration of two matters intrinsically threaded throughout this subject:

- *the wider European perspective;*
- *the future for nurses.*

These themes are not addressed separately because they are elements of all the issues referred to. Also, they are not addressed as individual items for a much more important reason. For too long, Europe has been addressed as if it is separate to the UK. It is not: the UK is Europe's offshore islands and as such, sits on the same continental shelf as the rest of Europe. The UK is part of Europe and all its social policy, including health policy, and needs to be considered in that framework. Regarding nursing, the same principle applies. It is impossible to determine what nursing is required or how it will need to change, unless it is considered as an integral, and indeed central part of all health care provision. At the conclusion of the chapter, however, an agenda for consideration is drawn up which permits the two issues to be addressed as prime focus.

THE COST OF CARING

To me, old age is always fifteen years older than I am.
Bernard Baruch, *New Reports,* **August 21, 1955**

I love everything that's old: old friends, old times, old manners, old books, old wines.
Oliver Goldsmith, She Stoops to Conquer (1773)1

The 1980s saw governments becoming more cost conscious. In the UK and other European countries, it became government policy to control spending in the public sector. Health care did not escape this. Paradoxically, it did not mean that less money was spent, rather the reverse. A greater demand for care emerged and in almost every European country the

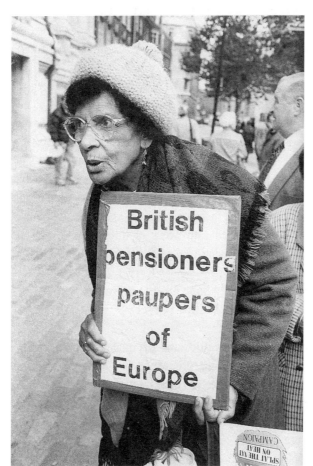

Fig. 13.1 *Meeting the cost of their own care is politicizing older people as never before*

burden for this fell upon the state (Levitt and Joyce, 1987; Leathard, 1990). This paradox of a wish to exercise constraint and yet a reality of increased need and increased spending, has not always been understood. The need to comprehend such policy tension underlies the analysis of possible future strategic directions.

Consider this as an example. In this data-ridden world, it is difficult to believe that the cost of caring for a client group like older people is not available. The reality is, that it is difficult even to achieve unanimity of view on what is an older person. This is for a number of reasons. Differences exist in the definitions of old for men and for women. There are variations in categorization with 60/65 years being used by some as the entry qualification for senior citizenship, others insisting it is 75+ and yet others 85+. The most recent twist is the emergence of health policy looking at young older people, i.e. 50–60/65 years.

If agreement on a definition of what constitutes 'elderly' by age band could be achieved, then a further complication arises in deciding what services are available for older people. Because responsibility for service provision has been delegated from central government to regional and local service providers, this creates difficulty as each area tends to count differently. Another is the extent of voluntary and informal service provision. A further complication arises from the fact that some of these services have to be paid for by the amount of money available to meet that demand, reduce staff movement, reduce training and development opportunities and disrupt previous strategic planning intentions. Knowing the number of people available to provide services therefore will, for the foreseeable future, remain uncertain.

Where more certainty exists is about the total population of older people. Using the definitions of older people as 65+, the OECD (1988) predicts an increase in the elderly population in the EC. As a percentage of the total population, the over 65-year-olds represented 9.3% in 1950, 13.7% in 1980, 16.6% in 2010 and 23.1% in 2040. The significance of this is two-fold. It means that the total proportion of the population available to contribute to the Gross National Product (GNP) from which all private and public resources are drawn, is decreasing. The second point is that the proportion of very old people in the population (i.e. those over 85 years) is also increasing. This is known as the double-ageing process because of the markedly increased care needs of this group (Bond and Carstairs, 1982; OPCS, 1989a,b; Family Policy Studies Centre and Help the Aged, 1991).

No-one's so old that he mayn't with decency hope for one more day.
Seneca, *Letters to Lucilus* **(1st c) 12.6, tr E. Philips Barker**

This means that the UK and Europe generally is looking at a qualitative change in the nature of our society. Since 1945, the ever-increasing proportion of wage earners in the population has ensured that, in real terms there has been an increase in the total wage-earning and therefore tax-paying populations. This means that the total resource available to provide care in either human resources or financial terms expanded. From the mid 1980s this reversed, and for the foreseeable future (i.e. post 2030) both resources will be diminished. A further aspect to this is that this problem is not worldwide. It appears that as a result of the fall in European population, and increase in Japan and the USA, the EC population will fall from 40 to 30% of the OECD (OECD, 1988) by 2050. This degree of change in the next half century could have profound effects on the quality of life for older people.

Contributing to the Cost of Care

It is clear, therefore, that changes in demography have direct impact on the resources available for caring. The economics of such change would suggest that the individuals who are in work will need to achieve ever higher levels of productivity. There will be much less social movement, and so the need to provide a much more comprehensive range of social facilities within neighbourhoods will be an issue. In a greying society which has more leisure time and unknown spending power (and presumably a reducing amount of savings) it is difficult to predict what the full social costs are going to be. In this country, as in all European countries, an increasing proportion of the care costs, (both medical, hotel and social) will be met from the individual's resources. Currently in the UK, access to benefits is controlled by assessment of earning and savings. This is a European-wide phenomenon. It will be interesting to see if this leads to greater empowerment of individuals as they come to terms with the reality of increasingly resourcing their own care. One expectation might be that cheaper forms of care will emerge with increasing volumes of informal and voluntary services. Currently, the UK has the largest voluntary sector in Europe (Home Office and Central Office of Information, 1992). Evidence of this is the way in which the 65–85-year-old cadre is developing, and providing various forms of social networks, supports or care for the 85+ age group (Smith, 1991).

The Role of the State

Consideration of demography and cost of caring leads to consideration of the role of the state. In the UK, as in all EC countries, three sources of income for older people exist. The largest component is the state pension. The other two, savings and earnings, might be significant for individuals, but represent a lower proportion of the total spending. It is accepted that the state spending will increase in the fields of state pensions, social services and health care (Family Policy Studies Centre and Help the Aged, 1991). This expectation has resulted in an increasing amount of policy work being done to evaluate options. In response to the increasing budgetary pressures, governments across Europe have delegated responsibility to service provision to regional and local levels. In the UK, this has been underway throughout the 1980s with 1993 being the year when local authorities had full responsibility for community care.

This devolution is usually associated with a removal of restrictions on decision-making, resulting in increased competition for resources. By delegating responsibility for services at a time when the demand for those services is increasing, the benefits of local responsiveness, closeness to decision makers and knowledge of local needs, are soon lost as the demand for service out weighs the resources available. It is then possible that the specialized care services represented by sheltered housing, specialist clinical care and customized public transport will

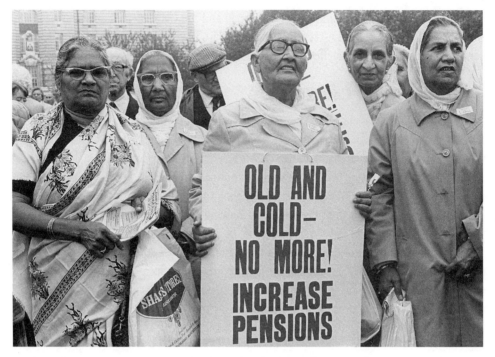

Fig. 13.2 *As the economics of health care bite, these are the demands that will occur more often*

not be provided at the level that is required. It is interesting to note that the individuals with sufficient resources tend to opt out and all EC countries indicate an expansion in the various care services utilized by older people in the private sector.

In considering the cost of caring, as a whole, the debate goes full cycle. The policy scenario is determined by:

- *the number of people in different age groups;*
- *how the cost of caring is met from the individual contributions and state provision;*
- *why the role of the state is changing.*

It is a European-wide change, and the only guarantee is that it will continue to change. Smith (1991) reports that the ratio between growth in expenditure per citizen on health and the per capita growth in the country's GNP increased in OECD countries by a ratio of 1.1 between 1975 and 1987. (The OECD countries are western Europe, Japan, USA, Canada and Australia.) This ratio, known as the elasticity between health expenditure growth and GDP was therefore showing health expenditure increasing 10% faster than the GDP.

However, since 1987, the figure has begun to reverse and in some countries, notably Germany and Sweden, it is now a negative figure. This adds strength to the strategic scenarios painted earlier. The foreseeable future is of increased demand for care but with decreasing financial and human resources to meet the demand.

REFORMING CARE SERVICES

In the UK, throughout this century, health services have been a profoundly political issue. It is often asserted that the pre-First World War legislation was prompted by the difficulty in finding enough healthy men to fight in the Boer War (Ham, 1985) Post-1919, history records dozens of reports, inquiries, investigations and reforming packages. Some were more memorable than others. The creation of the NHS in 1948 was an innovation which has remained unique. Recent history of reform in NHS really begins in 1974 with the creation of regions, areas and districts. 1984 saw the introduction of general management, and 1989 the concepts of purchasers and providers. What is interesting about this is the speeding up of the frequency of reform initiatives. To some, this is evidence of the wish of politicians to have a more direct say in the running of the NHS. More properly, it is a reflection of the rate of change and the need to respond to increased demands and less available finance.

The UK is not alone in trying to reform the health services. For example, France is focusing on reducing the number of GPs and cutting hospital beds, all as part of a package in which public hospitals have been given their own budgets. The payments for service by patients have been increased. The Netherlands is currently implementing a system of competition between insurance companies and health care providers. Germany is revising its health service provision to integrate the former eastern Germany. Greece is trying to reform its system of payments to doctors as a black economy of about 2% of GDP exists to top-up doctors' salaries. Finally, Spain is moving towards a universal health care coverage through multiple financing which will include contributions from employers. These are all major reforms which, in many cases, seem to be addressing problems at a developmental stage earlier than our own.

The description of the UK as the leading health service is certainly true when considering aspects such as comprehensiveness of service and freedom from payment at the point of service delivery. However, certain problems remain, most notably the failure of the 1984 NHS reforms to tie medical practice to resource utilization. The need for further reform became increasingly apparent as the 1980s progressed because of the evidence of unmet needs and increasing health service demands, not least from older people.

Commissioners and Providers

The 1989 reforms hinge on a single notion and that is that the NHS can be divided into two functions, commissioning and providing health care services. The shaping of the service to achieve this separation is ongoing and demonstrates the following features:

- *Trusts and directly managed units providing a range of acute and community care;*
- *health authorities reconstructed as commissioners to determine health needs and set contracts which providers bid for;*
- *GP fundholders with their own money to purchase a range of services to supplement the services they provide;*

■ *regional health authorities redesigned to manage the health market by the setting management contracts and monitoring services contract compliance.*

This new NHS has major implications for the care of older people, nearly all of them positive. While many people have focused on the creation of Trusts, in health care terms this will turn out to have been a minor issue for older people. The real gain will be the emergence in increasing numbers of proactive, health conscious GPs. All Trusts have to offer in the reformed NHS is improvement in efficiency and effectiveness which may mean that an older person's care experience may be briefer and of a higher quality. What the proactive GP fundholder can offer is disease/illness avoidance guidance and support in the adoption of healthier lifestyles as well as a far higher level of care and treatment from a primary health care base before, and more often avoiding, transfer to care services provided by Trusts.

The great weakness in the UK health service for older people has been the treatment–disease orientation emerging from a service dominated by hospital consultants. Mitchell *et al.* (1987) described the development of hospital services for older people which demonstrated the futility of persisting with a medically dominated model of health care. They drew together the best of medical practice and sought to integrate that with the care services available in the community, be they local authority or privately provided. This demonstrated how to reduce admission times and frequency of hospital admission and how to use these periods of hospital admission differently. It demonstrated the need for hospital services to adopt an integrated and holistic approach.

The approach described raises another issue. The greater proportion of all adult admissions to hospital are people aged 65 years or over (Victor, 1987). In order to achieve appropriateness of care, therefore, physicians and surgeons need to act in partnership with gerontological physicians to achieve optimal outcomes. Further, there must be a question about the care of people over 65 years diagnosed as having a psychiatric condition. The duplication of role of psycho-geriatricians and traditional geriatricians in contrast to the integrated manner of working evolved by gerontological physicians points to the need for newer shapes of service to emerge.

The gerontological physician works closely with the patient's GP. Putting together the health-oriented work of the GP, how some of the GP fundholders are beginning to create care packages for individuals, using social workers as well as their own nurses, OTs, physiotherapists, dieticians and practice nurses, all suggests that the new arrangements should benefit older people enormously. Because the GP contract now includes more monitoring of GP performance than previously, much more control is emerging in the system. GPs themselves are interested in more health monitoring. They are providing much more by way of communication and information so as to raise people's awareness of health issues. This is having the profound effect of empowering people and helping them to be informed about the decisions to be taken. Public libraries report that health-related texts are the most heavily consulted of their books (Gann, 1991), a feature that seems to be associated with an increasingly older population.

This proactive approach is also characterised by GP fundholders refusing to hand over their patients, body and soul, to hospital consultants. Increasingly, patients are referred for consultation and the GP and patient then consider this before embarking on further treatment. This is motivated by GP fundholders wanting to manage the care process more but also being anxious about having to pick-up in human and financial terms, treatments that they might not be absolutely convinced about. This interaction between commissioners and purchasers in this form is having an immediate effect on the care of older people. The longer term effects of contracts set by district health authorities (DHAs) emerging from health needs assessment will take some time to follow. Achieving effective definition of health needs and determining monitoring mechanisms to observe changes will take some time and be difficult to work through for older people, because of the problems touched on in the section on the cost of caring. However, the White Paper *Health of the Nation* (DoH, 1992) commits the health service to such an exercise, but the results will be in the longer term.

Social Service Reforms

It is not just the health service that is being reshaped, the whole of local government is being reshaped and this is at a time when increasing responsibility for care is being devolved to them. The impact on local social service departments has been immense. The equivalent of the Briggs Report (DHSS, 1972) in nursing was the Seebohm Report (DHSS, 1968). The impact of both reports on their respective professions was similar. The current reforms in social services are the equivalent of the NHS reforms, and therefore the impact is similar. The parallel reforms of health and social services break the cycle of looking at the respective responsibilities of each agency in sequence, or in isolation. The same principles are being adopted; that is, the creation of a commissioner–provider split, the establishment of service contracts and devolution of management services. All this is being done when, for the first time, government has given the lead responsibility to health and social services for different client groups so forcing the two agencies to work together to provide services.

The significance of this for the delivery of care to older people should not be underestimated. They are changes that will influence both service delivery and expectations about service. For instance, the notion of joint client appraisal has been extant for some time (Challis and Davies, 1986; Riordan *et al.*, 1988). Increasingly, protocols for one of the joint teams to do the full assessment for the whole team are emerging. The consequence of the social service reforms is that the care package agreed represents a contract of service and failure to deliver the health or social service side of that package is a breach of the contract. The consequences of this in the era of Citizen and Patient Charters are much more than simply sending a letter of apology. It will mean that the care services are not achieving the publicly set standards, that is a publicly acceptable standard of care is not being delivered, and clients and their carers will have recourse to procedures to achieve recompense and enforced compliance with the standard.

Other consequences of these reforms include the reviewing of the competing roles of community auxiliary nurses/health care assistants (HCA) and social services home helps. The role overlaps need to be clarified in order to ensure an extension of service provision. Similarly in the field of training and education. While the problems of achieving joint preregistration training seem insurmountable with only three joint training courses being approved and evaluated by the English National Board (ENB), the Central Council for Education and Training in Social Work (CCETSW) withdrawing from discussion on HCA training, the scene at postregistration training level looks more promising. Shared and joint training is beginning to occur as is shared/joint staff placement. The benefits of these approaches are a shared and clear focus on client needs and the development of mutual regard for the performance of colleagues in other professions. From an EC perspective, it will be interesting to see if those experiences translate to other countries. This is especially pertinent as the EC approach to training and education becomes clearer. The EC memorandum on Higher Education (Commission of the European Communities, 1991) made it clear that the greatest investment would be in skills training for well-defined functions. This is in contrast to the focus on conceptual development which is pursued by higher education in the UK. This is important in health care and social care terms because the health services have traditionally seen social services as a less well developed service than themselves while social services, stereotypically have seen the health service as focusing only on illness and the abnormal.

The memorandum on Higher Education could well be the lever that breaks down these positions and encourages both the ENB and CCETSW to recognize the commonality of their skills and knowledge base, and in so doing recognize the opportunities for common learning. Certainly the work underway through the National Health Service Training Directorate (NHSTD) to facilitate the implementation of care in the community, should help this.

Across Europe, the sort of health and social service reforms being implemented in the UK, are being pursued. The relationships between health and social services are not dissimilar across northern Europe, but as one moves south through Europe, the scene becomes increasingly disjointed. The need for a unified approach to the total care package required by older people becomes that much greater. This is increasingly so in countries where the GNP is already low and the bulk of the care is given by lesser skilled carers and nurses. Reforms of health and social services which help care to be focused on the care group of older people, must be welcomed.

Care Groups

The notion of care groups is a concept that has emerged with force in the last decade. Essentially, it means that services are constructed/provided in a total care package. It arose from an understanding that, as indicated in the previous section, care needs can only be delivered effectively, efficiently, economically and holistically, in a multi-agency manner. This is particularly the case where there are multiple reasons for dependence (e.g. physical, social, psychological or financial) and where the care has to be individually packaged in order to have its optimal impact.

The evolution of care packages has been a consequence of both technological and social changes. Longer life expectancy, the ability to treat the diseases of older age more effectively and the wish to retain the independent status of older people have all come into play. The result has been a more flexible approach to care which uses at the most effective, but most minimal level, the most expert, costliest and best available resources. Behind this is the realization that institutional care was not a high-quality experience. Also that institutional care put the full cost of care on to the state while intermittent support based around the individual's own home with occasional institutional care was a higher quality and more effective care experience (DoH, 1989).

In terms of care delivery, this requires a multidisciplinary approach to care with good communication and shared goals. This is evolving gradually for older people and has required a different response from the nursing profession. This has been manifested by role redefinition amongst district nurses, health visitors and hospital-based nursing staff. This has been supported by developments in education (UKCC, 1986) and the involvement of a wider range of paramedics in the care process. This process has been a dynamic one focused around this new definition of care.

It has brought a number of facets of care under review – first the question of the appropriate environment for care with a general assumption that, wherever possible, care at home is the preferred option; second, that the individual should have an increasing say in the nature of care to be delivered; and third, the establishment of joint review and joint recording systems. All of these have broken down traditional; barriers and ensured that the care delivered has been individualized. The knock on effect from this has been the need to develop new ways of managing that care delivery. This has taken the form of case-management, key workers and primary nursing. These new care management processes reciprocate the individual empowerment by identifying the person who is individually accountable for the delivery of that care.

This reshaping of care delivery and care management to provide a better quality service is an international phenomenon. It has opened up a new agenda which reflects the new thinking on empowerment and accountability. It has meant that in the minds of policy makers and strategists, new ways of delivering care to older people are possible. Certainly, it means that the resource for care giving goes further. In the light of the evidence in the first part of this chapter, it is clear that the dynamism which has produced these changes will need to continue to improve further thinking and experimentation if the quality of service for this care group is to evolve in tandem with the available resources. One answer to this may rest within the new thinking on primary care.

Primary Health Care

The thinking on primary health care is evolving so rapidly across the whole of Europe, that it is fair to say that whenever two experts on the subject meet, three definitions will emerge! It is probably safer to recognize the continuum that is understood to be primary health care. Again, a crude north–south divide exists in Europe. Primary health care can be best described as community care and disease epidemiology in northern Europe and environmental health and disease prevention in southern Europe. This is a crude generalization, but it demonstrates the very different understandings of public health that can exist. This continuum is worth considering because the different aspects of primary health care that it encompasses and therefore what the models of care for older people are, that these different notions predicate.

The primary health care movement that emerged from the Alma-Ata Conference in 1978 (WHO, 1978) has taken many forms. The recent work on the *Health of the Nation* in the UK is one example of this. Overall, it represents an attempt to improve the health of all nations and identifies the need for more widespread information about how to avoid disease, and the need for more information about disease incidence with the expectation that health care could be better targeted. This has challenged certain suppositions. For example, the belief that the best care was always hospital care, that health care must always be delivered by health care professionals and that increasing life expectancy was a concern for the third world only. The challenging of these suppositions is important for all care groups, but equally so for older people.

The debate about the venue for the delivery of care to older people has already been addressed. However, it has not been addressed across the whole of Europe. State institutional care still exists in many countries as a major plank in the national health care policy. International comparisons can be drawn with our own local government and private sector provision. In primary health care terms, the principle of independence, involvement in decision-making and empowerment, all suggest that the older person should have a wider range of options. Equally, the provision of health care does not necessarily require a professional care giver. The reality is that the diminishing GNP and human resource plotted against the increasing demand for health care expressed by ageing populations results in the need for a wider range of carers to be employed.

Because the realization of these changes has come earlier to northern Europe, the emphasis on the community care aspects of primary health care are much more developed. It addresses the need for integrated services, the use of people with a range of skills and different levels of skill to deliver care, and the focus on the diseases of old age. Perhaps the most important element of this in the UK was the focusing on the diseases of old age. Of real note is the change of title of those doctors concerned with care in this area. Formally geriatricians and psychogeriatricians they are increasingly known as physicians for older people. This is important when the vast majority of admissions to medical and surgical beds are people over the age of 65 years. Specialist physicians and surgeons are increasingly entering into a partnership with physicians for older people to achieve the best quality of care.

Behind this change, care developments in the public health field have challenged the traditional view of disease and health in old age. Post First World War in the UK, the view was that old age was a period of increasing disability and dependency. The study of lifestyles and disease incidence has challenged this fundamentally. The picture now is one of comparative good health and real independence as the lifestyles and financial status of older people change.

This picture of primary health care is at marked variance to the southern European approach which has much more in common with what in the UK would be seen as the shared focus of public health and environmental health. Here the interest is in monitoring the health of the population and influencing the state of the environment to ensure that health threats are avoided or removed. The development of work on *Health of the Nation* in the UK has begun to move this kind of thinking to centre stage. The implications for older people are for the first time concerned about roads as an obstacle to daily living, the quality of pavements and signs, and the importance of food of good quality at reasonable prices and accessible locally. The realization that the environment is important for older people and can be a deadly enemy, has been long in coming. Concerns in the past have always been focused around children and adults at work. The need for a safe environment, and the social costs for older people for not having a safe environment is now being calculated as the older population makes consequential claims on health and social service provision.

This range in understanding of the notion of primary health care is enriching. There is clearly no single view and the range of views has meant that the views have become more sophisticated. The need for self-reliance and independence in a resource limited world is enhanced by extending the work on primary health care. There is a need to recognize how different and newer thinking on primary health care has had an effect on service provision, in particular in the private and voluntary sector. The link between the two is rarely addressed.

The Private and Voluntary Sector

Increasingly, strategists are suggesting that the only way to meet the health care demands of the ageing population is for the private and voluntary sectors to expand to meet the shortfall (Levitt and Wall, 1992). The implications of this are two-fold. First, individuals will have to commit increasing proportions of their own wealth to their health care, and that health care will be provided by non-state funded services. Second, the voluntary care sector will need to expand even more rapidly than it has. This view about the expansion of voluntary services is one that is gradually spreading across Europe.

Consideration of the role of the private sector in health care is quite complex. This is because across Europe, there is a wide variety of services available, some state funded in one country are paid for directly by the consumer in another. In some countries, the scene is even more complex with part payment schemes in operation and individuals having to reclaim payments either against taxes or directly from the state. As this sort of complexity begins to emerge in the UK health market, the challenge for older people is to make the most of their savings while enjoying the best of health care. The expansion of the private sector in the UK occurred from the early 1980s onwards with the increasingly rapid programmes of health care reprovision for older people and those with a learning disability or non-acute mental illness. This was only possible because, with the help of state benefits, the private sector developed to meet this new health need.

A similar picture was true in the voluntary sector. Here again the financial picture is complex with a mixture of paid and unpaid staff being dependent on differing degrees of support from the public and from the state in order to provide a service. Interestingly, the services available are increasingly considered to be indispensable. Also, the people providing these services are increasingly expert. Given that the UK has the largest voluntary sector in the developed world, this means that we are observing a very marked shift in the resource focus. It adds to the complexity of determining what health care resources can be obtained by older people, but also requires health care professionals in general and nurses in particular to be constantly up-dating their knowledge of services available and building links between the care services offered by full-time professionally trained care staff and the voluntary services. Equally it means that there are an increasing number of openings for retired nurses to get involved in such voluntary services. Indeed, the voluntary services are increasingly made up of retired professionals intent on continuing to apply their skills.

In concluding this section on reforming health care services, it is worth reiterating that it is a dynamic process which has no final end. The changes in societies across Europe will continue to demand and bring forth new responses. This response will be a combination of resource availability, state involvement, new thinking and new techniques from the caring professions, and the willingness of those not in full-time employment to make a contribution to caring for others. It is a complex set of changes to monitor, but one that requires close attention.

EMPOWERMENT

Before you contradict an old man my fair friend, you should endeavour to understand him.
George Santayana, *Dialogues in Limbo* (1925), 1

The term has many meanings and is now more of a movement than a concept. Across the developed world it is reflected in consumers of health care wishing to be involved much more in decision-making about the nature and quality of health care provision. This implies an increased level of knowledge and understanding, and in many cases this is true. Equally, people are committing themselves to a greater level of involvement both in indentifying their health needs and in acquiring services to meet them. For older people, empowerment can be considered under a number of headings;

- *notions of old age;*
- *role of the media;*
- *post-retirement education and activity;*
- *social contribution;*
- *creativity;*
- *the influence of family/partner.*

Some of these have been touched on already but obtain a new focus when considered from the view point of empowerment.

Notions of Old Age

> *Old places and old persons in their turn, when spirit dwells in them, have an intrinsic vitality of which youth is incapable; precisely the balance and wisdom that comes from long perspectives and broad foundations.*
> **George Santayana, *Persons and Places: My host the World* (1953) 7**

Earlier, the problems of definitions of old age were addressed. That is one influence on what makes someone be considered to be old. There are others. For instance, people with disabilities are often considered to be older than they are (Vischer, 1978). Another phenomenon is that immigrants in any population are frequently considered to be older than the indigent population (Victor, 1987). These suppositions obscure some really important differences about how, and when, someone is considered to be ageing, and how their dependency and needs are assessed. Those who are perceived to age fastest are also perceived to be least able in determining their health needs and contributing to the decision-making process. Even more interesting is how women are considered to be less able than men in making such decisions and to be older than their equivalent male cohorts (Victor, 1987).

The contradictions only become apparent when surveying the attitudes of older people. Even those with severe disabilities or illnesses rarely claim to feel as old as their chronological age. Rather, the process of adaptation, which is an important part of the ageing process, seems to result in a high level of acceptance of the diminishing physical resource (Smith and Jacobson, 1991). Not enough is known about the older person's views on old age. The quotations scattered throughout this chapter give a sense of the range of view held. However, behind these notions lies a mass of prejudice and therefore barriers. The modern term for people who ascribe to these notions is 'ageists'. Even the profession of nursing has prejudicially alluded to the services for older people as the Cinderella services, so giving evidence of those negative attitudes (Wells, 1980). A powerful influence in both confirming and disaffirming these notions is the media.

The Role of the Media

> *Old age has its pleasures, which though different are not less than the pleasures of youth.*
> **W. Somerset Maugham, *The Summing Up* (1938), 73**

Much has been written in recent years about the image of ageing portrayed in newspapers and journals and on radio and TV (Victor, 1987; Heath, 1989; Young, 1991). The question of whether the media's imaging has led the views of the public about older people or that the public perception determines the perceptions projected in the media is undetermined. The truth probably rests somewhere in between. Certainly, campaigns run in recent years by organizations whose concerns are about the public imagery of older people appear to have had an impact in so far that soap operas, comedy programmes and plays now incorporate older people. Newspapers and journals increasingly carry material about older people and items relevant to older people

There is a realization in the financial pages of the newspapers that older people have an increasing amount of disposable assets. Older people are photographed kissing and enjoying a level and form of intimacy which even a decade ago would have been a subject of public comment and even ridicule.

This change in media projections is important to note because not only is it an indicator of public perceptions but also a great influence on it. Certainly, the increasing size of the older population will act as a major determinant of these perceptions as the media responds to market pressures. However, at another level, the media has yet to be fully exploited by those wishing to influence both older people, and the perceptions about ageing, positively. This includes the widespread use of health promotion/disease prevention material, the reviewing of activities and events in terms of benefits or costs to older people and the development of an awareness in the wide field of politics that older people's decisions count. The link between politics and the media is a close one as both feed off each other, and the turning point in media perception and projection about ageing will come when a major influence on the political decision-making is the concerns and agendas of older people.

Post-Retirement Education

I grow old ever learning many things.
Solon, *Poetae Lyrici Graeci* (ed. Berg, K.) 18

One example of activism among older people has been the massive increase in the use of educational facilities. This has included everything from the development of the University of the Third Age, through to the increased use of night school and distance learning facilities by older people. This may in part be people simply learning new hobbies but even so it suggests a different level of intellectual awareness and activity than has always been attributed to the retired population. Certainly the university of the Third Age and the Open University courses cannot be considered light or insubstantial. This represents the most fundamental challenge to the notion that people over the age of 65 years are less than intellectually capable.

The future would seem to demand that this intellectual acuity be built upon. The issue to be faced is how to maximize this capacity. Older people have different learning styles to younger ones, seeming to demonstrate higher levels of tenacity with their studies, a more reflective style and a greater ability to work on their own (Victor, 1987). Shaped properly around health information and education this would suggest there is room for a dramatic impact on health. The evidence is that even among older people, changes in lifestyle can effectively extend life and improve the quality of life, let alone reduce the demand for health care. The ability and interest in learning exhibited by older people needs to be drawn on, especially if the social contribution of older people is to be maximized.

Social Contribution

Earlier, reference was made to the potential contribution older people could make to the care of others. This is undoubtedly true. Indeed many people in the 60–80 years age range are working in volunteer schemes which either deliver care directly or assist care delivery services. The possibilities, however, are becoming even greater. Support services are springing up across Europe and older people are drawing on their organizational and life experiences to work in these. A new phenomenon, however, is the contribution of the older person to GNP. An increasing number are working beyond the retirement age, both full and part-time and so paying taxes. This has the knock on effect of delaying the withdrawal of savings which in effect leaves capital in the system for investment. In an era when fewer people are working, this will be of great significance. Equally, the presence of older people means that there is an increasingly available population available for recreational activities. This is the boom industry of the future and so makes a real social contribution.

This picture is true across Europe. The increasingly large older population is both generating and utilizing resources as never before (Nitjkamp *et al.*, 1991). Working the impact of this through is very complex as it has never been necessary previously to consider systematically the older generation as a resource and service generator. The different cultures that predicate the attitude to older people in different parts of Europe have a part to play here. Different regions have different beliefs and expectations about older people. This is reflected in how older people operate as resource users and generators. The media and education will be big influences in mediating this and both effecting and reflecting changes.

Creativity

> *What (Time) hath scanted men in hair, he hath given them in wit.*
> **Shakespeare, *The Comedy of Errors* (1592–93) 2.2.81**

The previous comments on education and social contribution lead logically to a view about creativity among older people. Again regional cultures produce different pictures. The historic view of older people sitting in rocking chairs reading and knitting is passing fast. This too is due to the different resource base generated through pension schemes and post-retirement earning potentials. It is also being influenced by the increasing demand for older workers to continue to work (Walker, 1989). This reflects changes emerging from the business world where senior and older staff are not expected to exhibit the same level of energy and expenditure that younger, aspiring staff are expected to demonstrate but are retained in the company. This change is important.

It is important at a number of different levels. First, because it extends the earning period, and second, and perhaps more importantly, because it reflects an awareness of the intellectual change exhibited in older people. Research in the last decade has refuted the long-standing studies about intellectual prowess peaking in the third decade and then decreasing slowly thereafter. Rather, it is clear now that from the sixth decade onwards new intellectual skills come into play (Foxall, 1991). These are now referred to as wisdom, the ability to assess information and reflect a preferred range of outcomes, which show a deeper awareness of what is practical and possible. It is suggested that this is the product of extensive life experience. This wisdom factor is now more widely appreciated and reflects a traditional cultural appreciation of grandparents' views. Wider understanding of this could change the perceptions about older people very significantly.

Family and Partners

An old man loved is winter with flowers.
German Proverb

Finally, a few thoughts on another changing phenomenon. Traditionally old age has been associated with loneliness as a result of one of the partners in a relationship dying. This belief arose from a European experience of war over many centuries where one generation of young men after another was killed in recurrent conflicts. For western Europe at least, it looks as if the last five decades of peace have broken that recurrent cycle. As a result, it is only when considering the over 85-year-olds that this becomes a real issue. The 65–85 age group are better perceived to be in a pairing and to have surviving families, even if those families are quite distant. It could well be a phenomenon of the next two decades to be watched carefully, as people even in their seventies are caring for dependent parents.

Equally, it is necessary to consider the changes in expectation about quality of life. Extended families are a great influence on these expectations. Health care will need to be responsive to this, as will social policy generally, as decision-makers maximize the developments in technology, especially telematics to ensure closeness of contact and availability of support. It is exciting to see the development of recreational activities based around older people. These no longer amount to glorified singles clubs. Rather they recognize that older people have partners and want the choice of involving their wider family or not. These changes reflect a wish to live the 'mature' part of the life cycle to the full and suggests that along with much that has been written before, the views on older people and ageing are changing and need to change.

CONCLUSION

This chapter has been written with the specific intention of raising some thoughts and some questions. It has also attempted to place this thinking in a European and a nursing context. It is trite but true to note that the future is uncertain. Nurses need to contribute to resolving this uncertainty not just be developing and delivering ever better models of health care, but by contributing to the thinking on policy development and actively engaging other agencies in that decision-making. The experience of the profession in this area is immense, there is a need to ensure that a proper contribution is made.

SUGGESTIONS FOR FURTHER READING

Body, R, (1990). **Europe of Many Circles – Constructing a Wider Europe.** New European Publications, London

Landsberger, B. (1985). **Long-Term Care for the Elderly: A Comparative View of Layers of Care.** Croom Helm, London

Pacolet, J. and Wilderom, C. (Eds) (1991). **Economics of Care of the Elderly.** Avebury, Aldershot.

Pinder, J. (1991). **European Community: The Building of a Union.** Oxford University Press, Oxford.

Wade, B., Sawyer, C., and Bell, J. (1983). **Dependency with Dignity Different Care Provision for the Elderly.** Occasional Papers on Social Administrations No. 68. Bedford Square Press/National Council for Voluntary Organisations, London.

REFERENCES

Bond, J. and Carstairs, V. (1982). Services for the elderly, a survey of the character and needs of a population of 5,000 old people. **Scottish Health Service Studies 42.** Scottish Home and Health Department, Edinburgh.

Challis, D. and Davis, B. (1986). **Case Management in Community Care: An Evaluated Experiment in the Home Care of the Elderly.** Gower, Aldershot.

Commission of the European Communities (1991). Memorandum on Higher Education in the European Communities, Com (91) 349 Final. Office for Official Publications of the European Communities, Luxembourg.

Conroy, M. and Stidston, M. (1988). **2001 – The Black Hole NHS. An Examination of Labour Market Trends in Relation to the NHS.** South West Thames Regional Health Authority, London.

Department of Health and Social Security (DHSS) (1968). Report of the Committee on Local Authority and Allied Personal Social Services, (Ch. F. Seebohm Esq), Cmmd 3703. HMSO, London.

Department of Health and Social Security (1972). Report of the Committee on Nursing (Ch. Prof. Asa Briggs) Cmmd 5115. HMSO, London.

Department of Health (DoH) (1989). **Caring for People:** Community Care in the Next Decade and Beyond. Cmmd 8(49) HMSO, London.

Department of Health (1992). **The Health of the Nation: A Strategy for Health in England.** Cmmd 1986. HMSO, London.

EUROSTAT (1988). **Demographic Statistics, (Theme 3: Population and Social Conditions. Series C: Accounts, Surveys and Statistics).** Office for Official Publications of the European Communities, Luxembourg.

Family Policy Studies Centre and Help the Aged (1991). **An Ageing Population** (Fact Sheet No. 2). Family Policy Studies Centre, London.

Feller, B. A. (1986). **Americans Needing Home Care, United States.** US Department of Health and Human Services, National Center for Health Statistics, Public Health Service, US Government Printing Office, Washington, DC.

Finch, H. (1986). Health and Older People. Research Report, No. 6. Health Education Council, London.

Foxall, N. J. (1991). Health education of the older client. In: M. G. Baines (Ed.) **Perspectives on Gerontogical Nursing.** Sage, Newbury Park, CA.

Gann, R. (1991). **The Health Care Consumer Guide.** Faber & Faber, London.

Grocott, T. (1989). A hole in the black hole theory. **Nursing Times, 85**(41), 65–67.

Ham, C. (1985). **Health Policy in Britain: The Politics and Organisation of the National Health Service,** 2nd edn. Macmillan, Basingstoke.

Heath, H. (1989). Old: almost a four-letter word? **Nursing Times 85**(31), 36–37.

Home Office and Central Office of Information (1992). **The Individual and the Community – The Role of the Voluntary Sector.** HMSO, London.

Leathard, A. (1990). **Health Care Provisions – Past, Present and Future.** Chapman & Hall, London.

Levitt, M. S. and Joyce, M. A. S. (1987). **The Growth and Efficiency of Public Spending.** (Occasional Papers. The National Institute of Economic and Social Research. No. 41) Cambridge University Press, Cambridge.

Levitt, R. and Wall, A. (1992). **The Reorganised National Health Service.** Chapman & Hall, London.

Mitchell, J. Kafetz, K. and Rossiter, B. (1987). Benefits of effective hospital services for elderly people. **British Medical Journal, 295,** 980–984.

Nitjkamp, P., Pacolet, J., Spinnewyn, H., Vollering, A., Wildero, C. and Winters, S. (Eds) (1991). **National Diversity and European Trends in Services for the Elderly.** University of Leuven, Higher Institute of Labour Studies, Leuven, Belgium.

Office of Population, Census and Surveys (1989a). **General Household Survey, 1986.** OPCS, London.

Office of Population, Census and Surveys (1989b). **General Household Survey, 1987.** OPCS, London.

Organization for Economic Co-operation and Development (OECD) (1988). **Ageing Populations – the Social Policy Implications.** OECD, Paris.

Ory, N. G. and Bond, K. (Eds) (1989). **Ageing and Health Care: Social Science and Policy Perspectives.** Routledge, London.

Riordan, J., Bramhall, B. and Backhouse, T. (1988). Teamwork to serve the elderly. **Health Service Journal, 98**(5101), 564–566.

Smith, A. and Jacobson, B. (Eds) (1991). **The Nation's Health: Strategy for the 1990s.** King's Fund Centre, London.

Smith, T. (1991). European health care systems. **British Medical Journal, 303,** 1457–1459.

Stone, R., Cafferata, G. C. and Sangl, J. (1987). Caregivers of the frail elderly, a national profile. **The Gerontologist 27,** 616–626.

United Kingdom Central Council for Nursing, Midwifery and Health Visiting (1986). **Project 2000 – A New Preparation for Practice.** UKCC, London.

Van Mannen, H. M. Th. (1988). Being old does not always mean being sick: perspectives on conditions of health as perceived by British and American elderly. **Journal of Advanced Nursing 13**(6), 701–709.

Victor, C. R. (1987). **Old Age in Modern Society: A Textbook of Social Gerontology.** Croom Helm, London.

Vischer, A. L. (1978) On growing older. In: V. Carver and P. Liddiard (Eds) **An Ageing Population: A Reader and Source book.** Hodder & Stoughton, Sevenoaks, Kent in association with Open University Press.

Walker, A. (1989). Fine words that could widen the great divide. **Guardian, 10 May.**

Wells, T. J. (1980). **Problems in Geriatric Nursing Care.** Churchill Livingstone, Edinburgh.

World Health Organization (1978). **Alma-Ata 1978: Primary Health Care: Report of the International Conference.** WHO, Geneva.

Young, P. (1991). As I was saying .... **Nursing the Elderly, 5**(1), 41.

Appendix:

Useful
Addresses

Every effort has been made to ensure that the following addresses and telephone numbers are current and correct, but the Publishers will be most grateful for information regarding any recent changes, along with suggestions for new inclusions in future editions.

These organizations may have local groups and may provide information for your area:

Age Concern
England: Bernard Sunley House
60 Pitcarn Road
Mitcham
Surrey CR4 3LL

N. Ireland: N. Ireland Old People's Welfare
    Council
128 Gt Victoria Street
Belfast, BT2 7BG

Scotland: Scottish Old People's Welfare
    Council
33 Castle Street
Edinburgh EH2 3DN

Wales: 1 Park Grove
Cardiff CF1 3BJ

Age Exchange Theatre Trust
Age Exchange Reminiscence Centre
11 Blackheath Village
London SE3 91A

Age-Link
Suite 5
The Manor House
The Green
Southall
Middlesex UB2 4BR

Alzheimer's Disease Society
158–160 Balham High Road
London SW12 9BN

Arthritis Care
6 Grosvenor Crescent
London SW1X 7ER

Arthritis and Rheumatism Council (ARC)
41 Eagle Street
London WC1R 4AR

Association of Continence Advisors
380–384 Harrow Road
London W9 2HO

British Association for Counselling
37a Sheep Street
Rugby
Warwickshire CV21 3BX

British Council of Organizations of
    Disabled People (BCODP)
St Mary's Church
Greenlaw Street
London SE18 5AR

British Deaf Association
38 Victoria Place
Carlisle CA1 1HU

British Diabetic Association
10 Queen Anne Street
London W1M 0BD

British Geriatric Society (BGS)
1 St Andrew's Place
Regents Park
London NW1 4LB

British Heart Foundation
102 Gloucester Place
London W1H 4DH

British Red Cross Society (BRCS)
9 Grosvenor Crescent
London SW1X 7EJ

British Sports Association for the Disabled
Haywood House
Barnard Crescent
Aylesbury Park
Bucks HP21 9PP

Cancer Link
17 Britannia Street
London WC1X 9JN

Carers National Association
29 Chilworth Mews
London W2 3RG

Centre for Policy on Ageing
25–31 Ironmonger Row
London ECN3 QPY

Christian Council on Ageing
The Old Court
Greens Norton
Nr Towcester
Northants NN12 8VS

Credenhill Ltd
10 Cossall Industrial Estate
Ilkeston
Derbyshire DE7 5UG

Council for Voluntary Service
(See local telephone directory)

Crossroads (Association of Crossroads Care
    Attendant Schemes)
10 Regent Place
Rugby
Warwickshire CV21 2PN

Cruse (National Organization for the
    Widowed and their Children)
Cruse House
126 Sheen Road
Richmond
Surrey TW9 1UR

Disabled Living Foundation
380–384 Harrow Road
London W9 2HU

Dial UK (Disablement Information Advice
Line)
117 High Street
Clay Cross
Chesterfield
Derbyshire S45 9DZ

Equal Opportunities Commission
Overseas House
Quay Street
Manchester M3 3HN

Family Welfare Association
501–505 Kingsland Road
London E8 4AU

Health Visitors' Association (HVA)
50 Southwark Street
London SE1 1UN

Help the Aged
16–18 St James's Walk
London EC1R 0BE

Hospice Information Service
St Christopher's Hospice
51–59 Lawrie Park Road
Syndenham
London SE26 6DZ

Institute for Complementary Medicine
21 Portland Place
London W1N 3AF

Jewish Bereavement Counselling Service
1 Cyprus Gardens
London N3 1SP

Marie Curie Cancer Care
(Mare Curie Memorial Foundation)
28 Belgrave Square
London SW1X QG

MIND (National Association for Mental
Health)
22 Harley Street
London W1N 2ED

Minority Rights Group
379 Brixton Road
London SW9 7DE

National Association of Bereavement
Services (NABS)
122 Whitechapel High Street
London E1 7PT

National Association of Citizens' Advice
Bureaux
115–123 Pentonville Road
London N1 9LZ

National Association of Widows
54–57 Ellison Street
Digbeth
Birmingham B5 5TH

National Council for Civil Liberties
21 Tabard Street
London SE1 4LA

National Ethnic Minority Advisory Council
(NEMAC)
2nd and 3rd Floors
13 Macclesfield Street
London W1V 7HL

North West Nurses Leg Ulcer Special
Interest Group
c/o Vascular Studies Unit
Withington Hospital
Nell Lane
Withington Manchester

Nuffield Nursing Homes Trust
Nuffield House
1–4 The Crescent
Surbiton
Surrey KT6 4BN

Parkinson's Disease Society
36 Portland Place
London W1N 3DG

Partially Sighted Society
Queen's Road
Doncaster
South Yorks DN1 2NX

Royal National Institute for the Blind
(RNIB)
224 Great Portland Street
London WIN 6AA

Royal National Institute for the Deaf
(RNID)
105 Gower Street
London WC1E 6AH

Royal Society for the Prevention of
Accidents (ROSPA)
Cannon House
The Priory
Queensway
Birmingham B4 6BS

SPOD (Association to Aid the Sexual and
Personal Relationships of People with a
Disability)
286 Camden Road
London N7 0BJ

The University of the Third Age
1 Stockwell Green
London SW9 9JS

Womens Royal Voluntary Service (WRVS)
234–244 Stockwell Road
London SW9 9SP

Index

Note: All references are to *gerontological nursing* and *older people*, which are therefore largely omitted as qualifiers. Similarly, most references are to the *United Kingdom* unless otherwise specified.

abnormal grief 154–5
acceptance of loss
   of another 150, 158, 159
   of own life 140
access to services and race 117
accident and emergency services 200
accidents and tragedies 154
accountability 285
acquired (experiential) prior learning 198
acute illness 39
Addison's disease 56
addresses 320–3
adrenal glands 57
advanced nursing practice and leg ulcers
   266–71
advertising 39–40
advocacy 281–319
   'best interests' concept 285–7, 290
   'care to advocate' 282–3
   doctors knowing best 283–5
   freedom to choose 289–92
   limits of 292–4
   'patient child' 287–9
Advocacy in Action (1991) 22
affection *see* friendship; love; relationships
Africa 32, 111
age 40–1
   appropriate practice 10–11, 197
   chronological 68–70
   problems of definition 301–2
   see also ageing; ageism; older people
Age Concern
   address 320

on AIDS 61
on bereavement 161
on continuing care units 213
Age Exchange 18, 320
ageing 32
   and gender 127–8
   and leg ulcers 261
   and rehabilitation 222, 224, 226
   theories of 50–5
      biological 51–3
      psychological 55
      sociological 53–5
   see also impact of ageing
ageism 30–2, 39, 262, 313
   form of 30–1
   'Golden Age' mythology 31–2
   see also images
Agenda for Action (1988) 202, 203
AIDS 64
aims and goals
   of groups 94, 95, 97, 98, 99
   in life 69
allergies 273
Alma Ata Conference (1978) 310
alone, living 32, 124, 140, 156
ambition 69
ambivalent grief syndrome 154
Ampthill 190
anaemia 268
anger
   about own death 140
   and grief 140, 144, 146, 147–8, 158
   and leg ulcers 267, 269

ankle pressure index 265, 278–9, 280
antecedents delineated and concept development 220
antibiotics 274
anticipatory grief 143
anxiety and fear 138, 155
    and leg ulcers 267, 271–2
apathy and grief 149–50
APL/APEL *see* acquired (experiential) prior learning
Arabs 142
arterial insufficiency 263
arterial leg ulcers 261, 262, 274
arthritis 261, 268
    addresses 320–1
Asian people 111–12, 114–15, 117–18
    see also race
assessment and leg ulcers 267, 268–9
attachments *see* relationships
Attendance Allowance 140
attention getting stage of theory building 219, 221–3
attitude to health 75
attractiveness *see* beauty
Audit Commission: *Making Reality of Community Care* (1986) 202
audits, clinical 18
Australia 304
authoritarian style of communication 84
autoimmune diseases 17, 61, 261
autonomy respected 290
awareness, cones of 139

bandaging, four-layer compression 263–4, 265, 270, 271–3
bargaining stage in dying 140
barriers to communication 82–5
beauty and attractiveness, ideas of 63, 121, 128
beliefs 69, 75–6

bereavement 128–9, 142–55
    and group care 99–100
    and health promotion 83
    helping older people cope with 155–64
    and relationships 144–6
    taboo about death 142–3
    see also grief and mourning; loss
'best interests' concept 285–7, 290
Beth Johnson Foundation 22, 87
Beveridge Report (1942) 196
biological clock theory of ageing 52
biological theories of ageing 51–3, 55
    see also functional ageing
Birmingham 23, 117–18
black economy 305
Black Report (1982) 81
bladder 57
blame for death 148
'Blitz' programmes 200
body shape and size 64, 67–8
bones *see* osteoporosis
Bosnia 32
brachial pressure index 265, 278–9
brain: decline in size 59
'brain storming' 91
breast care and disorders 17, 127, 198
Briggs Report (1972) 163, 307
British Geriatric Society 215, 243, 321
British Library 38
British Psychoanalytic Society 155
building theories, strategies for 218–23
    concept development 220
    description 219
    explicating assumptions 220
    and gerontological nursing 221
    labelling 219–20
    sharing and communicating 221
    statement development 220
    taking in 219, 221–3
'buzz groups' 91
'buzz words' 285

calcium loss 58
   see also osteoporosis
Canada 77–9, 304
cancer 16, 40, 137, 270
   addresses 321, 322
   and gender 127
   screening 17
car ownership 29
cardiovascular system and diseases 16, 17,
      55–6, 137
care
   groups concept 308–9
   plan contracts 271–2
   see also gerontological nursing
carers (mainly voluntary) 39
   age and gender 42
   and bereavement counselling 161–2
   and costs 42
   and dying 138, 161–2
   and gender 42, 125–6, 169–84
   and group 98–9
   and individual responses 169, 170,
      171–6, 182
   in past 189, 192
   and theories 225–6, 228–9
   and theories of nursing 225–6
   types of 228–9
   see also community care
Caring for People (1989) 202, 309
carry-on role of nurses 251–3
cataracts 200
causes
   of ageing *see* ageing, theories of
   of death 16, 137
   of leg ulcers 260
Central Council for Education and Training
      in Social Work (CCETSW) 308
Central Office of Information 303
cervical screening 17
chairs, arrangement of 90
change
   major *see* retirement

reaction to 69
   see also future *and under* National Health
      Service
chemical cross-link theory of ageing 52
Chicago, University of 35
child, patient treated as 287–9
choice, freedom of 289–92
chronic disease 16, 17, 193
   and theories 224–5, 226
   see also leg ulcers
chronic grief syndrome 154
chronological age and self image 68–70
Citizen's Charter 307
city life 35, 42, 269
class 129, 193
client-centred care *see under* individual
clinging 144
closing process in bereavement counselling
      163–4
clubs, social 36
   see also groups
cognitive changes 61–2, 222
collaboration *see* cooperation and
      collaboration
collective
   responsibility 194–5
commitment in caring 171
communication
   empowering local community *see*
      community health promotion
   and gender 129
   and health promotion 82–5
   and race 115–16, 118–19
   stage of theory building 221
community 35–7
   care
      Community Care Acts (1990 & 1991)
      113, 114, 169, 226,
      266
      early 190–2
      European perspective 307–8, 309–11
      leg ulcers 262, 263, 264

community (*cont.*)
  care (*cont.*)
    in past *see* Poor Laws
    and race 113, 114
    and theories 225–6, 227
    see also carers; primary care
  health promotion 85–93
    activities evaluated 92–3
    local media 88
    market stall 87
    one-to-one 92
    shops 86–7
    see also groups
  networks *see* relationships
  'tuning-in' to 82
  see also social world
compassion 171, 182
  compassionate ageism 30
competence in caring 171
compression bandages 263–4, 265, 270,
  271–3
concepts and definitions 19
  development 196–7, 220, 227–8
  of gerontology and geriatrics 5, 8, 196,
    213, 215
  of health 74–5
  of old age 5, 8, 43, 313
    problems of defining 301–2
    see also images
  of race and ethnicity 109
  of rehabilitation 241–2, 244
  of theories 50–1
  see also theories
confidant, need for 149
  see also friendship
confidence
  in caring 171
  loss of 149
confidentiality in groups 90–1
conflictual ageism 30
conscience in caring 171
'consent, informed' 289–90

consequences delineated and concept
  development 220
consumerism 77, 201
contamination 274
continence promotion 250–1, 321
continuity
  of care 19
  theory of ageing 53
contracts 307
  care plan 271–2
contradictory messages in communication
  84
convoy theory 35
cooperation and collaboration 18, 35, 39,
  228, 307–9
  lacking 264
core themes 10–23
  age-appropriate practice 10–11, 197
  healthy older person's 15–16, 224
  and lifespan perspectives 13–15
  quality 17–19
  therapeutic interventions 19–21
  see also dependency; gender;
    gerontological nursing; illness;
    political; social world
costs *see* finance
counselling and loss 155–7, 321
  bereavement 157–64
creativity 315–16
crime 120
  fiction 36
Cruse 161, 321
crying 144, 151
cultural/culture
  gap in communication 83
  needs of dying 141–2
  norms 111
Cushing's disease 56

day
  centres 118

Day Service Task Force 200
  surgery 200
death and dying 137
  and advocacy 293–4
  causes 16, 137
  death rate 121–3
  and emotions 140, 146–54, 158
    see also grief
  loss by dying people 138–42
  suicide 129, 147, 285
  type of death and grieving problems 152,
    153
  wartime 316
  see also bereavement; grief and mourning;
    loss
decision making
  interactive 23
  see also power, lack of
decline 69
  see also ageing
deep vein thrombosis 260, 261
defended personality 62
definitions *see* concepts
delayed grief 154
democratic style of communication 85
demography *see* population
denial
  of grief 142–3, 147
  of own death 140
Department of Health
  Advocacy in Action (1991) 22
  Caring for People (1989) 202, 309
  on community care (1992) 36
  Health of Nation (1992) 224, 307,
    310–11
  on leg ulcers 275
  on promotion 81
  Quality compendium 271
  Vision for Future 17
dependency 16–17
  chosen 82
  dependent personality 62

enforced *see* retirement
  and gender 124–6
  and institutional care 196–7, 240–1
  and myth 32–3
    resources drain 31, 32, 120
  in relationships and grief 144–6, 152, 154
  theories 216
  see also power, lack of
depression
  and gender 128–9
  and grief 149–50
  and leg ulcers 269
  and own death 140, 293–4
description stage of theory building 219
deskilling 240
despair
  and disgust 68
  and grief 140, 149–50
development stages in life 68–9
developments in nursing care 187–209
  history *see* past
  contemporary 197–9
  future *see* future developments
DHAs (district health authorities) 307
diabetes 56, 321
  and diet 14–15
  and leg ulcers 261, 268, 270
diagnostic aids, lack of 262–3
diet 42, 311
  and diabetes 14–15
  and health promotion 81
  and leg ulcers 274
  meals on wheels 36, 41
  past 193
differentiating and concept development
  220
disability 156–7, 228, 313
  addresses 321–2, 323
  disablement effect of hospital care 240
disbelief and grief 140, 147
discrimination within patient care 40
disease *see* illness and disease

disempowerment *see* power, lack of

disengagement theory of ageing 53–4, 139

disorganization

    disorganized personality 62

    and grief 140, 149–50

district health authorities 307

district nurses 117, 262, 267, 269

doctors 195–6, 242

    and change 306–7, 310

    and power 283–9, 291–2

    salaries of 305

    see also geriatric medicine

double jeopardy 110

double-ageing process 302

Down's syndrome 53

dreams 147

Drug Tariff 263

drugs

    addictive 29, 123

    therapeutic 161, 268, 270, 274

DSS *see* social services

Dunn Nutritional Unit 17

DVT (deep vein thrombosis) 260, 261

dying *see* death

earnings *see* income

Eastern Europe 32

EC (European Community) 111, 300, 302–4, 308

    see also Europe

economic aspects of practice 6

education and training

    changes 308

    counselling 158

    developments 198

    of doctors 284

    Education and Training (1989) 67

    and empowerment 314, 315

    and gender 126

    health 18, 67, 79, 81, 268

        see also promoting health

    higher 35, 62, 308, 314, 323

    and leg ulcers 272–3

    of nurses 286, 308

    and race 112

    and rehabilitation 254

    see also learning

ego integration 68

Eire 111

elderly *see* age; older people

elections and vote-catching 66–7

EMI (elderly mentally ill) 113

emotions/emotional

    and bereavement 140, 146–54, 158

        see also grief

    costs of being carer 42

    and gender 120

    inability to express 142, 154

    and leg ulcers 262, 267, 268–9, 271–2

    needs of dying person 138–40

    see also depression; friendship; grief and mourning; love; sexual activity

empathy, need for 110

employment

    and age 40–1

    and empowerment 315

    and gender 124–5

    loss of 155

    and race 112

    termination *see* retirement

empowerment 82, 117, 282, 286, 306, 312–16

    of local community *see* community health promotion

    see also advocacy

ending

    groups 91, 93

    life *see* death

    saying goodbye 159

endocrine system *see* hormones

English National Board (ENB) 198, 308

Ensuring Equity and Quality of Care for Elderly people (1994) 225

environment 35, 249, 311
epidemiology 309
    and leg ulcers 259–60
equal opportunities 39–40, 322
equipment 8
ergonomics of equipment 8
ethnicity 109
    see also race
eugenics 196
Europe 32, 299–319
    costs 301–4
    and empowerment 312–16
    and leg ulcers 260
    and race 108, 110–11, 116
    reforming care services 305–12
    self help 201
evaluation
    of groups 92–3
    of leg ulcers 272
everyday
    aspects of practice 6
    life, skills for 240
evolution 69
exaggerated grief 154
excellence, recognizing 19
exchange theory of ageing 54
excretory system 57
exercise and fitness 16, 59, 99, 201, 274
experience 69
    reflecting on 7–10
experiential learning 198
explicating assumptions stage of theory
        building 220
extrinsic theories of ageing 51, 53–5
eyes/sight 59, 200, 323

facilitators in groups 88, 91, 202
'failure to thrive' 227
family and kinship 194–5, 322
    see also carers; home; relationships
Family Policy Studies Centre 302, 303

'feedback system' 204
feelings see emotions
fiction
    crime 36
    images in 63–4
    see also television
finance/costs of caring 42, 81, 190, 271,
        301–5
    see also pensions
'finishing' see stopping
food see diet
formal groups 89
France 108, 110, 116, 305
free radical theory of ageing 52
freedom to choose 289–92
Freud, S. 149, 155
friendship 33–4, 35, 36
    and gender 129–30
    and grief 145, 149, 158
    new 151
functional ageing 55–63
    cardiovascular system 16, 17, 55–6, 137
    cognitive changes 62–3, 222
    endocrine system see hormones
    excretory system 57
    gastrointestinal system 58
    immune system 17, 58, 61, 261
    musculoskeletal system 58–9
        see also osteoporosis
    nervous system 59
    reproductive system 59–61
    respiratory system 16, 61
    skin 61–2, 274
    see also illness
funerals 142, 143
future
    developments in nursing care 199–204
        integrated care pathways or maps
            203–4
        nursing-led initiatives 200
        rehabilitation 253–4
        self care and self-help groups 200–2

future (*cont.*)
    developments in nursing care (*cont.*)
        social and medical policies 202–3
    National Health Service 33
Future of Professional Practice (1994) 225

gall stones 57
Galton, Sir F. 195–6
'gaming' 91
gastrointestinal system 58
GDP (Gross Domestic Product) 304
Gemeinschaft 35
Gemesellschaft 35
gender differences 5, 29, 119–30, 131, 132
    and age definitions 302
    and bereavement 149
    and carers 42
    and dependency 124–6
    and diseases 57
    and health 126–7, 130
    and images and stereotypes 39, 119–21,
        313
    and independence 124–6
    and leg ulcers 269–70
    and pensions 40
    and Poor Law 194, 195
    and primary and secondary ageing
        127–8
    and psychological wellbeing 128–9,
        130
    and retirement age 54
    and sexual activity 34, 59–60, 120, 121,
        128
    and statistics and trends 121–4
General Household Survey 300, 302
General Practice Research Framework 17
general practitioners 21
    and European perspectives 305, 306,
        307
    as gatekeepers 117
    visits to 127

generations
    interdependence 13–14
    intergenerational tension 32–3
genetics
    of ageing 52, 53
    of mortality 122–3
geriatric medicine and nursing, definition
        and development of 5, 196–7, 213,
        215, 239
    see also doctors; gerontological nursing
Germany 32, 304, 305
Gerocomy/Gerocomist 226
gerontological nursing
    individual responses to 168–86
    see also advocacy; bereavement;
        developments; Europe; gender;
        impact of ageing; leg ulcers; loss;
        new perspectives; promoting
        health; race; rehabilitation; social
        world; theories
gerontology defined 5, 8, 196
Gestalt psychology 8, 159
giving and receiving theory of ageing 54
gloom *see* depression; despair; grief;
        pessimism
GNP *see* Gross National Product
goals *see* aims and goals
'Golden Age' mythology 31–2
goodbye, saying 159
government/state
    and departments *see* Department of
        Health
    expenditure 301–5
    see also local government; National
        Health Service; pensions
GPRF (General Practice Research
        Framework) 17
GPs *see* general practitioners
Granuflex bandage 263
Greece 305
grief and mourning 137, 143, 146–55,
        157–9

abnormal 154–5
normal, process of 140, 146–54
    factors affecting 152–4
    stages described 147–53
and staff 162–3
see also bereavement
Griffith Report 202, 203
Gross Domestic Product 304
Gross National Product 302, 304, 308, 310,
    315
groups
    and bereavement counselling 161
    and care groups concept 308–9
    and facilitators 88, 91
    and gender 129
    and health promotion 87–91
        active couple 100, 101
        aims 94, 95, 97, 98, 99
        bereaved 99–100
        carers 98–9
        examples 93–101
        menopause 89–90, 95–6
        outcomes 91, 93, 95, 96, 97, 99, 100
        process 90–1, 94–100 *passim*
        and retirement 94–5
        sheltered housing 96–7
        structure 89–90, 94, 95, 97, 98, 99
    and leg ulcers 275
    and self help 95, 200–2
Guidelines for Assessment of Elderly People
    (1990) 6, 20
guilt and grief 140, 146, 148–9, 153
Gulf War 142

HALE (Healthy Active Life Expectancy)
    16
handicap 228
Harrow Health Authority 261
Hayflick limit 52–3
HCAs (health care assistants) 307–8
healing 17, 61

health
    beliefs 75–6
        Health Belief Model 268
    care assistants 307–8
    concepts of 74–5
    education *see under* education
    and gender differences 126–7, 130
    Health and Lifestyle Survey (1984–85)
        75
    Health of Nation (1992) 224, 307,
        310–11
    Health of UK's Elderly People (1994) 11,
        16
    healthism 75
    Healthy Active Life Expectancy 16
    healthy older person 15–16, 224
    loss of 136, 137
    needs 224–5
    needs assessment 307
    promotion *see* promoting health
    service *see* National Health Service
heart *see* cardiovascular system
Help the Aged 32, 302, 303, 322
heterogeneity 216, 221, 224–5
high technology 203
higher education 35, 62, 308, 314, 323
historical perspective *see* past
History Society of Royal College of Nursing
    38
HIV 64
holistic approach 216–17
    see also integrated services
home
    dying at 138, 162
    helps 36, 41, 307
    Home Accident Surveillance Survey
        (1988) 200
    leaving *see* residential care
    loss of 136, 137
    as preferred option 309
    preparation for going *see* rehabilitation
    see also carers; community care

Home Office 303
homes *see* residential care
homogeneity presumed but non-existent 5,
    12, 216, 222, 224
homosexuality 35, 61, 128
hormones 56–7
    hormone replacement therapy 80, 95–6,
    127
hospice 138, 322
hospitals
    admission 137, 140, 306
    care in 215, 226, 243
    death in 138, 142
    discharge from 40
    and leg ulcers 262, 263
    and rehabilitation 240–1
    returning to 147
    and theories 213, 222
    see also geriatric; residential care
housing
    and gender 125, 126
    and group 96–7
    and health promotion 81
    and race 112
    and social world 42, 65
HRT (hormone replacement therapy) 80,
    95–6, 127
hypertension 260
hyperthermia 62
hypothalamus 57
hypothyroidism 56

iatrogenesis 200
ice-breakers in groups 90
ignorance about leg ulcers 262
illness and disease 16–17, 39, 193, 195, 310
    acceptable 75
    and gender 127
    and grief, physical reactions to 146, 147,
        149–50, 154, 156–7, 159
    prevention 79–80

    see also promoting health
    and theories 222
    see also chronic disease; functional
        ageing; leg ulcers
images and stereotypes
    ageing 63–4
        impact of 65–6
        see also ageism
    and gender 39, 119–21, 313
    positive 36
    and race 110, 117
    and rehabilitation 240
    see also ageism; myths
immigrants *see* race
immobility 261
immune system 17, 58, 61, 261
immunological theory of ageing 52
impact of ageing 49–72
    self image 67–70
    social integration 63–7
    see also ageing, theories of; functional
        ageing
Improving Care of Elderly People in Hospital
    (1991) 215, 226
Improving Geriatric Care in Hospital (1975)
    243
income/earnings 303, 305
    see also pensions; poverty
incontinence 16
independence
    and gender 124–6
    and health promotion 85
    regaining *see* rehabilitation
individual
    care 17, 19, 215
    level of health promotion 82
    responses to caring 168–86
inequalities
    and attitudes *see* gender; race
    in health care 16–17
    in income *see* poverty
    see also power

infection 274
informal groups 89
informal sector 37
    see also carers
information exchange in groups 91
'informed consent' 289–90
innovation 18
Institute on Hearing (MRC) 17
Institute of Personnel Management 41
institutionalization 196–7
    see also residential care
insulin 57
integrated personality 62, 68, 242
integrated services 197, 203–4
intelligence 61–2, 83
interactive decision making 23
interdependence of generations 13–14
interdisciplinary activity *see* cooperation and
        collaboration
intergenerational tension 32–3
International Nursing Index 222
intrinsic theories of ageing 51–4
introspection 68, 156
Ireland 261
ischaemic ulcers *see* arterial leg ulcers
isolation *see* loneliness

Japan 303, 304
Jewish grieving 143, 144, 322
joint approach *see* cooperation
Joseph Rowntree Foundation 42–3

Kent Community Care Project 37
King Edward's Hospital Fund 78, 81
kinship *see* family
knotting 52
knowledge
    of death 138
    lack of 262
    see also education; learning; theories

labelling 227–8
    doctors 310
    as non-compliance 267, 269
    stage of theory building 219–20
    see also images
language barriers in communication 84–5,
        112
Laplace's Law 273
learning 61
    contracts 272
    see also education and training
Leeds 112
leg ulcers 258–80
    advanced nursing practice 266–71
    and ageing 261
    arterial 261, 262, 274
    causes 260
    and epidemiology 259–60
    Manchester Royal Infirmary Leg Ulcer
        Clinic 271–5
    nursing workload 262–6
    venous 260, 262, 270, 272–3
legislation 81, 305
    community care 113, 114, 169, 226,
        266
    see also Poor Laws
leisure 16, 123
lesbians 128
'leveller, age as' 110
liaison *see* cooperation and collaboration
life
    expectancy 31, 121, 124
    loss of *see* death
lifespan
    maximum 53
    model 155
    perspectives and theories 13–15, 68,
        69–70
limitations of communication 83
Lions Clubs 200
lipofuscin 53
listening 158

liver 57
lobbying 81
local area *see* community
local government 303, 307
  see also social services
local history 38
location of groups 89
loneliness and isolation 39, 40, 316
  of bereaved 152, 157, 160
  of death 138–9
  lack of *see* social world
loss
  acceptance of 140, 150, 158, 159
  of life *see* death
  types of 136–7
  see also bereavement
love 34–5, 314, 316
  loss of loved person *see* bereavement
  see also sexual activity
lung cancer 127
lymphocytes, decline in number of 52
lymphoid tissue 58

Macmillan nurses 138, 198
magazines and journals *see* newspapers
Making Reality of Community Care (1986)
  202
Manchester Royal Infirmary Leg Ulcer
  Clinic 271–5
maps, integrated care 203–4
'Marasmus Senilis' 195
marital status 124–5, 128
market stall 87
masked grief 154
maximum species lifespan 53
meals on wheels 36, 41
media 39–40, 64
  and empowerment 313–14, 315
  and gender 120
  local 88
  see also images and stereotypes

medical ageism 31
Medical Research Council 17
  Health of UK's Elderly People (1994) 11,
    16
medical students 284
medicalization of nursing care *see* doctors;
    geriatric medicine
memory
  and learning 61
  loss 83, 96–7
    and grief 150, 156
  oral history 37–8
  see also past
men *see* gender
menopause 79
  group 89–90, 95–6
mental impairment and illness 39, 113, 157,
    306
  address 322
metabolism, insufficient 57
migration *see* moving home; race
MIND (National Association for Mental
    Health) 157, 322
'mixed economy of care' 223
mixed ulcers 262–3, 265
morning: getting patients up 252–3
mortality *see* death
mourning *see* bereavement; grief and
    mourning
moving home 28–9, 35
MRC *see* Medical Research Council
multidisciplinary activity *see* cooperation
    and collaboration
musculoskeletal system 58–9
  see also osteoporosis
mutation theory of ageing 53
myths 29–30
  dependency 32–3
    resources drain 31, 32, 120
  'Golden Age' 31–2
  see also images
myxoedema 56

names
  named nurse concept 19
  naming systems of immigrants 115–16
National Association for Mental Health
        (MIND) 157, 322
National Association of Widows 161, 322
National Corporation for Care of Old
        People 243
National Health Service
  creation 194, 196, 305
  changes and reform 67, 113–15, 305–6
  and community care 169
  Directorate 308
  and expenditure 223
  and future 33
  and inequalities 16–17
  and informal sector 37
  see also gerontological nursing
National Insurance 130, 195
national policy on health promotion 81
National Sound Archives 38
'natural helping' see informal sector
NDUs (nursing development units) 198
needs 202, 204, 224–5
negative attitudes 83
  see also ageism; gloom; images
neoplasms 16
nervous system 59
Netherlands 305
networking
  personal see relationships
  professional 275
new ageism (scapegoating) 30
New Commonwealth and Pakistan
        (NCWP) see race
new perspectives 3–26
  experience, reflecting on 7–10
  and reflective practice 6
  see also core themes
newspapers and magazines 39, 88, 313–14
NHS see National Health Service
NI see National Insurance

night time care 241, 252
Nightingale, F. 192, 194
normal grief see under grief
North West Nurses Leg Ulcer Special
        Interest Group 275, 322
numbness and grief 140, 147
nursing see gerontological nursing; staff
nursing development units (NDUs) 198
nursing homes see residential care
nutrition see diet

occupational therapists, 'carry-on' work for
        251–3
OECD 302, 303–4
oestrogen 127
older people, definitions of 5, 8, 43, 301–2,
        303, 313
  see also age; gerontological nursing
one-to-one community health promotion 92
Open University 61, 314
optimism 31, 126, 213
oral history 37–8, 190–2, 193
Organization for Economic Cooperation
        and Development 302, 303–4
organization and theories of nursing 226
osteoarthritis 268
osteoporosis 16, 17, 127
  prevention 79–80
Ottawa Charter for Health Promotion
        (1986) 77–9
outcomes of groups see under groups

packages, care 308–9
pain
  alleviation 193
  of grief 142, 147, 151
  and leg ulcers 267, 269–70
  less awareness of 59
pancreas 57
parentalism 287–9

partnerships 18, 81
passive dependent personality 62
past
    collective responsibility 194–5
    community care 190–2
    frameworks 192–3
    and institutions 196–7
    medicalization 195–6
    nursing 188–97
    oral history 37–8, 190–2, 193
    practice 31–2
    rehabilitation 239–40
    relinquishing 159
    Victorian 189–90, 193–4
    see also memory
'patch' provision 37
paternalistic style of communication 84–5
pathways, integrated care 203–4
Patient's Charter 18, 264, 307
pensions 40, 54
    introduction of 124
    costs of 303
    and gender 130
    need to change 67
    Poor Law 189–90, 194, 195
    and race 110
    seen as charity 110
    see also retirement
permission
    permissive style of communication 85
    to grieve 158
    to stop grieving 149, 159
personality types 62–3
personalized care 17, 19, 215
pessimism 126–7, 212, 213, 215, 262
pets, loss of 136–7, 288
philosophy of nursing 226–7
physical ageing *see* biological theories;
        functional ageing
physical costs of being carer 42
physical effects *see* illness and disease
physical fitness *see* exercise

physiotherapists, 'carry-on' work for
    251–3
Piercy Report (1956) 241–2
pining and grief 140, 147
pituitary gland 57
planning 39, 81
pluralism, welfare 169
political/politicization 21–3
    aspects of practice 6
    and ideology and impact of ageing 66–7
    and interactive decision making 23
    and issue of health 305
    perspective on ageing 54
    see also advocacy
Poor Laws and workhouses 124, 189–95
    passim, 204, 213
population/demography
    changes (particularly ageing) 32–3, 123,
        182, 302, 303, 315
    and improved quality 196
    theories of nursing 223–4
positive stereotyping 36
poverty 42–3, 81, 125
power, lack of 228
    nurses 283–5, 291–2
    patients 285–9, 291–2
    removed *see* empowerment
    see also dependency
practical suggestions for dealing with
    bereavement 169–90
preconceptions *see* images and stereotypes
pregnancy 260
prejudice *see* images and stereotypes
premature ageing 53
presbyopia 59
pressure sores 193, 251
Prevention of Recurrence Clinics 265
primary ageing 127–8
    see also biological theories of ageing
primary care 19, 198, 199, 202, 226,
    309–11
    see also community care

primary disease prevention 79, 80
primary memory 62
private sector 225, 304, 311
   and individual responses 169, 170,
      176–82
problem orientation and solving 215, 222,
      225
   and ageism 30
Professional Conduct Report on Nursing Homes
      (1994) 11, 67
professionalization of nursing 216–17, 223,
      267, 275
progeria 53
programme theory of ageing 52–3
Promoting Better Health (1988) 202
promoting health 73–103
   Ottawa Charter 77–9
   sexual 64
   understanding 74–80
   see also strategy *and also under* groups
prostate gland 40, 57
protectionism, professional 217, 223
protest and grief 140, 149
psychiatric problems *see* mental
      impairment
psychoanalysis 155
psychology/psychological 222
   Gestalt 8, 159
   theories of ageing 55
   wellbeing and gender 128–9, 130
psychosocial assessment 268–9
psychosocial development 68
psychotherapy 155
public health 310
pyoderma gangrenosum 270

quality
   compendium 271
   as core theme 17–19
   of life 316
   of population improved 196

race, racism and ethnicity 5, 40, 108–19,
      130–1, 132, 313
   address 322
   and bereavement 141–2
   current context 113–15
   defined 109
   nurse's responsibilities 115–18
radio 88, 313
rationality 35
RCN *see* Royal College of Nursing
reactivation 242
realities 41–2
receptiveness, limited 83
recovery and grief 140, 150–3
recurring leg ulcers 265–6
Red Cross 200, 321
reductionism, professional 217
referrals, reduction of 21
reflection 6, 7–10
reforming care services 305–12
      see also changes *under* National Health
      Service
refusal of bereavement counselling 162
rehabilitation 19, 227–9, 238–57
   defined 228, 241–2, 244
   development of 239–40
   and future 253–4
   and hospital care 240–1
   not contemplated in past 195
   research 243–9
   role 250–3
reintegration 242
relationships 33–5, 316
   and bereavement 144–6
   and health promotion 82
   lack of 216
   and leg ulcers 269
   see also carers; friendship; love; sexual
      activity; social world
relief about death 149
religion 194
   and death 139, 143, 144

reminiscence therapy 90
reorganization and grief 140, 150–3
reproductive system 40, 57, 59–61
    see also menopause; sexual activity
research
    clinical 19
    and health beliefs 75–6
    and rehabilitation 243–9
    and theories 218
resentment and grief 140, 149
residential care and nursing homes
    admissions 137
    death in 138, 142
    and gender 121
    and individual responses 169, 176–82
    as last resort 229
    past 196–7
    and race 117
    reforms 310
    report on professional conduct in 11, 67
    and theories 225, 229
    workhouses *see* Poor Laws
    see also hospitals
resocialization 242
resources
    centre 37
    drain, older people seen as 31, 32, 120
    generators of, older people as 315
    health as 75
    lack 36–7, 41, 110, 302–4
    for leg ulcers lacking 262–6
    management 18
    and rehabilitation 244–9
    rehabilitation 248–9
respiratory system and disorders 16, 60
responsibility 285
    collective 194–5
    and race 115–18
retail trade 65
retirement
    age enforced 54
    as critical event 55

and gender 120, 125
group 94–5
migration 35
status lost with 109–10
    see also pensions
Review Clinics 265
rheumatoid arthritis 261, 268
risk taking by older people 28–30
ritual mourning 143–4
    lack of 142
role
    'carry-on' 251–3
    'play' 91
    positive 216–18
    report on 228, 243, 254
    sick 268, 269
    theory of ageing 55
*Role of Nurse in Rehabilitation of Elderly
        People* (1991) 228, 243, 254
Romania 32
routine care 193, 214–16, 240, 249
Royal College of Nursing
    Guidelines for Assessment of Elderly People
        (1990) 6, 20
    History Society 38
    *Improving Care of Elderly People in
        Hospital* (1991) 215, 226
    Improving Geriatric Care in Hospital
        (1975) 243
    *Role of Nurse in Rehabilitation of Elderly
        People* (1991) 228, 243, 254
    Standards of Care: Rehabilitation Nursing
        (1994) 228, 243, 254
    *Value and Skill of Nurses Working with
        Older People* (1993) 212–13, 218,
        229–30
Royal College of Physicians: *Ensuring Equity
        and Quality of Care for Elderly people*
        (1994) 225
Royal College of Psychiatrists 215
rust out concept 227
Rwanda 32

savings 303, 315
Scandinavia 260, 304
scapegoating 30
scleroderma 261
Scope of Professional Practice 199, 271
screening 17, 80
searching and grief 140, 147
seating arrangements 90
secondary ageing and gender 127–8
secondary care 226
secondary disease prevention 79, 80
secondary memory 62
Seebohm Report (1968) 307
self disclosure by women 129
self esteem and self image 30, 38
    and impact of ageing 67–70
    low 54, 83
self help
    groups 95, 201–2
    Self Help Care in Old Age Project (1986)
        22, 87
selfishness allowed 158
'senile purpura' 61
Senior Health Shop 87
sentence stem evaluation 93
sexual activity
    and gender differences 34, 59–60, 120,
        121, 128
    and health promotion 64
    importance of 34–5
    and incontinence problem 16
    loss of 155, 160
sharing stage of theory building 221
sheltered housing 96–7
shock and grief 140, 147
shops 86–7
shops, 'pop-in' health 16, 87
sick role behaviour 268, 269
sight 59, 200, 323
single people and people living alone 32,
        124, 140, 156
size of groups 89

skills
    creativity 315–16
    development, social support 38–9
    removed 240
    see also dependency
skin 61
    grafting 274
sleep disturbance 150
smell, sense of 58
smoking 29, 93, 123
social aspects of practice 6
social costs of being carer 42
social factors and grieving problems 152,
        153–4
social gap in communication 83
social hygiene/Social Darwinism 196
social images *see* images
social needs of dying 140–1
social policy and future 202–3
social pressures 69
social services 303
    and bereavement 140–1
    and carers 98–9
    reform 307–8
    Social Services Select Committee Report
        (1985) 202
    and social world 36, 37
social support skills development 38–9
social trends and impact of ageing 65
social world 11–13, 27–48
    and empowerment 315
    entering 37–42
    and leg ulcers 267
    new issues 42–3
    population changes 32–3
    restored *see* rehabilitation
    and risk taking 28–30
    social integration and impact of ageing
        62–7
    see also ageism; carers; community;
        gender; race; relationships
socialization 54, 242

sociological theories of ageing 53–5
solitary people *see* loneliness; single people
somatic mutation theory of ageing 53
Soviet Union/Russia 111, 196
Spain 305
Special Rules 140
staff and bereavement counselling 162–3
stages
    of dying 140
    of grief *see* normal *under* grief
    of knowledge building 219–21
    in life 68–9
standards 18, 218
    Standards of Care: Rehabilitation Nursing
        (1994) 228, 243, 254
state *see* government
statement development stage of theory
        building 220
status
    lack of 30
    lost with retirement 109–10
    in past 31–2
    restored *see* rehabilitation
    see also images
stereotyping *see* ageism; images; myths
steroids 268, 270
stopping grief process 149, 159
strategy, health promotion 80–93
    communication 82–5
    individual level 82
    local *see* community health promotion
    national policy 81
stress adaptation theory of ageing 53
strokes 16
structure of groups *see under* groups
styles of communication 84–6
subservience *see* power, lack of
suicide 129, 147, 287
Sun City 65
support systems
    and bereavement counselling 160–1
surgery 21, 200, 263

Sweden 304
systemic lupus erythromatosus ulcer 261

T cells 58
    imbalance 52
taboo
    about death 142–3
    about male carers 42
taking in stage of theory building 219,
        221–3
Task Force, Day Service 200
taste, sense of 58
technical
    aspects of practice 6
teeth 58
television 39–40, 88, 158, 313
    images 64, 110, 120
temperature, less awareness of 59, 61
tertiary disease prevention 79, 80
tests
    for arterial insufficiency 263
    theories 220
theories
    of ageing *see under* ageing
    defined 50–1
    of nursing 210–37
        context of care 225
        demography 223–4
        description, labelling and concept
          development 227–8
        and health needs 224–5
        model, need for 212–14
        new 229–30
        organization 226
        philosophy 226–7
        positive role and way forward 216–18
        providers of care 225–6
        value of 212
        see also building theories; concepts
therapeutic interventions 19–21
therapeutic reciprocity concept 227

thirst, less awareness of 59
thrombosis, deep vein 260, 261
thymus 58
thyroid gland 56, 57
time
    biological clock theory 52
    and listening 158
    span of leg ulcers 264
    timing groups 90
    see also past
traditional therapies of ethnic minorities 115
training *see* education and training
triple jeopardy 110
Trusts, NHS 67, 226, 305, 306
'tuning-in' to community 82
Turkey 111

UKCC *see* United Kingdom Central
        Council
ulcers *see* leg ulcers
understanding, limited 83
unexpected grief syndrome 154
uniforms 194
United Kingdom Central Council
    Code of Professional Practice (1992) 282
    Future of Professional Practice (1994) 225
    *Professional Conduct Report on Nursing
        Homes* (1994) 11, 67
    Project 2000 (1986) 309
    Scope of Professional Practice (1992) 199,
        271
United States
    advocacy 303, 304
    communities 35–6
    death and bereavement 146, 162–3
    knowledge base 222
    race 111
    rehabilitation 254
    relationships 34, 37
    self help 201
    social trends 65

standards 218
University of Third Age 314, 323

*Value and Skill of Nurses Working with Older
        People* (1993) 212–13, 218,
        229–30
venous leg ulcers 260, 262, 270, 272–3
very old people 302, 303
'victim'
    blaming' 75
    nurse as 284
Victorian nursing practice 189–90,
        193–4
'villages' for older people 65
vision 59, 200, 323
Vision for Future 17
vitamin deficiency 58
voluntary care 18, 169, 170
    see also carers
voluntary sector 302, 303, 311–12

'warehousing' 214, 216
wartime 316
    Wartime Hospital Survey 196–7
waste product theory of ageing 53
wear-and-tear theory of ageing 52, 53
weight gain and loss 150
Welfare State 169
Well Women/Men Clinics 16
Welsh Office 224
White Papers 202, 307
WHO *see* World Health Organization
widowhood 124, 128, 194–5
    associations and addresses 161, 321,
        322
    see also bereavement
wisdom 68, 316
withdrawal of support in bereavement
        counselling 163–4
women *see* gender

Women's Royal Voluntary Service 99, 200
workhouses *see* Poor Laws
Working for Patients (1989) 202
World Health Organization 74, 310
wounds
    healing 17, 61

    see also leg ulcers; pressure sores
WRVS 99, 200

yearning and grief 140, 147
young old people 302